Psychiatric Inpatient Care of Children and Adolescents: A Multicultural Approach

**WILEY SERIES IN CHILD
AND ADOLESCENT MENTAL HEALTH**

Joseph D. Noshpitz, Editor

FATHERLESS CHILDREN
by Paul L. Adams, Judith R. Milner, and Nancy A. Schrepf

**DIAGNOSIS AND PSYCHOPHARMACOLOGY OF CHILDHOOD
AND ADOLESCENT DISORDERS**
edited by Jerry M. Wiener

**INFANT AND CHILDHOOD DEPRESSION:
DEVELOPMENTAL FACTORS**
by Paul V. Trad

**TOURETTE'S SYNDROME AND TIC DISORDERS:
CLINICAL UNDERSTANDING AND TREATMENT**
edited by Donald J. Cohen, Ruth D. Bruun, and James F. Leckman

**THE PRESCHOOL CHILD:
ASSESSMENT, DIAGNOSIS, AND TREATMENT**
by Paul V. Trad

DISORDERS OF LEARNING IN CHILDHOOD
by Archie A. Silver and Rosa A. Hagin

CHILDHOOD STRESS
edited by L. Eugene Arnold

PATHWAYS OF GROWTH: ESSENTIALS OF CHILD PSYCHIATRY
Volume 1: NORMAL DEVELOPMENT
by Joseph D. Noshpitz and Robert King

PATHWAYS OF GROWTH: ESSENTIALS OF CHILD PSYCHIATRY
Volume 2: PSYCHOPATHOLOGY
by Robert King and Joseph D. Noshpitz

**PSYCHIATRIC INPATIENT CARE OF CHILDREN AND
ADOLESCENTS: A MULTICULTURAL APPROACH**
edited by Robert L. Hendren and Irving N. Berlin

Psychiatric Inpatient Care of Children and Adolescents: A Multicultural Approach

Edited by

Robert L. Hendren, DO
Irving N. Berlin, MD
University of New Mexico School of Medicine

A WILEY-INTERSCIENCE PUBLICATION
JOHN WILEY & SONS, INC.
New York • Chichester • Brisbane • Toronto • Singapore

In recognition of the importance of preserving what has been
written, it is a policy of John Wiley & Sons, Inc., to have
books of enduring value published in the United States
printed on acid-free paper, and we exert our best efforts
to that end.

Copyright © 1991 by John Wiley & Sons, Inc.

All rights reserved. Published simultaneously in Canada.

Reproduction or translation of any part of this work
beyond that permitted by Section 107 or 108 of the
1976 United States Copyright Act without the permission
of the copyright owner is unlawful. Requests for
permission or further information should be addressed to
the Permissions Department, John Wiley & Sons, Inc.

This publication is designed to provide accurate and
authoritative information in regard to the subject
matter covered. It is sold with the understanding that
the publisher is not engaged in rendering legal, accounting,
or other professional services. If legal advice or other
expert assistance is required, the services of a competent
professional person should be sought. *From a Declaration
of Principles jointly adopted by a Committee of the
American Bar Association and a Committee of Publishers.*

Library of Congress Cataloging-in-Publication Data

Psychiatric inpatient care of children and adolescents : a
  multicultural approach / editors, Robert L. Hendren, Irving N.
  Berlin.
      p.   cm. — (Wiley series in child and adolescent mental
  health)
   Includes bibliographies and index.
   ISBN 0-471-51509-4   620052956 X
   1. Child psychotherapy—Residential treatment. I. Hendren,
Robert L., 1949–   . II. Berlin, Irving N., 1917–   . III. Series.
   [DNLM: 1. Mental Disorders—in adolescence. 2. Mental Disorders—
in infancy & childhood. 3. Mental Disorders—rehabilitation.
4. Residential Treatment. WS 350 P9745]
RJ504.5.P783 1991
362.2′1′083—dc20
DNLM/DLC
for Library of Congress   90–13117

Printed in the United States of America

91 92 10 9 8 7 6 5 4 3 2 1

To our wives,

Mary Noële Hendren and Deane L. Critchley Berlin,

for their support and patience during the many extra hours we had to take from our activities at home to complete this volume.

Contributors

E. James Anthony, M.D., Director of Psychotherapy, Chestnut Lodge, Rockville, MD

Irving N. Berlin, M.D., Professor of Psychiatry and Pediatrics, Senior Consultant to the Division of Child and Adolescent Psychiatry, University of New Mexico School of Medicine, Albuquerque, NM

Scott Blackwell, Ph.D., Clinical Assistant Professor of Psychiatry, Division of Child and Adolescent Psychiatry, University of New Mexico School of Medicine, Albuquerque, NM

Virginia A. Cavalluzzo, Ph.D., Director of Education, Children's Psychiatric Hospital, Assistant Professor of Education and Psychiatry, University of New Mexico School of Medicine, Albuquerque, NM

Deane L. Critchley, Ph.D., R.N., Assistant Clinical Professor of Psychiatry, Division of Child and Adolescent Psychiatry, University of New Mexico School of Medicine, Albuquerque, NM

Thomas L. Givler, D.S.W., Director of Social Work Services, Children's Psychiatric Hospital, Assistant Professor of Psychiatry, Division of Child and Adolescent Psychiatry, University of New Mexico School of Medicine, Albuquerque, NM

Robert L. Hendren, D.O., Associate Professor of Psychiatry and Pediatrics, Director, Division of Child and Adolescent Psychiatry, University of New Mexico School of Medicine, Albuquerque, NM

Daniel Kerlinsky, M.D., Director, Psychopharmacology Program, Children's Psychiatric Hospital, Assistant Professor of Psychiatry, Division of Child and Adolescent Psychiatry, University of New Mexico School of Medicine, Albuquerque, NM

Lynn E. Ponton, M.D., Associate Professor of Psychiatry, Langley Porter Neuropsychiatric Institute, Adolescent Unit, San Francisco, CA

Natalie Porter, Ph.D., Director, Programs for Children, Assistant Professor of Psychiatry, Division of Child and Adolescent Psychiatry, University of New Mexico School of Medicine, Albuquerque, NM

Ellen Flaherty Rindner, R.N., M.S., C.S., Program Coordinator, St. Vincent's Day Hospital Program, St. Vincent's Hospital, Harrison, NY

Frederick L. Stearns, M.S.W., Clinical Social Worker, Children's Psychiatric Hospital, Instructor of Psychiatry, Division of Child and Adolescent Psychiatry, University of New Mexico School of Medicine, Albuquerque, NM

Luis Vargas, Ph.D., Chief Psychologist, Children's Psychiatric Hospital, Assistant Professor, Division of Child and Adolescent Psychiatry, Department of Psychiatry, University of New Mexico School of Medicine, Albuquerque, NM

Series Preface

This series is intended to serve a number of functions. It includes works on child development; it presents material on child advocacy; it publishes contributions to child psychiatry; and it gives expression to cogent views on child rearing and child management. The mental health of parents and their interaction with their children is a major theme of the series, and emphasis is placed on the child as individual, as family member, and as a part of the larger social surround.

Child development is regarded as the basic science of child mental health, and within that framework research works are included in this series. The many ethical and legal dimensions of the way society relates to its children are the central theme of the child advocacy publications, as well as a primarily demographic approach that highlights the role and status of children within society. The child psychiatry publications span studies that concern the diagnosis, description, therapeutics, rehabilitation, and prevention of the emotional disorders of childhood. And the views of thoughtful and creative contributors to the handling of children under many different circumstances (retardation, acute and chronic illness, hospitalization, handicap, disturbed social conditions, etc.) find expression within the framework of child rearing and child management.

Family studies with a central child mental health perspective are included in the series, and explorations into the nature of parenthood and the parenting process are emphasized. This includes books about divorce, the single parent, the absent parent, parents with physical and emotional illnesses, and other conditions that significantly affect the parent–child relationship.

Finally, the series examines the impact of larger social forces, such as war, famine, migration, and economic failure, on the adaptation of children and families. In the largest sense, the series is devoted to books that illuminate the special needs, status, and history of children and their families, within all perspectives that bear on their collective mental health.

Joseph D. Noshpitz

Washington, DC

Preface

Our involvement (I.N.B. since 1978 and R.L.H. since 1986) in the development of an effective psychiatric inpatient program for Anglo, Hispanic, and American Indian children, adolescents, and families has given us insights about the problems in providing such care and the methods that are most successful in solving them. From participating in a number of meetings on how to train mental health professionals to work effectively with minority populations, we discovered that little seemed to be known about interacting with these groups, and resources to guide the director, administrator, and staff of child and adolescent inpatient settings were scarce. Yet, psychiatric hospitals are ever more involved with youth and families of various minorities. We decided that a book describing our own experiences and those of our faculty and staff in the development of the multicultural aspects of inpatient treatment would be a valid and useful contribution.

Our personal experience has led us to an acute awareness of the needs of minority populations and the problems they encounter with various Anglo agencies, especially during psychiatric hospitalization of their children and adolescents. We hope this book will help to crystallize the thinking and efforts of the mental health professionals and staff at other inpatient settings where minority youth and their families are treated and will add to the necessary prescription of care a greater degree of mutual understanding.

Albuquerque, New Mexico   Robert L. Hendren
March 1991   Irving N. Berlin

Acknowledgments

We are grateful to our Program Coordinator, Vanessa Willock of the Division of Child and Adolescent Psychiatry, and to Shirley Putna, Division Secretary. Both have given unstintingly of their time and effort in preparing and correcting chapter manuscripts.

We also appreciate the support of the Division of Child and Adolescent Psychiatry faculty who collaborated in this effort.

We are especially indebted to the Hispanic and American Indian children, adolescents, and families who have taught us so much and have been so patient as we have continually tried to improve our work with them.

R.L.H.
I.N.B.

Contents

Foreword   xvi

PART I
INTRODUCTORY CONCEPTS   1

Chapter One
A Philosophy of Inpatient Care   3
Robert L. Hendren and Irving N. Berlin

Chapter Two
Culturally Responsive Inpatient Care of Children
and Adolescents   14
Luis A. Vargas and Irving N. Berlin

PART II
PRETREATMENT CONSIDERATIONS   35

Chapter Three
Determining the Need for Inpatient Treatment   37
Robert L. Hendren

Chapter Four
Effective Treatment Planning   66
Irving N. Berlin and Robert L. Hendren

PART III
TREATMENT MODALITIES AND ISSUES   89

Chapter Five
Integrating Interdisciplinary Team-Centered Treatment   93
Daniel Kerlinsky

Chapter Six
Inpatient Group Treatment of Children and Adolescents   112
Frederick A. Stearns

Chapter Seven
Working Therapeutically with Parents of Hispanic and
American Indian Children and Adolescents in the Hospital   127
Thomas L. Givler

Chapter Eight
Working with Resistance in Families: A Cross-Cultural
Perspective   143
Natalie Porter and Scott Blackwell

Chapter Nine
The Educational Process as Ego Enhancement in
Inpatient Settings   161
Virginia A. Cavalluzzo

Chapter Ten
Short-Term Psychiatric Hospitalization of Children
and Adolescents   176
Lynn E. Ponton

Chapter Eleven
The Therapeutic Matrix in the Inpatient Treatment of
the Adolescent   194
E. James Anthony

Chapter Twelve
Multicultural Aspects of Countertransference with
Children and Adolescents in Milieu Settings   207
Deane L. Critchley

Chapter Thirteen

Multicultural Issues in the Milieu Treatment of Violent
Children and Adolescents   221
Irving N. Berlin

PART IV
PROFESSIONAL ISSUES   233

Chapter Fourteen

Recruiting, Developing, and Training Staff for Work in
a Multicultural Setting of a Children's Psychiatric Hospital 235
Ellen C. Rindner

Chapter Fifteen

Nursing's Contributions to a Psychiatric Inpatient
Treatment Milieu for Children and Adolescents   250
Deane L. Critchley

Chapter Sixteen

Administrative Issues in Present-Day Inpatient Care   264
Robert L. Hendren and Irving N. Berlin

Chapter Seventeen

Some Principles of Clinical Administration Derived from
Therapeutic Insights   278
Irving N. Berlin

Chapter Eighteen

Evaluating Outcome in a Multicultural Inpatient Setting   289
Luis A. Vargas

PART V
CONCLUSION   311

Chapter Nineteen

Current Issues and Future Directions for the Psychiatric
Hospitalization of Children and Adolescents   313
Robert L. Hendren and Irving N. Berlin

Author Index   321

Subject Index   325

Foreword

This work brings together two fields that seldom find apposition. It is at once a major study of the philosophy and methodology of the inpatient care of adolescents, and an important contribution to the tactics and strategy of handling racial and ethnic issues in psychiatric treatment. Although an edited work, a number of the chapters were written by one or both of the two editors.

A word about these author/editors: Irving Berlin has been a senior child psychiatrist for some 50 years, and the flavor of his extraordinary experience informs every part of this work. Robert Hendren is one of the brilliant younger professionals who are moving toward the forefront of the field. His energy, imagination, and creativity offer a beautiful complement to Berlin's seniority. Together, they have produced an extraordinary work.

Although it was not designed to do so, inpatient treatment for adolescents had been largely devoted to the management and treatment of youngsters with character disorder. Hence, in considering the offerings in this remarkable book, it seems appropriate to say something about character disorder as a psychiatric concern. There is probably no mental health condition more typical of 20th century society than this one. All the din of broken homes, child sexual abuse, violence toward children, reconstituted families, parental alcoholism and substance abuse, neglected children, spousal violence, and abandoning parents come together in this final common pathway: They warp the growth of personality in the affected children.

Many children can negotiate a certain amount of this trauma and come through relatively unscathed; they may be hurt but the family experience does not destroy them. All too many children, however, are either inherently more vulnerable or are simply faced with too much pain. They then become traumatized to an overwhelming degree. Presently, some form of character deviance ensues. These youngsters may become avoidant, paranoid, aggressive, or uncontrollable. They are frequently a danger to society at large or to themselves—or, commonly enough, to both.

All the social ills—poverty, cultural alienation, substance abuse, criminality, and mental illness, to name only a few—can find expression in the rearing of children, and the products of such rearing may in turn continue the saga of despair and destruction generation after generation.

One of the powerful connecting links in this matter of character disturbance, with its attendant cluster of destructive symptomatology: paranoid projection, unrealistic grandiosity, dishonest manipulativeness, deviant sexuality, involvement in theft and exploitation as the primary source of income, proneness to violence in the face of even minor social stress, and inability to tolerate tenderness or closeness. Such patterns are generated early in life, usually in infancy and the preschool years, and they produce an individual who has great difficulty adjusting to society, whether it be home, classroom, schoolyard, or neighborhood. By their teens, the presence of character disorder bears heavily on everyone and the quest for relief often begins to involve one agency after another. Special education, mental health, welfare services, protective services, the various echelons of the penal system, all become embroiled. Frequently the youngsters pass from one setting to another until, when they are old enough, their depredations and desperate lashings out earn them a long term prison sentence. The end of it all is a miserable saga of blighted families and wasted lives that transmit damage to generation after generation.

For society at large, and for the mental health practitioner in particular, the constant question is how to deal with all of this. Let us assume that one is forced to begin late, as late as puberty, when the problems are already all too evident, or even later, in the latter years of adolescence. What should we do? How to contain such youngsters? How to work with them? What can offer surcease for their torment, and for the pain they inflict on those with whom they live? For, once character disorder is established, the single most abiding element that accompanies the course these youngsters pursue through their lives is pain. On the one hand, there is their own sense of emptiness, alienation, chronic anger, and self-hatred; and on the other hand, the impact on their surroundings of the feelings they generate: the fear, the distrust, the sense of group disruption, personal violation, and systematic destructiveness that touches family, friends, peers, lovers, teachers, and professionals with whom they interact.

In many instances, our best answer is long-term, inpatient care. Admittedly a formidable response, but the problem is an awesome one, and, often enough, nothing less has a chance. It is a difficult work, and one not loved by many practitioners. The patients are sly, uncooperative, resistant, threatening, and sometimes dangerous; at best they respond slowly and grudgingly to treatment. Special skills are required, and these are not widely disseminated in our culture. Much more attention, research, and preparation are needed. Which brings us to the material presented in the ensuing pages.

This book is one of the few that seeks to illuminate the philosophy underlying such care, the methodology which such work requires, the special techniques that must be developed to implement it, the nature of the staffing pattern that carries out this approach, the training such staff requires to learn tolerance for what these youngsters do to begin with, and then how to respond appropriately and therapeutically as necessary. This is one of the great frontiers of our time. In a larger sense, the challenge of the 21st century will be to come to understand, and to learn to cope with, human aggression. We have developed our technological capacity for destruction to the point that high levels of energy have become increasingly portable. The handgun was one great leap forward, the automatic weapon was an order of magnitude greater, and we can look forward to hand-held lasers, or who knows what kind of armament, in the years to come.

In effect, as time goes on, a single disturbed person will have more and more lethal power at his or her command. We do not have any choice; we must learn how to deal with character disorder. And the study, the struggle, the interface at which much of this is taking place is precisely in the inpatient setting.

To be sure, only a small fraction of these youngsters are being cared for in such mental health communities today. The large majority are either out on the streets or contained in some fashion by the juvenile justice system. But all too often the penal type setting is merely a holding environment. At best, a temporary respite for the youth and for society; at worst, a school for learning to hone and sharpen one's criminal proclivities and to make the network contacts that will ensure future depredations of even more serious character. So we have to learn from men like the editors and authors of this work, and encourage and foster what they do. They are the front line.

A second major focus of this book is the matter of the great cultural and ethnic gaps with which our society is riven. If character disorder is inadequately attended to in our research and methodology, understanding the nature of cultural differences and devising strategies to permit optimal work across these gaps lags even further behind. Berlin and Hendren are almost unique in America in the depth of their commitment to work with the mental health problems of native Americans; their book is replete with examples of how their specialized efforts have borne fruit when responding to the needs of this group. In similar fashion they have studied work with Latin Americans and have many far-reaching implications for work in this field.

It is of special importance to note the changing character of the American population. The 20th century has seen an ever-growing trickle of inhabitants from the third world finding their way into the more affluent first world. As the 21st century unfolds, this trickle will very likely become a flood, and the mix of cultures and populations is likely to proceed at an extraordinary pace. We hear daily stories of Pakistanis who have come to England; North Africans to France; Vietnamese to Hong Kong; Cubans, Haitians, and Mexicans to the United States; and so on for a long and growing list of substantial migrations. We are told, for example, that soon the longstanding position of blacks as the largest U.S. minority will be eclipsed by the increasing number of Latins. The need to deal with these new arrivals and, among other things, to meet their mental health problems is critical. Some of the preliminary work is being done by these authors, and the culture has much to learn from them.

Given the several interfaces at which they are working, the authors present us with a set of rich and vital issues. They have much to teach us.

JOSEPH D. NOSHPITZ, M.D.

Part I

Introductory Concepts

Multiple forces affect the practice of the inpatient psychiatric treatment of children and adolescents. In Chapter 1, we provide a historical perspective of the hospital treatment of young people with mental disorders and we review the ways in which inpatient psychiatric treatment is changing. We explain the reasons for these changes, which include improved evaluation and treatment methods, increased use of less restrictive settings, and pressures from insurance carriers and other payers to decrease or eliminate costly inpatient care. Effective or successful treatment depends on making the facilitation of relationships the primary focus of an inpatient program. This focus is especially important as the treatment population becomes more culturally diverse.

The concept of the centrality of relationships, introduced in Chapter 1, is repeated throughout the volume. Significant relationships encompass the family's interactions with the hospital staff, the staff's interactions with each other and with the patient, and the communications among the clinicians doing individual, family, and group psychotherapy, pharmacotherapy, or behavior therapy. The quality of these relationships determines the effectiveness of any treatment modality.

Respect for the cultural background of the patient and the patient's family requires that staff members have at least a working understanding of each culture's way of viewing the world, family relationships, and mental illness. The chapter describes the traditional attitudes of Hispanic and Navajo cultures toward mental illness and offers a table that compares Anglo with Hispanic and Navajo views of the healing process.

In Chapter 2, Vargas and Berlin highlight the importance of cultural responsiveness among hospital personnel. They describe the Hispanic and native American cultures in the Southwest, to illustrate the importance of cultural knowledge and understanding for effective inpatient psychiatric treatment. The problems that arise from variations in acculturation among minority groups are discussed, as are the issues that require clarification so that the staff can plan how to work with the patient and coordinate staff efforts. The importance of an extended family and of the community to the therapeutic process is described and illustrated in vignettes.

CHAPTER ONE

A Philosophy of Inpatient Care

Robert L. Hendren
Irving N. Berlin

This volume attempts to integrate current basic therapeutic concepts applicable to the inpatient care of children and adolescents with the effective involvement of an ethnically diverse population in such treatment. The book's basic philosophy is that the curative ingredient in treatment is the relationships developed among the child or adolescent patient, the patient's family, and the staff, by which we mean both the therapists and the milieu staff. When using techniques such as pharmacotherapy or behavioral management, the quality of the relationships among staff, patients, and families often determines whether a medication is taken appropriately and whether side effects are accurately reported so that any necessary modification of the medication or the dosage can take place. The spirit of caring that permeates a behavioral program and its interpretation to the patient and family will determine the effectiveness of a point system, a level system, or consequences imposed for uncooperative behaviors. The nature of this relationship is important in all therapeutic interactions.

Throughout, this volume emphasizes the particular kind of empathy required at all levels in work with ethnic minorities, to help them learn to trust and work with the child/adolescent hospital staff. Effective treatment depends on the quality of the staff's understanding of a particular culture's traditions and the staff's ability to make that awareness clear. An improved understanding of the issues affecting ethnic minority populations will lead to the provision of the best possible child and adolescent psychiatric inpatient care.

Many minority individuals and families have special problems in relating to Anglo institutions, but we are fully aware that "Anglo" children, adolescents, and families represent a variety of European backgrounds and foreign cultures that they retained after immigration. Special circumstances also exist in various regions of our country. New England, the South, the Midwest, the Southwest, and the various regions of the West all exert special cultural influences on their Anglo population. Socioeconomic class is well recognized for its influence on attitudes and behaviors. In very recent times, we have become concerned with the most deprived Anglo population—the homeless adults, and especially their children and families, who are forced by economic circumstances to leave a home base and wander over our land looking for better circumstances. Thus, to render the most helpful and comprehending psychiatric care, we need to be sensitive to the life experiences and special circumstances of both Anglo and minority children, adolescents, and families from other ethnic backgrounds.

IN THE BEGINNING

Inpatient psychiatric care for children and adolescents was first established in the 1920s and 1930s, primarily for the care and behavioral management of postencephalitic children and for the treatment of autistic and schizophrenic children (American Psychiatric Association, 1957; Barker, 1974; Berlin, 1990). From providers of custodial care and specialized care to autistic children, these hospital units evolved into multimodal, integrated programs with a therapeutic milieu for children whose psychiatric disorders could not be treated on an outpatient basis (Berlin, 1978). The programs were usually long-term, psychodynamically oriented units with complex and far-reaching goals (Redl, 1959). Inpatient treatment was often very similar to residential treatment, both in length of stay and in philosophy (Jemerin & Philips, 1988). Since the 1970s, hospital-based programs have grown enormously in number, and changes have occurred in their philosophy (Harper & Geraty, 1987).

RECENT CHANGES IN INPATIENT CARE

A number of recent developments have resulted in expansion of inpatient treatment programs for children and adolescents who have a variety of psychiatric disorders and in changes in the philosophy of evaluation and treatment. The field of knowledge in child and adolescent psychiatry has grown rapidly in the past 20 years. Experience, research, and an increasing number of mental health professionals who work with child and adolescent disorders have improved our understanding of the serious emotional disturbances that require inpatient care.

The DSM III and DSM III-R (American Psychiatric Association, 1980, 1987) added significantly to our ability to diagnose psychiatric disorders in children and adolescents. Compared to previous classification systems, the DSM offered greater reliability and general uniformity. It contributed to the rapid expansion of literature describing effective treatment interventions based on these more reliable diagnoses and on the utilization of sound research designs.

Probably the most significant development in the field of knowledge has been in the use of psychopharmacologic agents. The current widespread use of medications in both inpatient and outpatient settings reflects not only this increased knowledge but also the growing interest in and need for rapid and safe interventions to modify dysfunctional behavior (Jemerin & Philips, 1988). Attention is being focused especially on severe depression, severe obsessive-compulsive disorders, certain personality disorders, and disorders with violence as a symptom. These disorders did not previously respond to milieu treatment and psychotherapy alone (Berlin, 1990).

We need also to recognize the increase in actual numbers, in recent years, of infant and child victims of sexual abuse and severe physical abuse. The etiology of violent behavior in children and adolescents, of multiple personality in adolescent girls, and of serious depression in both sexes can be attributed to the great increase in incidence of both kinds of abuse (Egeland, Sroufe, & Erickson, 1983).

The influence of third-party payers has contributed to the growth of and change in inpatient treatment programs in recent years. The number of psychiatric beds has expanded because of increased awareness of psychiatric disorders in children and adolescents, open-ended insurance reimbursement, and the easing of regulations for creating additional psychiatric beds. Private insurance companies, in the face of rising costs and increased numbers of adolescents hospitalized, have lowered and limited their coverage for inpatient treatment (Harper & Geraty, 1987). In many states, Medicaid coverage for inpatient treatment is also being limited. Shorter hospital stays and efforts at more intensive inpatient treatment are resulting from these limitations.

Linked to the recently increased emphasis on hospital-based care is a refocusing of resources that will have a strong impact on inpatient programs in the future. The number of child and adolescent discharges from private psychiatric hospitals approximately doubled between 1980 and 1985 (National Association of Private Psychiatric Hospitals, 1985, 1986; National Institute of Mental Health, 1987) and seems to be steadily increasing (Weithorn, 1988). There is also a growing public and professional perception that the level of utilization of psychiatric hospitalization, especially for adolescents, is inappropriate ("Committed youth," 1989; Weithorn, 1988). The American Academy of Child and Adolescent Psychiatry (AACAP), among other mental health organizations, has responded to this perception by publishing criteria and guidelines for appropriate hospitalization (AACAP, 1989). Although some people believe that the increasing rate of psychiatric hospital treatment represents overuse of inpatient care (Butts & Schwartz, 1991), children and adolescents who need psychiatric hospital care but who do not have insurance coverage often have trouble finding a public or private facility that will accept them without an excessively long wait. This delay appears to represent a maldistribution of resources.

Another influence that is changing the philosophy of treatment in inpatient programs is a strong movement toward community-based, less restrictive psychiatric care. The National Institute of Mental Health (NIMH) awards monies to states to develop comprehensive community-based service systems through a Child and Adolescent Service System Program (CASSP) grant. Public Law 99-660 authorized grants to states to develop and implement statewide comprehensive mental health plans for community-based mental health services. Family members, through such influential organizations as the National Alliance for the Mentally Ill (NAMI), are also strong supporters of less restrictive care becoming available in their home or community. A recurrent source of concern, however, is the lack of funding to train competent child and adolescent mental health professionals to provide these community services.

An important component of this movement toward community-based services is greater emphasis on culturally relevant care. The nonwhite population in the United States is growing at a much faster rate than the white population, because of higher birth rates and immigration ("Beyond the melting pot," 1990). As they increase in size and strength, minority populations are requiring greater sensitivity to and support for the cultural background of their patients who need psychiatric care. Caregivers must understand the child and the family's cultural beliefs and practices, which may associate a mental illness with a stigma and self-devaluation. One must also be aware of each minority's world view, religious background, indigenous healing practices and beliefs, values of interpersonal interdependence, kinship structure, family support, and ways of relating to health care providers and to the health delivery system in the United States (Lefley, 1990). There is beginning to be a literature and extensive experience supporting the concept that cultural knowledge and sensitivity of service providers improve the patient's acceptance of treatment (Lefley, 1986) and ultimate prognosis. (For a summary of the cultural beliefs and values of Hispanic and Navajo Indian communities, see pages 9–11.)

TREATMENT MODELS

Treatment philosophy and length of stay are intimately related and are central to the treatment model used. Short-term or acute-care inpatient units typically have an average length of stay of 30 to 60 days. Treatment goals are usually confined to crisis stabilization, diagnosis, focused intervention with the patients and their families, and preparation for referral to outpatient or residential treatment.

Intermediate-term inpatient treatment varies in length from 1 to 6 months and has more ambitious goals for both the child and the family (Harper & Geraty, 1987). An initial goal of developing more intense interactions with the staff of the therapeutic milieu of the inpatient unit may lead to expectations that a behavioral program will help modify patients' problem behaviors. A longer separation from a dysfunctional family, while intensive family therapy attempts to create a healthier family system, can be critical. Structure and containment effect an avoidance of potentially destructive problems with impulse control. There is time for careful evaluation of appropriate pharmacotherapy and for treatment of severe emotional disturbances that could not be safely or effectively treated in a less restrictive or shorter-term setting.

Long-term inpatient treatment refers to programs lasting longer than 3 to 6 months. Long-term care may be advised for young patients in the following five groups:

1. Those who have not experienced an adequate decrease in the severity of their psychiatric symptoms, to allow treatment in a less restrictive setting;
2. Those with severe personality and/or developmental disorders;
3. Those with severe major affective disorders or psychotic disorders in addition to severe personality disorders;
4. Those who are intensely and repetitively self-destructive;
5. Those who are chronically psychotic or severely impaired due to a psychiatric condition (Blotcky & Gossett, 1988).

Long-term treatment often uses a combination of behavioral and psychodynamic or developmental models.

RELATIONSHIPS AS A COMPONENT OF TREATMENT

This book's underlying treatment model is based on the therapeutic use of a variety of relationships and is generally applicable to short-, intermediate-, or long-term treatment. The goal of treatment is to improve the young person's ability to relate to others and the capacity of others to relate to him or her. Staff–patient relationships focus on increasing the number of mutually satisfying interactions. Group therapy and family therapy focus on developing the necessary trust in others so that the interpersonal relationships and systems of which the young person is a part can be altered and improved. Individual treatment may focus on intrapsychic issues with the child, but only within the context of past and current relationships, including the relationship to the therapist. When psychotropic medication is utilized, its purpose is to improve behavior, cognition, or emotional regulation in such a way that the child's reciprocal interaction with others also improves.

The centrality of relationships goes beyond the direct relationship with the child. The manner in which the hospital administration relates internally to the staff and externally to the community is an important parallel process that ultimately impacts on the efficacy of treatment. Essential components of this internal and external relatedness, and determinants of the effectiveness of treatment processes, are the sensitivity to cultural issues and the cultural awareness that the hospital staff brings to every phase of the patient's evaluation, admission, treatment, and aftercare.

THE HISPANIC TRADITIONS

The purpose of understanding as much as possible about a particular ethnic culture is to use that understanding to help develop the most effective therapeutic relationship. This section describes briefly some of the basic beliefs of traditional Hispanic families. In the next section, the Navajo Indian traditions are presented, to illustrate some of the values held by many American Indian communities. These descriptions may make it easier to understand the issues raised in other chapters and the vignettes that describe clinical interactions with various Hispanic and American Indian families and their communities.

Time and acculturation have greatly lessened the belief in and the practice of *curanderismo*, the traditional Hispanic folk medicine system. However, because *curanderismo* is still used among certain Hispanic groups, a brief preliminary description may be helpful. Wide variations of the practice exist among Hispanic communities—an important fact to remember in clinical situations. An individual's culture is never the only determining factor of his or her behavior, but it is often the most important ingredient in intercultural interactions, especially between patient and healer. For example, even such a simple thing as failing to vigorously shake a Hispanic patient's hand in an initial interview may be interpreted by the patient as indicating a lack of concern; being overly admiring and complimentary, even though unintentionally, about an infant or young child creates a potential for *mal ojo* (evil eye) (Mull & Mull, 1983).

The Hispanic communities of northern New Mexico are quite different from other Hispanic communities in the United States. Hispanics there are in the majority and exert considerable cultural and political dominance over both the Pueblo Indians and the Anglos (Scheper-Hughes & Stewart, 1983). In many of these Hispanic families, the emphasis on respectful behavior is so strong that the normal word for you (*usted*) is used to address persons whose degree of intimacy elsewhere in Spanish-speaking cultures would result in the use of the intimate form of you (*tu*). *Usted* is often used between spouses, siblings, and close friends (Quintana, 1980).

Hispanic beliefs about health and illness hold that the mind and body are inseparable and not dichotomized as in Western thought; balance and harmony in all areas of life are crucial. Patients see themselves as innocent victims of malevolent environmental or supernatural forces such as infection, poverty, evil spirits, or angry saints. The body and soul, however, can be separated: one's soul can travel in dreams or one can lose one's soul. Curing requires the participation of the family, which reflects the great importance of interdependence in the culture. An ill person needs to be resocialized, to have greater acceptance of the more traditional Hispanic world view (Maduro, 1983).

In working with Hispanic patients, one must recognize these beliefs and their influence on the patient and must show respect for family hierarchy, in which the father is the major decision maker and the most powerful family member.

Because *curanderismo* is a holistic system, people seek help for physiological, psychological, and social disturbances. If the psychiatric practitioner is willing to work with folk healers when requested by the patient's family, the patient and family can be helped more effectively because the cultural relevance of the treatment is enhanced.

AMERICAN INDIAN CULTURE AND TRADITIONS— AN EXAMPLE

In both the Hispanic and Navajo cultures, preservation of social and familial harmony and suppression of conflict take priority over individual rights and needs. The Navajo communities reinforce avoidance of a verbal analysis of one's emotional states and negative feelings. The existence of harmony in the family and clan or social group is valued over personal autonomy and individual achievement. These cultures have family constellations rather than the nuclear family that is most common in the Anglo culture. An extended-family social group may live in close proximity and has responsibility for the behavior of its members. An individual's behaviors reflect group attitudes and have an impact on the entire social group.

Mental disturbance may be stigmatized. It is usually attributed to the bad luck of familial inheritance, to possession by evil spirits, or to accumulated misdeeds in past lives. Because of these beliefs, mental illness is commonly feared and denied. Care for emotional problems is first sought through medical professionals rather than psychiatric practitioners.

Mental health services that have been successful have focused on prescribing medication, giving advice, and attending to practical problems, advocacy, and family involvement. Less successful interventions are those that emphasize communication, interpersonal feelings, introspection, and egalitarian role relationships.

Therapies that emphasize family dependence and role structures rather than independence and individualism are most beneficial. They focus on restoring the patients' interpersonal equilibrium with the significant people in their lives. Concentration is on the here and now, on behavior rather than moods and feelings, and on interdependence among people. These interventions discourage verbal exploration of problems, a search for origins, and disclosure of inner feelings and emotions, which are considered private.

Culturally appropriate clergy and traditional (folk) healers can be extremely helpful. These resources permit expression of somatic and spiritual complaints, use of a shared language, culture, and terminology, and identification with common beliefs regarding the causes and relevant treatment of an illness.

The degree of acculturation in Hispanic and American Indian individuals and families needs to be determined early in treatment. An understanding of how traditional their beliefs are may indicate how comfortable they may be in family, group, and individual therapy. Table 1.1 characterizes Anglo, Hispanic and Indian ethnic cultural attitudes toward healing.

Table 1.1.   Characteristics of Western and Cultural Healing

Category	Western Healing	Cultural Healing
Classification of Illness (Nosology)	Based on empirical facts and scientific principles; rational	Based on the mythology or belief system of a particular culture; not rational
Healing Techniques	Based on anatomical and physiological principles; can be effectively applied transculturally	Based on cultural values and beliefs; can be used only in the area of cultural influence
Healer	Physician or other scientifically trained personnel	Shaman, medicine man, priest or healer grounded and trained in cultural lore (myth and ritual)
Patient	Must passively follow directions; doctor is responsible for the cure	Must actively believe in the therapy, carries most of the responsibility for the cure
Social Function of Healing	Small; sometimes almost nonexistent	Large; many persons may actively participate
Prestige of the Healer and Size of Fee	Relatively large	Relatively large
Drawbacks	Ignores the patient's humanity; neglects the effects of cultural symbols on the harmony of mind and body	Ignores the patient as a biological organism; neglects the simplest rules of physical therapy and organic cause

Adapted from D. Sander, *Navajo symbols of healing*. New York: Harcourt Brace Jovanovich, 1979.

SUMMARY

A rational philosophy of child and adolescent psychiatric inpatient care must take into account the insights derived from historical and recent events, which contribute to our current therapeutic thinking; the recent changes in thinking about the etiology and treatment of psychiatric disorders of childhood and adolescence; and the systemization of diagnostic categories. An additional influence is the advent of many privately funded hospitals built in response to a great increase in the number of children and adolescents requiring inpatient care. The role of insurance companies in determining what kinds of care will be paid for, and for how long, has altered treatment methodologies involved in short-, intermediate-, and long-term care and brought greater emphasis on the use of psychotropic medication. These factors influence the way in which the milieu staff functions and weigh heavily on our philosophy of care. Despite shorter lengths of stay and the use of more psychotropic medication, the most important element in our treatment philosophy centers on developing sensitive and supportive relationships among all elements in the hospital, our patients, and their parents. In this spirit, we need to work with individuals and families of different cultures who may be alienated from Anglo institutions and who are in need of our care.

REFERENCES

American Academy of Child and Adolescent Psychiatry. (1989). *Policy statement: Inpatient hospital treatment of children and adolescents.* Washington, DC: Author.

American Psychiatric Association. (1957). *Psychiatric inpatient treatment of children.* Baltimore: Lord Baltimore Press.

American Psychiatric Association. (1980). *Diagnostic and statistical manual of mental disorders* (DSM). Washington, DC: Author.

American Psychiatric Association. (1987). *Diagnostic and statistical manual of mental disorders* (3d ed. rev.) (DSM-III-R). Washington, DC: Author.

Barker, P. (1974). History. In P. Barker (Ed.), *The residential psychiatric treatment of children* (pp. 1–26). New York: Wiley.

Berlin, I. N. (1978). Developmental issues in the psychiatric hospital treatment of children. *American Journal of Psychiatry, 135,* 1044–1048.

Berlin, I. N. (1990). The history of the development of the subspecialty of child/ adolescent psychiatry in the United States. In J. Weiner (Ed.), *Textbook of child and adolescent psychiatry.* Washington, DC: American Psychiatric Association Press.

Beyond the melting pot. (1990, April 9). *TIME,* pp. 28–31.

Blotcky, M. J., & Gossett, J. T. (1988). Psychiatric inpatient treatment for adolescents. *The Psychiatric Hospital, 20,* 85–93.

Butts, J. A., & Schwartz, I. M. (1991). Access to insurance and length of psychiatric stay among adolescents and young adults discharged from general hospitals. *Journal of Health and Social Policy.*

Committed youth. (1989, July 31). *Newsweek,* pp. 66–72.

Egeland, B., Sroufe, L. A., & Erickson, M. (1983). The developmental consequences of different patterns of maltreatment. *Child Abuse and Neglect, 7,* 45–69.

Harper, G., & Geraty, R. (1987). Hospital and residential treatment. In R. Michels & J. Cavenar, Jr. (Eds.), *Psychiatry* (Vol. 2, ch. 64). New York: Basic Books.

Jemerin, J. M., & Philips, I. (1988). Changes in inpatient child psychiatry: Consequences and recommendations. *Journal of the American Academy of Child and Adolescent Psychiatry, 27,* 397–403.

Lefley, H. P. (1986). Evaluating the effects of cross-cultural training. In H. P. Lefley & P. P. Pedersen (Eds.), *Some research results in cross-cultural training for mental health professionals.* Springfield, IL: Thomas.

Lefley, H. P. (1990). Culture and chronic mental illness. *Hospital and Community Psychiatry, 41,* 277–286.

Maduro, R. (1983). *Curanderismo* and Latino views of disease and curing. *Western Journal of Medicine, 139,* 868–874.

Mull, J. S., & Mull, D. S. (1983). A visit with a *curandero. Western Journal of Medicine, 139,* 730–736.

National Association of Private Psychiatric Hospitals. (1985, 1986). *Annual survey.* Washington, DC: Author.

National Institute of Mental Health. (1987). *Mental health, United States.* Rockville, MD: Author.

Quintana, F. L. (1980). Child rearing in Indian and Hispanic New Mexico. In I. N. Berlin (Ed.), *Children and our future* (pp. 34–41). Albuquerque, NM: University of New Mexico Press. (Monograph.)

Redl, F. (1959). The concept of a therapeutic milieu. *American Journal of Orthopsychiatry, 29,* 721–736.

Sander, D. (1979). *Navajo symbols of healing.* New York: Harcourt.

Scheper-Hughes, N., & Stewart, D. (1983). *Curanderismo* in Taos County, New Mexico—A possible case of anthropological romanticism. *Western Journal of Medicine, 139,* 875–884.

Weithorn, L. A. (1988). Mental hospitalization of troublesome youth: An analysis of skyrocketing admission rates. *Stanford Law Review, 40,* 773–838.

CHAPTER TWO

Culturally Responsive Inpatient Care of Children and Adolescents

Luis A. Vargas
Irving N. Berlin

Everything's part of the circle of life; everything is part of the song of the Great Spirit. That's the way I see things; it's probably the biggest difference between Native philosophy and the non-Indian philosophy, where ideas and actions are put into little boxes, where some things, some days, are thought of as holy, while most other things are not. (Sun Bear, 1983, p. 39)

The typical children's psychiatric hospital ostentatiously reflects the dominant culture in which it exists. The pictures on the walls, the style of the interior decorations and furniture, the layout of the rooms, offices, nursing station, and classrooms often represent the tastes and preferences of the dominant culture rather than those of the ethnic minority patients that it might serve. During the empty night hours, when the children have gone to bed and the busy interactions of the staff and the patients have ended for the day, the physical environment created for these young patients makes its strongest cultural statement. For example, a levels chart on the living room wall conveys the importance of achievement; the locked "cubbies" in the playroom, where the children store their valued possessions, underscore the value of ownership. To many young ethnic minority patients, the hospital's physical environment, intended to convey to them a genuine concern for their problems, speaks in a foreign tongue. The challenge of being culturally responsive must be confronted *before* children come to the hospital and must entail more than verbal efforts.

This chapter addresses the need to develop culturally responsive psychiatric inpatient milieus for ethnic minority children and adolescents. We have drawn primarily from our experience with Hispanics and American Indians in New Mexico to illustrate our points. The chapter is divided into two major sections: pre-admission considerations and treatment considerations.

PRE-ADMISSION CONSIDERATIONS

The Mexican . . . seems to me to be a person who shuts himself away to protect himself: his face is a mask and so is his smile. In his harsh solitude, which is both barbed and courteous, everything serves him as a defense: silence and words, politeness and disdain, irony and resignation. (Paz, 1985, p. 29)

The Presenting Problem

The family introduces itself to the hospital through the presenting problem. More than just a subjective description of what is "wrong" with the child, the presenting problem is a representation of the family's and child's understanding of how the world works (their beliefs and ways of thinking) and of solutions to problems of daily living.

The arrival of the family and child at the hospital does not imply that they accept the hospital's problem-solving approaches. Some minority families, particularly the more unacculturated ones, feel either directly or indirectly coerced to seek help because of pressures from schools, social welfare services, or the courts—referral sources that are likely to represent the dominant culture. Ethnic minority families that adhere to their cultures' traditional views and values enter the doors to the hospital with considerable trepidation. The hospital's physical surroundings give potent cultural messages. How do these families view such a mainstream-culture facility if the only minority staff present, if any are visible at all, are receptionists and clerical and maintenance staff? Cultural responsiveness begins with the efforts of the hospital to create a multicultural atmosphere that acknowledges its mainstream roots while conveying its receptivity to other cultural views and values. Creating this receptivity means having ethnic minorities represented in the clinical and administrative staff, reflecting in the decor the tastes of the patients' cultures, and offering literature and magazines that patients and their families like—to mention but a few ways of developing a welcoming environment.

When patients' families adhere to traditional views and values, we as clinicians must recognize the potential for implicit but potent clashes in conceptualization of the children's problems and, consequently, in the families' implicit and nonarticulated perceived solutions. The presenting problem is often stated by the child and the family with an implied parameter of potential solutions: "If you have an earache, you do not go to an orthopedist." The fact that a minority family presents itself to the hospital does not imply that family members accept our solutions at a fundamental, cultural level. When presenting mainstream solutions (a treatment plan) to American Indians, for example, it may be necessary to give particular attention to explaining the "whats," "hows," and "whys" (i.e., what the treatment plan will be, how we will carry it out, and why we believe it will work). In so doing, we are explicitly sharing and teaching our own basic ways of thinking and understanding as represented in the presenting problem. Additionally, we might acknowledge our openness to the family's seeking, parallel to our treatment, traditional cultural healing ceremonies. (They may or may not want to share them.) For instance, Navajo families tend to be much more open about their healing ceremonies than are some Pueblo families.

Levels of Acculturation

While our efforts must focus on empathically understanding the family's and child's conceptualizations of the presenting problems, such understanding requires that we, as clinicians, assess the levels of acculturation of the child and the family members. Wide discrepancy between parents, among generations (i.e., grandparents, parents, and children), and even among the child's siblings can be a significant contributant to the presenting problem and to the child's and family's acceptance of our treatment.

For example, Fred was a 14-year-old, psychotic, Pueblo Indian boy who was referred for possible hospitalization with considerable urgency by the Pueblo social worker. Knowing that Fred came from a traditional Pueblo Indian family, the intake staff at the hospital recognized that evaluation for hospitalization could not take place until the maternal grandmother, who was essential to any decision making in the family, returned from a visit to family members in a neighboring state. On her return, the grandmother, mother, father, patient, and patient's older brother, who acted as translator, all attended the evaluation. It was difficult to elicit the precipitating circumstances of Fred's psychosis until the grandmother described, using her grandson as an interpreter, how Fred had always been a very sensitive and insecure child, starting with several long hospitalizations, when he was 6 and 8 years old, for surgical correction to a club foot. The family then affirmed that Fred's recent problems appeared to be related to his transfer from the Pueblo elementary school to a high school in a nearby town where the students made fun of him because of his academic retardation, his large size, and his awkward walk. The grandmother stated through her grandson that a healing ceremony had been conducted without evident change in Fred. Had traditional solutions not been tried first, the family probably would not have been receptive to the prospect of psychiatric hospitalization for Fred.

In contrast to Fred and his family, some children and their families present problems associated with cultural marginality (Cervantes, 1976; Stonequist, 1961). These youngsters neither adhere to traditional values nor assimilate the American mainstream ways. Perhaps the best example, in the Hispanic culture, is the *cholo* and his post-World War II predecessor, the *pachuco*. Paz (1985) provided a good description of this marginal Hispanic youth:

> *Since the* pachuco *cannot adapt himself to a civilization which, for its part, rejects him, he finds no answer to the hostility surrounding him except this angry affirmation of his personality. . . . [I]nstead of attempting a problematical adjustment to society, the* pachuco *actually flaunts his differences. The purpose of his grotesque dandyism and anarchic behavior is not so much to point out the injustice and incapacity of a society that has failed to assimilate him as it is to demonstrate his personal will to remain different.* (pp. 15–16)

In his starched khaki or grey pants, sleeveless T-shirt, and bandana-tied or netted hair, the *cholo* represents more than a sartorial misfit in a unit. He is an angry jester who taunts both the traditional values and beliefs of his parents and those of the American mainstream culture. His caricatured presentation becomes a tragicomic statement of his intransigence in a struggle to assert his unique identity and to experience some ascendancy over others.

Another example of marginality, although usually without such adverse social consequences, is the Hispanic "low riders" whose flashy, low-lying, customized cars often provide a marked contrast to the status of their creators. Young Mexican Americans, often of limited financial means, work diligently and meticulously to create uniquely dazzling showpieces that ride within a few inches of the ground so that they can go cruising very slowly (low riding) down their town's or city's main street. Their banding together into low-rider clubs is one of the few ways in which they can feel some power in their powerless positions. Their cars become the symbol of what they aspire. Anaya (1978), in his essay "Requiem for a Low Rider," described an adolescent, Jessie, who was looking for excitement and meaning in life initially through cruising in his low rider. Jessie strove to be the ultimate "Mr. Cool" and was, at first, admired and esteemed by his friends, who enjoyed cruising with him. However, his almost compulsive effort to "cruise through life" looking for the best "high" eventually alienated him from his classmates and led him to drugs and death.

Another variation of the culturally marginal person is an adolescent or parent who has suddenly found ethnicity. For example, Alberto, who was baptized Albert, is a Mexican American father who is married to a New England Episcopalian woman and overespouses his and his children's "Mexican-ness." As a teenager he resented being so dark-complected and tried to lighten his skin by scrubbing himself with lemon juice on an *estropajo* (a scrubbing pad). He was very Americanized until the early 1970s, when he participated in the Chicano Movement in East Los Angeles while attending a prestigious private college in Claremont. Such overtraditionalization of cultural values and beliefs may often evoke anything from tolerant amusement to open protest among more genuinely traditional family members. It may also reveal a need to identify with a culture because, despite apparent acculturation, an adult still faces "hidden" or internalized discrimination, with its demoralizing effect on a core sense of self.

We must also be careful to recognize when psychopathology is masquerading as cultural differences (Montalvo & Gutierrez, 1984). Some of the ethnic minority families that present to the hospital may be in a state of cultural anarchy. For example, an American Indian family may have rejected traditional Indian beliefs and values. Family members may have discontinued participation in religious ceremonies and feasts as they attempt to "urbanize" or, worse yet, as they struggle with severe alcohol problems, unemployment, and generations of poverty and hopelessness, knowing that they were once a proud, independent, and productive people. Some families may use traditionality as a way of objecting to Western medicine, sometimes out of guilt or a sense of estrangement, as if to assert their cultural differences and their expectations of being misunderstood and not treated with respect. Parents who have been regarded as rejecting of their culture by other community members may angrily or resistantly assert their "traditional beliefs." Holding out these beliefs as being in conflict with Western or Anglo ways is sometimes their way of protesting the need for family therapy and other parental involvement in the hospital's treatment of their child.

Perception Toward the Hospital and Its Procedures

From the point of the initial evaluation for hospitalization, an appraisal of what the hospital represents to the family and the child or adolescent must be made. Where civil commitment is a requirement, how do the parents and other important family members feel about "giving up" some of their rights? Civil commitment and other aspects that we may regard as "procedural safeguards" may actually augment the minority family's feelings of alienation from their culture, relinquishment of parental authority, and ethnic or racial oppression. In American Indian families, there is often a conflict because the state courts do not recognize tribal court jurisdiction in many subject areas—an old wound for these families that has remained unhealed for centuries.

Involvement of Family Decision Makers

Our medical and legal systems assume that all families are set up the same way: a family is nuclear and is headed by a parental dyad or a single parent. Thus, consents for hospitalization and medication and permissions for release of information must be signed by the custodial parent or parents, and, if the patient is over a certain age, by the patient. We are not likely to question the premise of these legal requirements and, when confronted with challenges to them, we may attempt to convince the family of the need for such protections for the patient and family.

However, in American Indian families, a decision to hospitalize a child or adolescent may require the approval of extended family members, such as a grandparent, uncle, or, as in Fred's case, the clan matriarch. In our press to hospitalize a child and to convince the accompanying parent of the necessity for hospitalization, we may force a family to not seek the input of important family members or to bypass them in the decision-making process. Our sense of urgency can lead to an erroneous assessment of the parents' reaction as being resistance to treatment. They may be struggling to make important decisions without crucial family members or to overcome a fear that important family members will blame them for taking this step. The family may interpret our actions as an indirect but potent sign of disrespect for the family hierarchy and as a callous disempowerment of the family.

We act legally and ethically, from the dominant culture's perspective; yet we give a loud message of insensitivity to the minority family. Should it come as any surprise when the child, parents, and extended family fail to develop trust in us and confidence in our efforts? The need to recognize which family members should be included in important decisions about a child or adolescent is imperative to developing a therapeutic alliance with the family, which might involve grandparents, aunts and uncles, and other extended family. These same family members might be included in the family therapy that is planned during the child's hospitalization. In Hispanic and American Indian families, it is not unusual to have more than two generations, and extended family members in each generation, participate in family therapy.

TREATMENT CONSIDERATIONS

Healing is a powerful, culturally endorsed ritual. There is no doubt that if you trust the practitioner and if you share the same cultural myths, healing is better achieved. In the final analysis, however, I must admit that the [crises] of modern life are no better alleviated by psychiatrists than by visionaries, for both attempt to provide explanations for questions that have no simple answers. (Hammerschlag, 1988, p. 17)

Carlos was an 8-year-old Hispanic boy who came from a very small mountain town in which no streets were paved, not even the road that led into it. The town was largely composed of one extended family; most households in the town had the same last names. Despite the fact that this family and generations before it had not had any contact with Mexico, the family members spoke Spanish that was interspersed with corrupted archaic Spanish words—the product of the isolation of generations of Spanish families in these mountain communities. Carlos lived with his parents and three siblings in a one-room adobe house. The dirt floor was covered by linoleum; there were no windows (they let in too much cold air during the harsh winters) and no gas or running water. The father was unemployed, reportedly because of a work-related back injury sustained several years before. His unemployment seemed, in part, related to his own despondency and hopelessness about his and his family's situation. But any suggestion of moving, to find a better way of life, evoked cold looks of disbelief at the speaker's audacity. This was home! This was family!

A bright, verbal child, Carlos proved to be a delightful and informative historian. He told the therapist (L.A.V.) of his Spanish lineage, of the resented Mexicans who had invaded New Mexico, of his ancestors' ownership of vast expanses of forest land, and of the hated *foresteros* (forest rangers) who had taken his ancestors' land. (The forest rangers represented the

United States' reclamation of land that had previously been owned by these old Hispanic families.)

Carlos was admitted to the hospital after several suicide attempts which included trying to hang himself, running in front of oncoming vehicles, and jumping from a tree. He had been a well-adjusted boy until he was sexually molested by several cousins and reported the abuse to his father. His father, angered and alarmed by this revelation, reported the abuse to the local police, which led the grandparents, who headed the families, to ostracize Carlos, his siblings, and his parents. The grandparents and family were enraged that Carlos's father had taken family affairs to outsiders and, much worse, to *Anglos!* Who was this father to take such self-righteous action? This was the same man whom the grandfather had rescued on numerous occasions from drunken brawls during which Carlos's father had threatened his combatants with various weapons. "I've saved you from getting killed or killing yourself and now you turn and kill us," the grandfather told his son in Spanish.

The ostracism proved a stress too great to bear for Carlos, who was already struggling with the consequences of his abuse. He felt overwhelmed with guilt, rage, shame, and despondency. The feeling that he was responsible for, essentially, the entire town's ostracism of his family was more than he could tolerate. His suicide attempts were his efforts to extricate his family from the shame he had brought upon them. Carlos entered the hospital in awe of all the conveniences and luxuries, the same ones that would later lead him to feel so selfish for being there when his family had so little at home. At the time of admission, the treatment staff could only wonder what the appropriate treatment would be.

Awareness of Treatment Staff Cultural Biases

When treating multicultural populations, hospital staff members need to continuously address their own cultural biases and "cultural countertransferences." Carlos was a very engaging youngster, but female staff members found his attitude toward women unenlightened at best and infuriating at worst. In his own eyes, Carlos was the perfect little gentleman, a tribute to his parents' upbringing. Unfortunately, the young female staff initially resented being treated as if they were helpless, second-class citizens. One young female staff member resented this youngster's insistence on opening doors and helping her with heavy objects because his attitude seemed to imply that she was weak and helpless. Had we not directly addressed our staff's biases and culturally-based countertransferences, this child would have soon been resented for what he had been taught was good behavior.

In another case, the staff became angered at a 7-year-old Pueblo boy from the reservation who "refused" to stop taking other children's toys without their permission and was reluctant to "keep his place" in the dining room and in the room he shared with an Anglo roommate. When we addressed how our concept of ownership ran counter to the concept of sharing with which the child had grown up, staff members came to see him in a much more positive light. While the staff made overt efforts to teach the boy their views and values so as not to confuse him, they also began to see the positive aspects of his values. His willingness to share even made him an important role model for other children.

Similarly, the reluctance of Indian children to look into the face of an adult may pose problems, if not understood in its cultural context. In many Indian cultures, looking directly at the face of an adult, especially when being disciplined, is a sign of disrespect; to avoid looking directly at the face of the adult is considered proper. This behavior on the part of a child in American mainstream culture would draw a directly opposite reaction.

Universal Nature of Prejudice

With very few exceptions, most of us have prejudices against other races and peoples because we have been conditioned by our early experiences with immediate family, extended family, and the community environment in which we were raised. Those of us in mental health work need to become aware of the sometimes subtle prejudices we harbor; we may be revealing them in disguised ways.

Anglos, no matter what their convictions, are likely to have discriminatory feelings against all people of color; the intensity of those feelings depends on individual child-rearing circumstances. Most prejudice emerges in work situations. In psychiatric hospitals, Anglos may control hiring practices or find excuses for their inability to collaborate with minority persons. In one adolescent ward, an Anglo "old timer" and his Anglo colleagues described a recently hired Hispanic male mental health worker as not able to think fast enough to be of much help in containing aggressive adolescents. When a violent incident occurred, the Hispanic worker functioned quickly and effectively; yet it was passed off by the Anglo worker as a fluke. "Just wait," he said, undaunted in this challenge to his prejudice.

In another example, a very bright young therapist, of Jewish origin, repeatedly disclaimed any prejudice because, as an Anglo minority, he had experienced and suffered the effects of discrimination throughout his schooling and work situations. One day a very histrionic Hispanic girl, a young adolescent named Angie, was admitted to his unit. In her therapy hours and on the unit, she flirted shamelessly with every male. In the unit meetings, the therapist's comments about Angie made it clear that he was uncomfortable with her behavior. In a treatment conference two weeks after her admission, he explained that it was his conviction that such a narcissistic young woman was not treatable. He advised her discharge.

When the unit director and team disagreed and overruled him, he became very angry and left the meeting sulking. The therapist was asked to meet with the unit director and the hospital director to discuss the issues of his ability to continue to work with Angie. Fortunately, the therapist was in analysis and had begun to discuss his anger and the problems he had in working with this Hispanic adolescent. He discovered that he was dealing with an old stereotype, perhaps stemming from family attitudes toward Hispanic women. He could actually recall images from movies that featured the sexually overpowering Hispanic stars of the past and was contrasting them to the sexually repressive attitudes in his Orthodox Jewish household. He saw Angie as flamboyant, seductive, and sexually threatening, and he worried that he would not be able to maintain a therapeutic attitude toward her. Since he was beginning to deal with his previously unconscious prejudice, he continued to work effectively with his patient.

Hispanics, again based on childhood learning and experiences, are likely to be prejudiced against Anglos, who, in recent history, have been their primary oppressors in employment, land ownership, government, and education. Hispanics frequently have prejudiced feelings against Indians, who historically have viewed them as callous trespassers and cruel invaders and with whom they now may vie on the labor market, and against blacks, with whom they also now may compete for jobs. Of equal significance is the historical depreciation of Indians in Latin American countries and its generationally long-term effects on many Hispanics. It is important to recognize the divided identity of the mestizo in Latin American countries, particularly Mexico. Paz (1985) talked of the "developed Mexico" (headed largely by educated, affluent Mexicans who covetously esteem Western European values and life-styles) versus the "other Mexico" (the poor, underdeveloped, mestizo/Indian populace who not only do not share such values but may actually disdain them).

Vázquez (1978) cited others who referred to hierarchical societal distinctions in Mexico. He described the distinction made by Agustín Yáñez, a Mexican philosopher, between *la gente decente* (literally, the decent people) versus *los pelados* (literally, something plumed or bared; connotatively, a nobody or penniless person). Notable Mexican leaders like Hidalgo, Juárez, Villa, Carranza, and Zapata emerged from *los pelados*. Yáñez's dichotomy was roughly equivalent to Paz's "developed" versus "the other" Mexico. Vázquez also discussed the classification developed by Ezequiel A. Chávez, a highly influential Mexican philosopher and educator at the turn of this century. Chávez described the Mexican hierarchy as composed of the Europeans, or *criollos*, followed by the superior mestizos, the vulgar mestizos, and, lastly, the Indians, or *indígena*. The superior *mestizos* espouse or aspire to espouse the beliefs, values, and attitudes of the *criollos*. The vulgar mestizos reject these beliefs, values, and attitudes; but, rather than be seen as capable of such intentional rejection, they may be dismissed by the upper societal echelons as incapable of such enlightened aspirations.

Such prejudice can be both subtle and intense, cemented by unspoken, ubiquitous societal and familial messages that these long-standing biased hierarchies are *not* to be challenged. The result is often a prejudice that is denied and is extremely resistant to change—all the more reason for a culturally sensitive therapist to be aware of it. Alberto, the parent who overespouses his Mexican-ness, can, in part, be understood in this context. His conflict is the internalized, personalized struggle between the "developed" and "the other" Mexico, *la gente decente* and *los pelados*, the superior mestizos and the vulgar mestizos. As Paz (1985) put it: "The other Mexico, the submerged and repressed, reappears in the modern Mexico: when we talk with ourselves, we talk with it; when we talk with it, we talk with ourselves" (p. 287). It is from this intrapersonally tormenting paradox that Alberto cannot escape.

Depending on the locations of their tribes or pueblos, Indians not only may feel anger and hatred toward Anglos and Hispanics, their oldest oppressors and now the administrators of their welfare and health services, but they may discriminate against Hispanics and blacks as labor competitors and illegal owners of land to which they lay claim.

Thus, while many prejudices have an economic basis in terms of who gets a job or an education or who can succeed in business, many convictions about race and color have become part of us early in life and are the products of beliefs and attitudes transmitted, not necessarily verbally, from generation to generation.

No matter how any minority or majority group regards other peoples, there is a universal prejudice against women. In all ethnic groups, including American Indian tribes that are matrilineal, there is constant discrimination against women. They are paid less than men for the same work, their advancement is thwarted, and their ideas and opinions are deprecated. These prejudices also have their origins in early learning within the family and community.

Cultural Quality of the Milieu

The cultural tone of the milieu can make the difference between engaging or losing the cooperation of the child and his or her family, even when the therapist is the paragon of cultural sensitivity. A seemingly simple way of facilitating cultural sensitivity is to have a culturally diverse staff that has a wide range in age and religious beliefs. This is not as simple as it sounds. The management of such a staff is likely to be a challenge to the unit chief, who must help the staff to recognize and appreciate each member's differences and contributions without devaluating or invalidating each other.

Only then can a therapeutically valuable and culturally responsive staff be developed.

A culturally diversified staff not only is likely to be culturally responsive but also is best equipped to deal with psychopathology masquerading as cultural differences. For example, a multicultural staff in one unit was able to appreciate the cultural implications of a Pueblo girl's reluctance to report in group therapy what she did while on a therapeutic absence to her pueblo, because she had engaged in a tribal ceremony that was not to be shared with outsiders. The same multicultural unit staff was able to therapeutically confront a hostile Hispanic boy and his mother, both of whom were insisting that their enmeshment was a cultural value that was not being taken into account by what the family perceived to be a culturally myopic staff. The staff's readiness to acknowledge the closeness of Hispanic families, in an effort to be culturally sensitive, had initially prevented staff members from recognizing how the mother–son relationship was leading to the son's massive anger at being denied individuality and independence, which are characteristic male values in Hispanic culture.

Development of a culturally responsive staff and milieu is not dependent on recruiting bright, educated staff members. A few of these are necessary; they add to the diversity. More important is recruitment of culturally diverse staff members who enjoy working with children, have prior relevant experiences (perhaps with children of their own), and have a talent or "intuitive feel" for understanding and working with children. In essence, the best recruits are *natural therapists* from different cultures.

Staff Attitudes Toward the Child and the Family

Hospitalization of any child can elicit intense conflict between the child's family and the staff. The parents may feel usurped by the staff and the staff may, unconsciously or otherwise, convey to the parents the message that they have been poor parents and that the staff is a much better parent substitute (Berlin, 1973). In a multicultural setting, the potential for conflicts between staff and family members is increased substantially. The required cultural sensitivity goes beyond the recognition of different cultural norms for certain behaviors of children, parental practices, and discipline: Staff members must recognize their own culturally based expectations. For example, a quiet Navajo mother who never questions the staff may be seen as slow and concrete and as requiring simple directives and short, if any, explanations. Yet, this mother may actually be an astute observer whose reluctance to involve herself in the workings of the unit milieu is increased by her sense of being cruelly treated by the staff as being retarded. Only because of her love for her child does she submit herself silently, each week, to such humiliation in the unit. Were staff members able to recognize the potential for such problems, they might make attempts to convey their appreciation for her devotion toward her child and involve her in ways that enhance her sense of efficacy and influence in the milieu. This mother may be a powerful person in her clan and extended family, and may feel powerless and without influence in the milieu, thus facing a double bind.

The role of milieu staff is not solely to be supportive; the staff must sometimes deal with very difficult behaviors of both the child and the family. Sometimes, a multicultural staff can deal intuitively with the resistance and challenges posed by minority children and their families. An example of this intuitive approach is illustrated in the case of an angry Hispanic father who had lost custody of his son while he was in prison and his son had been neglected and abused while under his mother's care. The father, who identified strongly with the *cholo* subculture, adamantly denied any role in his son's problems and resented greatly the son's hospitalization. In his visits to see his son, which were very important to the boy, the father assumed a hostile, taunting, and almost caricatured *cholo* stance which the staff resented, particularly since the boy tried to emulate his father to gain his affection. The father's *cholo* stance represented not only his disdain for the dominant mainstream culture of which the staff was a predominant symbol but also a rageful retaliation toward his parents, whose values he was attacking. In therapy, the father lamented furiously how his parents, especially his mother, had rejected and abandoned him and how his brother (the oldest of the family) had always had his mother's undaunted support and love, even though his brother had had more serious problems with the law.

After one particularly difficult therapy session, the father came to visit his son seething with anger that found disturbing expression in his indirect derisiveness toward the staff. A staff member, a strong-willed Hispanic grandmother whose dedication to the children was unwavering, called to the father to come into the kitchen where she was making *biscochitos* (Mexican Christmas cookies) with his son and other children. Experiencing the unspoken onslaught of the anger he evinced, which likely emanated, in part, from the frustrated yearning for his own mother's affection, she responded intuitively. She told him very frankly that she could tell how angry he was but that she simply would not allow him to express it so negatively in the presence of the children in the unit. She reiterated how important his visits were to his son and how she wanted him to have them. To the father's surprise, she told him to roll up his sleeves and come help her and the children cut the dough. The visit ended with all of them eating the *biscochitos*, the children with milk and the adults with the coffee she had made. Although the father continued to struggle with his unresolved anger and personal conflicts, he often sought out this staff member and preferred to visit when she was present. She continued, with the consultation of the therapist (L.A.V.), to impose limits on him when he became too angry or acted otherwise inappropriately.

Cultural Responsiveness of the Hospital

When treating multicultural populations, the potential for iatrogenic contributions can be significant. A Pueblo child, whose upbringing emphasizes sharing and disapproves of possessiveness, may be disciplined in the unit for failure to "respect" other children's ownership and may become the victim of iatrogenic, countertherapeutic interventions. A Navajo family that is, from the treatment staff's perspective, severely affected by the recent death of the maternal grandmother who largely raised the hospitalized child may refuse to talk about the death and its impact on the child and family. Unaware of Navajo sanctions against talking about the dead for fear that the decedent's spirit will invade the speaker or haunt his or her house, the therapist may pound the family with ever more refined and persistent "interventions" that both frustrate and anger the family. The struggle that ensues as the child and family resist these efforts to talk about the death of the grandmother becomes an iatrogenic conflict that diverts the focus from the reason the child is in the hospital. Furthermore, such a struggle may make it impossible to explore which other family members are important to the child and can provide important nurturance.

Recognition of the Navajo taboo, along with the realization that the death is important in the etiology of the problem that brought the child to the hospital, is imperative to effective treatment. Given such awareness, the therapist may find creative, indirect ways of addressing the death's aftermath, including consultation with and use of a medicine man who has learned how to deal with the taboo by providing comfort to the child and family through sings or ceremonies. A therapist and staff who understand that talking about death is taboo among the Navajo can express their awareness of both the taboo and how much pain the death must have caused. In other words, the therapist may talk about death in the third person, carefully cognizant to address death generically without personalizing it to the grandmother.

Development of interventions that make sense from the perspective of the ethnic minority child and family, and repeated reevaluations to ensure that the interventions are not a reflection of the staff's own ethnocentricity, should be integral parts of daily rounds and of case conferences.

Cultural Applicability of Interventions

Treatment milieus are predicated upon a set of beliefs and values that usually derive from those of the mainstream culture. As Americans, we value assertiveness, independence, and personal ownership; we believe that we control our own destiny; and we insist on the separation of self and other and of self and context. Our values and beliefs contribute to the diagnosis of problems in living, but they also can misdirect our treatment efforts.

For example, teaching a Pueblo boy to talk assertively and directly to his elders about his feelings, when such an approach is not likely to be accepted in his family or community, is evidently countertherapeutic and contradicts the child's cultural values and beliefs. Recognizing the mediating role of Pueblo elders may be one way of helping the boy to communicate his troubles to the family. The therapist might enlist the help of tribal elders and encourage the boy to communicate his concerns to them.

Misdirected treatment efforts may also be seen when treatment staff address issues of discipline with American Indian children. In a number of American Indian tribes, the mother's brothers and sisters (the child's uncles and aunts) are the family disciplinarians. The young person may turn to these individuals for help when there are problems with parents. Unless the therapist can utilize extended family, clan members, or tribal elders as advocates for the Indian child or adolescent, helping the patient to clarify and alter the conflict-inducing behavior of chaotic parents may be difficult.

Carlos, who was introduced earlier in the chapter, caused one of the authors (L.A.V.) to question whether the interventions in the milieu actually had practical applicability and relevance outside of the hospital setting. Carlos found refuge in our unit. Through the patience and guidance of a talented, self-assured, young black woman on our staff, Carlos came to view the female staff in a different light. He even told his therapist that through this woman he had come to see the strength his mother had, which he had never recognized. Carlos's relationship with his parents, which was already strong, was further strengthened. Such success was gratifying, but our staff was still left with the question of what we could actually do for this child to help him at home.

The therapist (L.A.V.) and the unit outreach worker, who are both Spanish-speaking, decided to plan a visit to Carlos's grandparents' home—a decision that was welcomed by the parents, who had on various occasions intimated such an effort might be helpful. Upon arriving at Carlos's father's home, both visitors were struck by the strengths of Carlos's family and the hardship and despondency that they confronted daily. As the visitors and Carlos's father walked down the dirt road to the grandparents' house, the father explained his trepidation about meeting with his father and his brother and sisters after having been ostracized for several months and his fear that the trip might be in vain. The group was met by an angry brother and sister who threatened Carlos's father. Yet, while they seemed to be ominous obstacles to the hospital staff's entry into their parents' home, they, like Carlos's father, seemed extremely pained by the tragedies that had beset their families. After some introduction by the therapist of the purpose of their coming, the hospital staff members were allowed entry.

A two-and-a-half-hour meeting followed. Conducted entirely in Spanish, it dealt with the accumulated anger of the grandparents and their children toward each other, their frustrated goals and dreams, and their despair about the worsening of their families' circumstances. This despair had found full expression in the sexual abuse incident, which was an extremely traumatic event to the entire extended family. It symbolized the most feared outcome: that generations of hard work, of proud ownership of valued, if now diminished, land, and of unwavering hope in the face of hardship and adversity had been for naught. The families, especially the grandparents, now faced dissolution, generations of shame, and a realization that they had been responsible for the failed end of the efforts of so many earlier generations. The meeting succeeded in reuniting the families and finding treatment for the perpetrators of the abuse, with the grandfather's support. More importantly, the meeting provided the families with a renewed sense of efficacy and empowerment.

Carlos's father announced the success of the meeting to his family and gave permission to renew visits with his parents. As Carlos happily ran down the dirt road to be reunited with his beloved grandfather, the therapist was impressed with the resolute efforts of the family members to deal with such personal and familial tragedies. At best, the therapist and the outreach worker could take credit for listening to Carlos's family's suggestions that perhaps the solution to Carlos's dilemma lay in mobilizing the extended family.

Carlos's case serves to remind us not to overvalue or depend too heavily on the impact of the milieu to meet a child's needs, at the expense of underrepresenting the fact that the child and the family will have to develop coping strategies that work at home in their community—apart from the hospital. This is not to minimize the role of the milieu; it can be extremely helpful, as in Carlos's case, in alleviating the presenting problems and stresses that the child experiences. Rather, the caution is intended to direct our efforts toward helping the child and family to have greater success where it is likely to count most—at home.

Openness of the Hospital Setting

For the ethnic minority family, the hospital's procedures and policies may seem like uncaring sentries that prevent access to information about the child's treatment and to the child. Openness must begin when the initial evaluation of the child is shared with the family, and an attempt is made to enlist the family's cooperation. Particularly because minorities' parenting styles are likely to be different from those of the mainstream culture, greater efforts should be made to enlist the family, in the milieu, as collaborators in the child's treatment.

Inviting the parents to be on the unit during times in which they typically have difficulty with the child (e.g., mealtimes or bedtime) or in the classroom may serve not only to acquaint them with the hospital and its staff but, equally important, may allow staff to teach the parents new skills that can help to restructure prior problematic relationships within the family. Inviting the families to share meals with the staff and patients; forming an active parents' support group and offering babysitting services, during meetings, for the parents' other children; arranging for occasional potluck dinners organized by the parents; and involving the families in the planning and execution of unit activities, such as camping trips, can further facilitate the development of trust among the child, the family, and the hospital staff.

Empowerment of the Child and Family

There is a seeming contradiction in the inpatient treatment of a child. A goal in treatment is to empower the child and the family, yet the constant evaluation of the child and family and the medical/legal system in which the treatment takes place often make them feel powerless. Staff members must be careful to avoid blaming the parents. Through the staff's efforts to empathize with the child and the parents, to understand the impact of culture and poverty, and to recognize and encourage any signs of parental tenderness and understanding toward the child, the foundation for empowerment is begun.

When medication is necessary for the child, there is considerable potential for empowerment of the family. For example, if staff members recognize that parents' fears and prejudices toward medication are derived from cultural taboos or beliefs, they can develop an educational process that allows native healers or clan patriarchs/matriarchs to intercede with the parents for a trial of medication. Thus, a situation that could have easily been the basis for disempowerment of the family can result in significant empowerment.

Enlistment of Community and Family Support

Sarah, a 14-year-old Pueblo Indian girl, was hospitalized for an acute paranoid schizophrenic episode. She was clearly hallucinating and told the staff that male and female voices were telling her that she would die. Both parents were bright, English-speaking individuals who worked at responsible jobs in the pueblo. They could not give the treatment staff any clues about the sudden onset of the psychosis. A week earlier, after school, Sarah had attended a clan meeting of adolescent girls. She was strangely silent that evening. The next day, she talked of hearing voices. Her mother, who was an important member of the clan, could not discover from the elders who ran the meeting and helped with the planning for some festivities any happening that might have been responsible for Sarah's problems.

Sarah was placed on Stelazine and was assigned to a young Anglo woman, her primary staff person on the unit; a female child psychiatry fellow was assigned to be Sarah's therapist. Slowly, Sarah adjusted to the unit, resumed her enjoyment of school, and began to relate to her primary staff person. After two weeks on medication, she began to evidence trust in her therapist and recounted the events that led to her illness—events that, she said, made it impossible for her to return to the pueblo.

At the adolescent group meeting of the clan, Linda, an 18-year-old girl whom Sarah very much admired and who was a model for her, had looked very depressed. Linda told Sarah that she had been offered a scholarship to a state university. Linda wanted very much to complete the undergraduate program in social work as a step toward obtaining a master's degree in social work. When Linda had told her parents about the scholarship, they looked upset. They told Linda that they had agreed to a proposal by her mother's clan that Linda spend the next year as a teacher in their expanded HeadStart program. Linda could begin college the following year. Her parents felt that there was no way they could go back on their word. Linda was very despondent and had thought of suicide, but felt that she could "sweat out" the next year and then get on with her career plans.

Sarah was terribly shaken by the unilateral decision. She was already a whiz in math, had become proficient in use of a computer at school, and enjoyed using it to keep the books for the Glee Club. Sarah had talked with her mother often about wanting to apply for a scholarship to attend business school, get an M.B.A., and return to the pueblo as an accountant, not a glorified bookkeeper like her mother. Her mother had always encouraged her in her plans. That night, Sarah had dreams of being tortured because she would not do the clan's bidding. The next day, she was certain that she would die because she wanted to "do her own thing." She was sure that her ideas and plans would be interfered with by the clan.

Of great interest to the therapist and staff was Sarah's certainty of not being given what she wanted, which she had actually *not* experienced and which seemed based on her mother's frequent stories about how she was frustrated at work. She had not been given the recognition and promotions she deserved because the men in the finance office, who were her superiors, were made uneasy by this very bright and competent woman. They did not want to be placed in direct competition with her. Thus, to have the important women of her clan, including her mother, spoil Linda's cherished plan and its imminent fulfillment made Sarah feel that she could not trust anyone.

The therapist's supervisor (I.N.B.), who had dealt with a similar situation, pointed out that the issues to be resolved were in the pueblo and the clan. A presentation to Sarah's parents, especially to her mother, by Sarah with support from the therapist and primary staff person would be the beginning. At the family therapy meeting, Sarah recounted the events preceding her illness. Her mother was surprised and said that the clan's job was to do what it could to develop the pueblo's programs; the impact of its decisions on the young clan members was rarely considered. She promised to raise the issue that week at a clan meeting. At the next family meeting, Sarah's mother described the discussion at the clan meeting and the decision that the education of the young women of the pueblo was of paramount importance. The decision about Linda was reversed and Sarah was promised every consideration when it was her turn to pursue her career education. As in the example of Carlos, the resolution of the conflicts essentially lay in the collaboration of the community. The hospital care had helped Sarah to overcome her psychosis and to clarify the issues with her mother that had led to her illness.

The cases of Carlos and Sarah illustrate the importance of developing and strengthening social supports while the child is still in the hospital. There is no substitute for outreach visits to the child's home and community, to a prospective school, or to the community mental health center that is to provide the follow-up care. The staff can also convey to the family its respect for culturally sanctioned healing, which may be enlisted by American Indians and some Hispanic families.

CONCLUSION

The efforts to be culturally responsive require constant evaluation and reevaluation, constant attention to every staff member, child, and family. To be successful, the process involves, above all else, continued self-examination and introspection and, because of this, a very special staff.

My work was to do good . . . I was to heal the sick and show them the path of goodness. But I was not to interfere with the destiny of any man. Ultima, the curandera (Anaya, 1972, p. 247)

Acknowledgments

I would like to express my appreciation to Carl Beaver, Maya Roeder, M.A., Donna Adkins, Larry Narvaez, Dixie Vigil, Jodi Rice-Hamm, Shirley Van Haren, M.S.W., Patricia Rivera, M.S.W., Wilhemina Tengco, M.D., Sr. Jude Moore, ACSW, and our unit volunteer grandmothers, Rosa Telles and Rita Moquino, for teaching me about being culturally responsive and for providing, through their work, many clinical examples of culturally responsive interventions. (L.A.V.)

I am very grateful to the variety of native American and Alaskan Native professionals, paraprofessionals, and indigenous native healers in health, mental health, and education who were patient and friendly in their repetitive efforts to help me learn how best to work with them and how much I could gain from their instruction if I did not hurry. (I.N.B.)

Both authors express their gratitude to the many Hispanic and American Indian children, adolescents, and families, the Albertos, Carloses, Freds, and Sarahs, who helped us learn the essentials of responsive and culturally attuned inpatient care and tolerated our blunders and insensitivities.

REFERENCES

Anaya, R. A. (1972). *Bless me, Ultima.* Berkeley, CA: Tonahtiuh International.

Anaya, R. A. (1978, February). Requiem for a low rider. *La Confluencia: A Magazine of the Southwest,* pp. 2–6.

Berlin, I. N. (1973). Parental blame: An obstacle in psychotherapeutic work with schizophrenic children and their families. In S. A. Szurek & I. N. Berlin (Eds.), *Clinical studies in childhood psychoses* (pp. 115–126). New York: Brunner/Mazel.

Cervantes, J. M. (1976). *A consideration of marginality and culture conflict: The Chicano perspective.* Unpublished manuscript, University of Nebraska—Lincoln.

Hammerschlag, C. A. (1988). *The dancing healers: A doctor's journey of healing with Native Americans.* San Francisco: Harper & Row.

Montalvo, B., & Gutierrez, M. (1984, August). The mask of culture. *The Family Therapy Networker,* pp. 42–47.

Paz, O. (1985). *The labyrinth of solitude.* L. Kemp, Y. Milos, & R. P. Belash (Trans.), New York: Grove Press.

Stonequist, E. V. (1961). *The marginal man: A study in personality and culture conflict.* New York: Russell and Russell.

Sun Bear. (1983). *Sun Bear: The path of power, as told to Wabun and to Barry Weinstock.* Spokane, WA: Bear Tribe Publishing.

Vazquez, F. H. (1978). *European ideas in Mexico: An analysis of the Mexican philosophical discourse.* Unpublished doctoral dissertation, Claremont Graduate School.

Part II

Pretreatment Considerations

Successful inpatient psychiatric treatment of children and adolescents depends on careful patient screening and on effective treatment planning that is based on sound theoretical models and cultural sensitivity. Chapter 3 reviews basic evaluation principles and guidelines for admissions and offers a format for the admission process, including the collection of relevant information. Evaluations must not only determine the symptom picture, but also describe the young person's level of development and how it affects his or her relationships with family, peers, general environment, and culture. Effective treatment planning, described in Chapter 4, depends on an integrated theoretical understanding of the development of psychiatric disorders. An integrated developmental and biopsychosocial model is presented. Specific components of treatment plans are suggested for short-, intermediate-, and long-term hospital stays. Cultural factors that must be addressed in planning are delineated.

CHAPTER THREE

Determining the Need for Inpatient Treatment

Robert L. Hendren

The decision to admit a young person to a psychiatric hospital is a serious one. Making this medical decision requires the careful consideration of a trained evaluator who has a complete knowledge of child and adolescent psychiatric disorders, treatment modalities, and available resources. Because hospitalization is at the most restrictive and most expensive end of the continuum of care and requires the patient's removal from the home, the best interests of the child or adolescent (and, where appropriate, his or her family) must be the paramount consideration.

Hospitals, like most other institutions, are usually part of a dominant culture. In North America, this means that the psychiatric hospital is associated with the white or Anglo culture. As a result, people from minority cultural backgrounds (including disadvantaged Anglos) have an additional reason for fearing and feeling uncomfortable with the idea of hospitalization for themselves or a member of their family. The nature of the meeting between the patient and the hospital's evaluators, who determine the need for hospitalization, is therefore extremely important in setting the tone for the family's engagement in treatment. Methods for evaluating in a culturally sensitive manner the need for psychiatric hospitalization are the topic of this chapter.

REFERRAL

Usually, a patient's family first encounters the psychiatric hospital during the contact with the intake worker. The nature of this contact often composes the opening theme for all subsequent meetings between the family and the hospital. Is the intake worker engaging and understanding or distant and judgmental? Does the worker seem culturally sensitive? Is the information gathered in a respectful manner? Is the evaluation process adequately explained?

The hospital must determine who referred the young person for hospitalization. Was the referral made by the child's parents, the school, the outpatient therapist, or, in the case of adolescents, was the young person self-admitting? Another important question is: Are all family members in agreement with the referral? Family members may resist referral for hospitalization or they may strongly favor hospitalization. Either of these responses can produce sometimes obvious and sometimes subtle influences on the evaluating clinician's decision to admit (Perlmutter, 1986). Notations on the family's attitude toward hospitalization are often useful as predictors of later resistance to treatment recommendations and/or to treatment. An example of a form for collecting pertinent information at the time of referral for hospitalization is shown in Figure 3.1.

The person making the initial contact with the family must learn the presenting symptoms and their duration and severity. Symptoms such as

Figure 3.1. Psychiatric Inpatient Referral Form

CHILDREN'S PSYCHIATRIC HOSPITAL
Adolescent Ward Referral Form

Name _____ Date of initial call _____

Date of birth _____ Age _____ Sex _____ Social Security no. _____-___-_____

Parent/Guardian _____

Address _____

Phone (res.) _____ (bus.) _____ County _____

Insurance

Medicaid _____ yes _____ no _____ Other_____

Private payer (name/address/phone) _____

_____

Referral source _____
                         (name)   (address)   (phone)

Current living situation _____

History

Suicide _____ Aggression _____

Substance abuse _____ Legal charges _____

Sexual abuse _____ Physical abuse _____

Evidence of psychosis _____

Other _____

Current presenting symptoms _____

_____

_____

_____

School _____ Grade _____ Reg. or special ed. _____

39

Figure 3.1. Psychiatric Inpatient Referral Form   (continued)

Previous and Current Treatment

Place	Date	Duration	Diagnosis	Meds.

Impressions

(family involvement, treatability, urgency) _____

_____

_____

_____

_____

_____

Records requested date _____

Interview schedule date _____

_____

Signature of initial intake person

Final disposition _____

suicidal behavior, evidence of psychosis, and aggressive or impulsive behavior are likely to represent an urgent need for expedience in arranging an evaluation. A history of sexual and/or physical abuse or of legal charges raises issues that require special attention in the evaluation process because governmental and judicial agencies may have to become involved. A history of previous and current treatment settings, and of the duration and nature of the treatment contact, helps to profile the effectiveness of less restrictive treatment settings and the patient's responsiveness to earlier treatment. All of this information, if gathered in a thoughtful manner, can lead to initial impressions regarding family issues, treatability, and urgency. The intake worker's impressions can be very helpful to the evaluating clinician in the development of a thorough and expeditious evaluation of the young person's suitability for inpatient psychiatric care.

When additional information is necessary to determine whether an evaluation should take place, or when an evaluation is scheduled, requests for collateral information should be communicated to the current and previous therapist(s), the current school placement, and, when appropriate, the family physician and/or the juvenile authorities.

SCREENING FOR ADMISSION

Most guidelines for evaluation for admission to a psychiatric hospital recommend that the assessment of children and adolescents be carried out by a child and adolescent psychiatrist. The American Psychiatric Association (APA) "believes that the health of children and adolescents will be served best if psychiatrists—preferably child and/or adolescent psychiatrists—are responsible for all psychiatric admission decisions, treatment planning, and discharge decisions" (American Psychiatric Association, 1989). The American Academy of Child and Adolescent Psychiatry (AACAP) defines a "properly qualified psychiatrist" to assess children and adolescents for hospitalization as a "fully trained child and adolescent psychiatrist." For patients 14 years or older, a qualified psychiatrist may be "a general psychiatrist with documented specialized training, supervised experience, and demonstrated competence in work with adolescents" (American Academy of Child and Adolescent Psychiatry, 1989). Further, the decision to admit a patient to the hospital should be "based upon either a direct examination conducted personally by the responsible physician or upon the physician's review of the findings of an appropriately trained and trusted clinician" (AACAP, 1986).

The clinician conducting the psychiatric assessment of a child or adolescent must have a working knowledge of child development, childhood psychopathology, and an accepted classification system (the Diagnostic and Statistical Manual III-Revised, DSM III-R, or the International

Classification of Diseases, ICD-9) (Lewis, 1986). The evaluating clinician must also be alert to cultural characteristics that could affect the patient's behavior, to cultural stereotypes and variations, and to transferences and countertransferences that may develop from class, cultural, or racial biases (Spurlock, 1985).

All of the components of a comprehensive psychiatric evaluation of a child or adolescent are not covered in this chapter. Readers who desire this information might consult Lewis (1982) or Simmons (1981).

Before meeting with the family or the patient, the evaluating clinician should review thoroughly the data gathered by the intake worker and the collateral information. In an emergency evaluation, the evaluating clinician should review the available information and identify the additional information needed to make a quick yet reliable decision regarding hospitalization. The urgency of the evaluation must be considered as well. When children or adolescents are clearly demonstrating behavior that endangers themselves or others and have a condition that might respond to psychiatric treatment, the initial evaluation should be briefer and more focused. When the need for psychiatric hospitalization is less clear, a more extensive evaluation is appropriate. The extent of the evaluation will also be affected by the hospital's length of treatment (acute, intermediate, long-term).

The interview with the child, family members, and other relevant people should take place in a comfortable and private setting that acknowledges the surrounding cultures in its room decor. When posters, pictures, objects of art, and furniture arrangement reflect the styles of the various cultural groups, the familiarity of the setting can help put the family at ease. Interviews of the patient and the family together as well as separately are desirable, to gather a complete history and to create a full picture of the functioning of each individual and of the family unit.

A sample questionnaire that assesses the family and the child or adolescent patient is shown in Figure 3.2. When there is ample time before the evaluation interview, this questionnaire can be sent to family members for completion and then used as an evaluation guideline during the initial interview. The form in Figure 3.3 is a questionnaire for recording the pertinent medical history.

THE ADMISSION DECISION

The decision of whether to admit a child or adolescent for psychiatric hospitalization is made after all of the information gathered is screened or reviewed by the admitting psychiatrist. The admitting psychiatrist may arrive at the decision alone, after reviewing the information he or she has gathered. Or, a team of one or more clinicians, diagnosticians, pediatricians, and/or trainees may present the information they have gathered

Figure 3.2. Family Information Form

CHILDREN'S PSYCHIATRIC HOSPITAL
Family Questionnaire

Child's name _____ Age _____ Birth date _____

Parents' name(s) 1. _____

2. _____

Address 1. _____

2. _____

Phone contact (res.) _____ (bus.) _____

Insurance company (name/address/phone) _____

_____

Other significant persons(s) 1. _____ / _____

and relationship   2. _____ / _____

Address(es) 1. _____

2. _____

Phone(s) 1. _____

2. _____

Presenting Problems

1. List the problems that you brought your son/daughter/ward in for.

a. _____

_____

_____

Figure 3.2. Family Information Form (continued)

b. _____

_____

_____

c. _____

_____

_____

d. _____

_____

_____

e. _____

_____

_____

Family

1. List everyone who lives in the child's home, including yourself.

	Name	Relation to Child	Age
a.			
b.			
c.			
d.			
e.			
f.			
g.			

Figure 3.2. **Family Information Form** *(continued)*

2. Please check (✓) the ethnic background of each of the following:

	Child	Mother	Father
Asian	——	——	——
Black	——	——	——
Hispanic	——	——	——
Native American	——	——	——
Anglo	——	——	——

3. Mother's occupation ————————————————————

   How far did she go in school? ————————————————

   Age ——————————————————————————

4. Father's occupation ————————————————————

   How far did he go in school? ————————————————

   Age ——————————————————————————

5. Total income of household residents: (check one)

   —— $ 0–$ 7,000

   —— $ 7,001–$14,000

   —— $14,001–$21,000

   —— $21,001–$28,000

   —— $28,001–$35,000

   ——   Over $35,000

6. What language is spoken at home most of the time? ————————

7. Does the child speak a language other than English? —— yes —— no

   If yes, what language? ——————————————————

Figure 3.2.   Family Information Form   (continued)

8. Do the parents speak a language other than English? _____ yes _____ no

   If yes, what language? _____

9. Religious preference (check one)

   _____   Catholic

   _____   Protestant

   _____   Jewish

   _____   Other _____

   _____   None

10. How important is religion to you?

    _____   Not at all

    _____   A little bit

    _____   Quite a bit

    _____   Extremely

11. List anyone in the family (including grandparents, aunts, and uncles) who has had a drug or alcohol problem.

    a. _____

    b. _____

    c. _____

12. List anyone else in the family who has had a mental disorder.

    a. _____

    b. _____

    c. _____

Figure 3.2. Family Information Form (continued)

13. List anyone in the family who has been in jail.

    a. _____

    b. _____

    c. _____

14. Were the parents abused as children? (check one)

	Mother	Father
Physically abused	_____	_____
Sexually abused	_____	_____
No	_____	_____

15. If one of the child's natural parents is not in the home now, where is he/she? _____

    _____

    Does the absent parent keep in contact with the child? _____

16. Do any relatives live in the same town as the child? (names and relationship)

    _____ / _____

17. Do any relatives help the child's parents with their children or give advice about them? (name and relationship) _____

    _____ / _____

18. Do the child's parents have any close friends? (names) _____

    _____

19. If you live with the child and you are married, please rate how satisfied you are with your marriage right now.

Very Unsatisfied				Average				Very Satisfied	
1	2	3	4	5	6	7	8	9	10

Figure 3.2.   Family Information Form   *(continued)*

School

1. What school was the child in before coming to the hospital? _____

   _____

2. What grade? _____   _____

3. Was he/she in special education? If so, check the appropriate box(es).

   _____ B-Level   _____ Behavior disordered

   _____ C-Level   _____ Learning disabled

   _____ D-Level   _____ Communication disordered

   _____ Mixed   _____ Mentally retarded

                              _____ Mixed

4. Has the child been tested for special education? _____

5. Has the child ever failed a grade? _____ yes _____ no _____ grade

Peers

1. Check one column for each question.   Yes   No

   a. Does the child have many friends?   _____   _____

   b. Does he/she have a best friend?   _____   _____

   c. Have any of his/her friends had a mental disorder? _____   _____

   d. Have any of his/her friends been involved with
      drugs?   _____   _____

   e. Have any of his/her friends been in trouble with
      the law?   _____   _____

Figure 3.2. *Family Information Form* *(continued)*

History

1. Check one column for each question.   Yes   No

   a. Were there any birth complications?   _____   _____

   b. Was he/she a happy baby?   _____   _____

   c. Was he/she an easy baby to care for?   _____   _____

2. When did he/she learn to talk? (age) _____

3. When did he/she learn to walk? (age) _____

4. When did he/she complete toilet training? (age) _____

5. Check one column for each question.   Yes   No

   a. Has he/she ever been treated for a physical disorder? _____   _____

      If so, give description. _____

   b. Has he/she ever been in an accident in which he/she was knocked
      out?   _____   _____

6. How many different moves has he/she made in his/her life? _____

   How many in the past two years? _____

7. Has he/she ever been in trouble with the law? _____ yes _____ no

   a. If so, what offenses brought him/her to the attention of the law?

      1) _____

      2) _____

      3) _____

   b. How old was he/she when he/she first was in trouble with the law? _____

   c. Who is the probation officer? (name and phone) _____

   _____

Figure 3.2. Family Information Form *(continued)*

8. Check one column for each question.   Yes   No

   a. Has he/she ever been physically abused?   _____   _____

   b. Has he/she ever been sexually abused?   _____   _____

   c. Has he/she ever been taken out of the home
      because of neglect?   _____   _____

9. Has he/she ever been treated before? _____ yes _____ no

   If so, by whom? In what year?

   a. _____ 19_____

   b. _____ 19_____

   c. _____ 19_____

10. Has he/she been on medication before? _____ yes _____ no

    What was it?

    a. _____ 19_____

    b. _____ 19_____

    c. _____ 19_____

11. When do you think his/her problems began? _____

    _____

12. Has he/she ever talked about suicide? _____ yes _____ no

    If so, did he/she have a plan? _____

13. Has the Department of Health and Human Services ever been involved in
    care of the child? _____ yes _____ no

    If so, who is the caseworker? (name and phone) _____

    _____

14. Has your son/daughter/ward ever used street drugs? What are they? _____

    _____

Figure 3.2.   Family Information Form   *(continued)*

15. What kind of discipline strategies have you tried in the past?

_____

_____

_____

_____

Person completing this questionnaire: _____

Relationship: _____

Figure 3.3.   Medical Information Form

CHILDREN'S PSYCHIATRIC HOSPITAL
Medical History

Patient name _____   CPH# _____
                                         (For hospital use only)
Address _____

Date of birth _____

Please put a check (✓) on *only* the lines that have information that applies to your child. Next to each check that you enter, use the space under "Describe" to give details.

1. PREGNANCY AND BIRTH HISTORY

Mother's age at child's birth _____

Length of pregnancy _____

Problems during pregnancy	Yes	No	Describe
Illnesses	___	___	_____
Medications	___	___	_____
Cigarette smoking	___	___	_____
Marijuana smoking	___	___	_____

Figure 3.3.   Medical Information Form   *(continued)*

Problems during pregnancy   Yes   No   Describe

Street drugs   _____   _____   _____

Alcohol   _____   _____   _____

Length of labor _____

Presentation: Head _____   Feet _____   Other _____

C-Section _____   Reason _____

Birth weight _____

Complications   Yes   No   Describe

Cyanosis   _____   _____   _____

Jaundice   _____   _____   _____

Respirator   _____   _____   _____

Intensive care   _____   _____   _____

Birth defects   _____   _____   _____

Breast-fed   _____   _____

Bottle-fed   _____   _____

Baby's age at discharge _____

2. DEVELOPMENT

List child's age for the following:

Sat alone _____

Walked _____

Words _____

Sentences _____

Problems _____

_____

Figure 3.3.   Medical Information Form   (*continued*)

3. IMMUNIZATIONS

Fill out the attached immunization record. A copy of the immunization record is required *at the time of admission.*
[document not shown]

4. MEDICATIONS CHILD IS CURRENTLY TAKING

Name of medication   Dosage   Date begun _____

a. _____   _____

b. _____   _____

c. _____   _____

d. _____   _____

e. _____   _____

5. HOSPITALIZATIONS AND OPERATIONS

Name of Hospital   City and State   Date   Problem

a. _____

b. _____

c. _____

d. _____

e. _____

6. ALLERGIES

	Yes	No	Describe
Medications	___	___	_____
Hay fever	___	___	_____
Asthma	___	___	_____
Foods	___	___	_____

Figure 3.3.   *Medical Information Form* *(continued)*

	Yes	No	Describe
Insects	_____	_____	_____
Other	_____	_____	_____

7. INJURIES

	Yes	No	Describe
Broken bones	_____	_____	_____
Head injuries	_____	_____	_____
Unconscious	_____	_____	_____
Frequent accidents	_____	_____	_____

8. SUBSTANCE ABUSE

	Yes	No	Describe
Cigarettes	_____	_____	_____
Alcohol	_____	_____	_____
Marijuana	_____	_____	_____
Drugs	_____	_____	_____
Inhalants	_____	_____	_____

9. INFECTIOUS DISEASES (check where appropriate)

_____ Chicken pox

_____ Infectious mononucleosis

_____ Mumps

_____ Tuberculosis

_____ Hepatitis

_____ Measles

Figure 3.3. Medical Information Form   *(continued)*

_____ German measles

_____ Other

_____ Recent exposure (describe) _____

_____

SEXUALLY TRANSMITTED DISEASES

_____ Gonorrhea   _____ Syphilis

_____ HIV (AIDS)   _____ Herpes

Recent exposure (describe) _____

_____

10. GENERAL (check where appropriate)

_____ General good health	_____ Chest pain
_____ Sleep problems	_____ Heart murmur
_____ Decreased appetite	_____ Bronchitis/Pneumonia
_____ Increased appetite	_____ Stomach pains
_____ Weight loss	_____ Constipation
_____ Weight gain	_____ Diarrhea
_____ Skin rashes	_____ Encopresis
_____ Headaches	_____ Urinary tract infection
_____ Visual problems	_____ Bed wetting
_____ Glasses	_____ Daytime wetting
_____ Hearing problems	_____ Sexually active
_____ Toothaches/Dental problems	_____ Bone or joint problems
_____ Sinus infections	_____ Depression

Figure 3.3. Medical Information Form (*continued*)

————— Earaches   ————— Suicide attempts

————— Physical abuse   ————— Sexual abuse

————— Neglect   ————— Other

Comments ——————————————————————————

————————————————————————————————

————————————————————————————————

If female:

Menstruation:

Age of onset ———————————— Regular ——————————

Date of last period ——————————— Irregular —————————

Length of menstrual period ———————————————————

Cramps ——————————————— Excessive bleeding —————————

Vaginal discharge —————————— Pregnancy ———————————

Vaginal infection ——————————— Abortion ————————————

Previous pelvic exam —————————— Birth control ————————

11. NEUROLOGICAL PROBLEMS

	Seizures	Headaches
Age of onset		
Duration		
Frequency		
Date of last occurrence		
Descriptions		

Figure 3.3. *Medical Information Form* *(continued)*

	Yes	No	Results
EEG _____	___	___	_____
CT Scan _____	___	___	_____
MRI _____	___	___	_____
Neurological consult (where) _____			
Comments _____			

_____

12. FAMILY HISTORY (check where appropriate)

_____ Diabetes   _____ Seizures (convulsions)

_____ Heart disease   _____ Depression

_____ Hypertension   _____ Alcoholism

_____ Kidney disease   _____ Schizophrenia

_____ Asthma/Allergies   _____ Mental retardation

_____ Anemia   _____ Physical disability

_____ Tics/Tourette's syndrome   _____ Other

Name of last school attended _____

Address of school _____

Grade in school _____

_____

Signature

_____

Relationship to Patient

_____

Date

for review by the admitting psychiatrist. The advantage of the team approach is that broader consideration can be given to all of the issues to be considered for hospitalization and for other interventions. The result is usually a shared decision that leads to greater investment from the multidisciplinary team. The disadvantages are that the team approach is time-consuming and, at times, gathering and considering everyone's input becomes cumbersome.

The first factor to be considered in determining the need for psychiatric hospitalization is *the nature of the presenting psychiatric disorder.* Most children or adolescents being considered for inpatient treatment present with at least one of the following:

1. A symptomatic picture suggesting an early or developing psychotic disorder;
2. Moderate to severe depression;
3. Aggressive and/or impulsive behavior that may be antisocial in nature;
4. Disorganized or ineffective family functioning (Blotcky & Gossett, 1988).

The severity and duration of the disorder, the degree of impairment it has caused, and the coping abilities of the child or adolescent, the family, and their social and cultural supports should all be assessed, as the first step in screening for admission. Can the condition be safely and effectively handled outside the hospital setting? Related to an assessment of the effectiveness of their coping skills is a consideration of the developmental level of the child or adolescent and the family. Are their primary defenses lower-level defenses such as denial, splitting, or projection or do they use higher-level defenses such as sublimation, humor, and repression? (See Table 3.1.) Is the child or adolescent functioning at an age-appropriate level cognitively (e.g., concrete or formal operations), psychosexually, and psychosocially? What level of moral development has been achieved? Young people who are significantly below their expected level in several areas are in need of more intensive interventions.

The capacity to relate to others is the second important variable to be assessed when considering hospitalization beyond crisis management. Children who have little capacity to relate to peers, adults, or groups are less likely to benefit from psychiatric hospitalization than are those who can develop relationships, because a large part of psychiatric intervention depends on an interpersonal relationship. The capacity to relate to others must be carefully assessed. Some children who are very quiet and reserved, due to their personal temperamental style or to cultural influences, may initially appear to have little capacity to relate to others. Potential reasons

Table 3.1 **Psychological Defense Mechanisms**

Mechanism	Example
EARLY DEVELOPMENTAL DEFENSES	
Denial is an unconscious mechanism that allows the adolescent to avoid awareness of thoughts, feelings, wishes, needs, or external reality factors that are consciously intolerable.	An adolescent denies any feeling of abandonment or rejection by the noncustodial parent after a divorce.
Projection is the unconscious mechanism whereby an unacceptable impulse, feeling, or idea is attributed to the external world.	An adolescent experiencing repeated trouble with the law claims all of the problems are due to law enforcement officers who "have it in for" him or her (projection of guilt).
Splitting occurs when the adolescent unconsciously views people or events as being at one extreme or the other.	A hospitalized patient views each of the medical staff as being all "good" or all "bad."
MID-LEVEL DEVELOPMENTAL DEFENSES	
Acting out occurs when unconscious emotional conflicts or feelings are expressed in an area different from the one in which they arose. Generally, acting out is a feeling expressed in actions rather than in words.	An adolescent girl who is angry at her family after being grounded runs away from home without verbally expressing her anger.
Regression is a partial or symbolic return to more infantile patterns of reacting or thinking.	An adolescent returns to childish and dependent behavior following a family move to a new city.
Counterphobia is seeking out experiences that are consciously or unconsciously feared.	An adolescent repeatedly engages in risk-taking behavior.
Identification occurs when a person unconsciously patterns himself or herself after some other person. (Role modeling or imitation is similar to identification, but is a conscious process.)	An adolescent identifies with a rock star or an athletic coach whom he or she admires.
Reaction formation unconsciously transforms unacceptable feelings, ideas, or impulses into their opposites.	An adolescent mother feels resentment toward the demands that caring for her child make on her. However, she repeatedly tells herself and others how wonderful motherhood is. At times, she worries unnecessarily that some harm will come to her child.

Table 3.1 *Psychological Defense Mechanisms* *(continued)*

Mechanism	Example
Repression (unconscious) and **Suppression** (conscious) occur when unacceptable thoughts, wishes, or impulses that would produce anxiety are pushed out of awareness.	An adolescent "forgets" to tell her parents of a failing grade in school.
Displacement occurs when emotions, ideas, or wishes are transferred from their original source or target to a more acceptable substitute.	An adolescent who is angry with a teacher berates a sibling for no apparent reason.

LATER DEVELOPMENTAL DEFENSES

Isolation of affect is the separation of ideas or events from the feelings associated with them.	An adolescent, in a cool, unemotional manner, describes the circumstances of a serious automobile accident in which he received multiple injuries.
Rationalization uses reasoning and "rational" explanations, which may or may not be valid, to explain away unconscious conflicts and motivations.	An adolescent explains her drug abuse by saying that "everyone" does it.
Intellectualization controls affects and impulse by analyzing through excessive thought without experiencing the feeling.	When asked about the automobile accident in which his father was killed, an adolescent begins discussing the mechanics of trauma, velocity of impact, safety rules, and changing trends in life expectancy.
Sublimation unconsciously replaces an unacceptable feeling with a course of action that is personally and socially acceptable.	An adolescent whose father recently died from a myocardial infarction begins a vigorous exercise program.
Humor is used defensively to relieve anxiety caused by the discrepancies between what one wishes for oneself and what actually happens.	An adolescent laughs about an embarrassing encounter with her teacher.
Altruism is a seemingly unselfish interest in the welfare of others.	An adolescent whose parents are divorcing volunteers to work as hospital aide.

for reserved or distancing behavior should be considered before concluding that these children are incapable of forming relationships.

In addition, a child's ability to relate to others may be increased through the use of medications or the sensitive and empathic interventions of the hospital team. If a child's ability to relate is difficult to determine or if it seems possible that the hospital intervention could change the presenting behavior, hospitalization should be considered on a trial basis.

A 16-year-old Navajo boy, Daniel, was referred for hospitalization as a result of frequent runaways, school refusal, and depression. Daniel presented as a withdrawn boy who spoke only a few words. After suffering the loss of both of his parents in alcohol-related deaths, he had lived with various relatives and at Indian schools. He did not look up to make eye contact with any of the examiners. Reports from the school he had attended most recently described him as mildly mentally retarded. Because of his seeming inability to relate to others, his reported mild mental retardation, and his pattern of frequent runaways, hospitalization was not recommended and he was referred for outpatient treatment near his current home on the reservation. Several months later, he was referred once again with similar presenting complaints. An examiner who was sensitive to the boy's cultural training and lack of verbal expression and eye contact sought additional information about the boy's depression from other sources and by watching the boy on the playground. This time, hospitalization was recommended and, after several days to allow Daniel to become more comfortable with the cottage staff and to assess his depression, he was placed on antidepressant medication. Within three weeks, the combination of nondemanding expressive therapies, a supportive milieu, and medication led to a dramatic improvement in Daniel's depression. His performance at school suggested he was functioning in the average range of intelligence. While he remained quiet with others, he adjusted well to the unit and did not attempt to run away. As a result of his improved behavior, a stable foster home was located and he has been doing relatively well since discharge.

The capacity to benefit from treatment is a third variable to be considered when screening for hospitalization. To benefit from treatment, the young person must have a disorder known to improve from psychiatric treatment. Certain cases of mental retardation, organic brain disorder, or conduct disorder would generally be excluded. If the potential patient is not able to relate to others, the intense relationship therapies that are important in hospital programs cannot be utilized.

Finally, *the appropriateness of less restrictive settings* must be considered (see Table 3.2). Can the child or adolescent be safely and effectively treated in an outpatient, day treatment, or residential treatment setting? If so, are these resources available in the community where the young person lives? If not, should hospitalization be considered simply because it is the least

Table 3.2.   Continuum of Psychiatric Care

Outpatient treatment. Children and/or their families meet with mental health professionals in an outpatient setting one or more times per week for counseling, individual/group family therapy, and/or medication prescription and review.

In-home therapeutic services. Home-based crises-oriented interventions are provided on an outreach basis, to work intensively with children and families in their homes. The intervention is brief (2–5 months), intense, and family-focused.

Day or partial hospitalization. Day treatment or partial hospitalization provides an integrated set of educational, counseling, and psychotherapeutic interventions for the child and family for at least 4 hours per day in an out-of-home setting. Vocational skill building and crisis services are often included.

Therapeutic foster care. The child is placed with foster parents who have been specifically recruited to work with emotionally disturbed children. There are usually few children in the home, and foster parents receive special training and support as well as a special stipend.

Group home or residential treatment center (RTC). RTCs vary from highly structured, medically oriented treatment facilities to community based, socially oriented therapeutic living arrangements with a lower staff–child ratio than group homes. Typically, children are more emotionally disturbed in a RTC than in a group home and less disturbed than in an inpatient unit.

Inpatient psychiatric hospitalization. Inpatient care is typically the most restrictive, most expensive, and most intense form of psychiatric intervention, with a low staff–child ratio and a high percentage of medical staff. Some inpatient units are secure.

Adapted from B. A. Stroul & R. M. Friedman (1986). *A system of care for severely disturbed children and youth.* Washington, DC: CASSP Technical Assistance Center.

restrictive *available* setting? Less restrictive settings must also be considered when there is significant risk of separating the child from his or her community or culture. Removal of children from their cultural community can result in difficulties when they reintegrate upon discharge.

Denise, a 14-year-old Apache girl, became suicidal after her mother killed her stepfather and then herself; her mother had learned that the stepfather had been unfaithful to her and had sexually abused Denise over a period of several years. Denise was in therapy with an Anglo social worker at the time, and the therapist recommended hospitalization. Because Denise was assessed to have serious potential for attempting suicide by the staff at the hospital's crisis unit, hospitalization was determined to be essential. However, Denise's aunt, who now had custody, refused hospitalization, saying it was not the Indian way. She wanted Denise to stay within the tribe for native healing. When the hospital physician insisted that hospitalization was necessary to protect Denise and that he would not release her, the aunt and other extended family refused to have any more to do with the hospital or with Denise. Fortunately, the social worker who had been working with Denise and who practiced at a separate outpatient program was able to continue to see Denise's family. Denise was released from the hospital as soon as she was judged to be not eminently suicidal. Her release to her family and regular outpatient therapy occurred sooner than it would have if members of Denise's cultural community had been more receptive to working with the hospital.

ADMISSION CRITERIA

The essential criteria for admission to a psychiatric hospital include a diagnosis of a psychiatric disorder and the criteria for inpatient psychiatric hospitalization described in the AACAP's *Guidelines for Treatment Resources, Quality Assurance, Peer Review, and Reimbursement* (1986). These include having a significant risk of suffering, death, or significant injury; significant pain or distress; or significant disability or dysfunction in school performance, social interactions, or family relationships. Additional criteria include failure of treatment at a lower level of care as well as clarification of why a lower level of care is not appropriate. Young people who are admitted for psychiatric hospitalization should be demonstrating one or more of the following:

1. Danger to self, others, and/or property;
2. Bizarre behavior;
3. Need of high-dose, unusual medications or somatic and psychological treatment with potentially serious side effects;
4. A need for 24-hour skilled observation (National Association of Private Psychiatric Hospitals, 1989).

If the criteria for admission are met, the young person and the family should be prepared for admission through communication of the reasons for admission, the alternatives considered, an admission time, and a projected length of stay. The inpatient treatment recommendations should include a discussion of the possible treatment approaches (individual, family, group, and/or pharmacologic) as well as living, school, and payment arrangements.

If the child's or adolescent's symptoms do not meet the criteria for hospitalization, or if the family refuses inpatient treatment, the appropriateness and availability of other resources need to be considered. Table 3.2 suggests a continuum of care.

When inpatient psychiatric treatment is agreed upon by the family, or if the evaluating physician determines that the child's safety requires admission, regardless of the family's agreement, a legal commitment hearing may be necessary in some states. Although children are not found to fully understand the reasons for hospitalization (Roth & Roth, 1984), they may be asked for their consent to hospitalization in addition to their parents'.

The admission criteria must be carefully documented in the admission note. Accompanying reports must indicate results of an initial mental status examination, a physical examination, and a formulation and initial treatment plan. Referral sources and third-party payers should be informed of the admission.

SPECIAL PROBLEMS

It is not unusual for a child to present for hospitalization when his or her custody is not clear or determined. This ambiguity occurs in divorcing families, or when a child is living with extended family and the custodial parent or guardian is no longer involved with the child, or when the state is in the process of taking custody. Determining who is legally able to sign admission and treatment papers, who is financially responsible, and who will take the child upon discharge becomes difficult. Undetermined custody can prolong hospitalization and interfere with treatment progress. The child's confusion about a future caregiver is added to his or her feelings of not being cared about and not belonging. Until clarification occurs, the depression or acting out continues or increases. Discharge plans that are unclear result in a large investment of time and expense for the hospital. Whenever possible, hospital admission should be delayed until custody is determined. In an emergency involving a child whose custody is undetermined, the state can take temporary custody and the child then can be hospitalized. These arrangements always should be made prior to hospitalization.

At times, the family of a child who is from a minority cultural background and has been referred for hospital evaluation can appear very resistant to the recommendation for hospital treatment even though it is clear that the need exists. If the child is not an imminent danger to self or others, it may be constructive to prolong the evaluation process and ask the family to return at a later date. Pressure to hospitalize a child immediately may be interpreted as a lack of respect for the family's need to consult with important people and to utilize the services of native healers within their community, at a pace that is consistent with their culture. Before an important decision such as hospitalization is made, meetings with an extended family matriarch or patriarch and/or healers within the cultural community can insure more community support and parental participation. Easing the pressure on the family by prolonging the evaluation allows the family the time to arrive at a decision in a manner that is consistent with their cultural background.

CONCLUSION

The process of determining the need for hospitalization is a critical step in the successful treatment of children and adolescents who have serious emotional disturbances. The process is clearer when the patients are dangerous to themselves or to others. The steps that establish a treatment alliance with a variety of Anglo, Hispanic, or American Indian families are important in determining the families' accessibility to the treatment process.

The evaluation of the referral information, the information gathered during the interview with the child or adolescent and the family, and the information from other pertinent sources determines whether the criteria for admission have been met. The manner in which this evaluation is done is the initial step in establishing a treatment alliance with the patient and the family. Thus, the process must be sensitive to the cultural background of the family. Otherwise, the family's discomfort and feeling of estrangement from the hospital will predict either ineffective treatment or treatment refusal.

REFERENCES

American Academy of Child and Adolescent Psychiatry. (1986). *Guidelines for treatment resources, quality assurance, peer review, and reimbursement* (ch. 4, pp. 34–36). Washington, DC: Author.

American Academy of Child and Adolescent Psychiatry. (1989). *Policy statement: Inpatient hospital treatment of children and adolescents.* Washington, DC: Author.

American Psychiatric Association. (1989). *Statement on psychiatric hospitalization of children and adolescents.* Washington, DC: Author.

Blotcky, M. J., & Gossett, J. T. (1988). Psychiatric inpatient treatment for adolescents. *The Psychiatric Hospital, 20,* 85–93.

Lewis, M. (1982). *Clinical aspects of child development* (2d ed.). Philadelphia: Lea & Febiger.

Lewis, M. (1986). General psychiatric assessment of children and adolescents. *Psychiatry, 2,* 1–18.

National Association of Private Psychiatric Hospitals. (1989). *Guidelines for psychiatric hospital programs—children and adolescents* (pp. 1–7).

Perlmutter, R. A. (1986). Emergency psychiatry and the family: The decision to admit. *Journal of Marital and Family Therapy, 12,* 153–162.

Roth, E. A., & Roth, L. H. (1984). Children's understanding of psychiatric hospitalization. *American Journal of Psychiatry, 141,* 1066–1070.

Simmons, J. E. (1981). *Psychiatric examination of children* (3d ed.). Philadelphia: Lea & Febiger.

Spurlock, J. (1985). Assessment and therapeutic intervention of black children. *Journal of the American Academy of Child Psychiatry, 24,* 168–174.

CHAPTER FOUR

Effective Treatment Planning

Irving N. Berlin
Robert L. Hendren

GENETIC FACTORS AND ENVIRONMENTAL EXPERIENCES

Successful treatment planning begins with an awareness of the possible etiology of a disorder, whether due to genetic and/or environmental factors. Thus, the child's or adolescent's temperament and how it has influenced his or her acceptance within the family is an important variable. Is a "slow to warm up" or irritable temperament responsible, in part, for discordant reactions? Has it caused the parents to be unable to nurture and be supportive of the child's physical, cognitive, and emotional development? The degree to which a child's temperament is a factor in his or her inability to relate easily to the mother, thus making the mother–infant "fit" a poor one, may determine how that infant or child relates to the world. A history of a poor "fit" between mother and infant may indicate long-standing problems that cannot easily be resolved (Maziade, Caron, Cote, Boutin, & Thivierge, 1990; Thomas, Chess, & Birch, 1968).

Other childhood psychiatric illnesses—autism, childhood schizophrenia, severe depression, and, from recent evidence, obsessive-compulsive disorder—have a clear genetic base. All of these disorders have had a poor prognosis, but certain pharmacologic agents have proven recently to be very helpful and important in the treatment of depression and obsessive-compulsive disorder (Adams, 1985; Swedo, Rappoport, Leonard, Lenane, & Cheslow, 1989).

Other disorders, like attention deficit disorder, with or without hyperactivity, appear to be organic in origin and can often be treated effectively with central nervous system stimulants. ADD or ADDH results in behaviors, in school and at home, that alienate both adults and peers. The attentional problems make learning very difficult in every aspect of living as well as in school. The child develops defensive attitudes, avoiding responsibility by denying the effects on others of any troublesome behaviors. Angry, defiant behavior, negativism, and fighting increase both the alienation of others and the feelings of failure and hopelessness in the child. Treatment now available can reduce the attentional and hyperactivity problems, but the other psychological difficulties that have developed over time persist. A child or adolescent who avoids schoolwork, has poor social skills, and has not learned to take responsibility for tasks of daily living—helping with chores, taking care of his or her room, and/or cooperating with family or friends in any planned activities—will continue to have a poor self-image and feelings of not being cared about. Psychotherapy with the child or adolescent and the parents is important. The family must help the youngster to learn anew how to "fit into" the home and school environment. Since adults have done many of the child's tasks for him or her, the relearning process is difficult and often painful.

Environmental experiences may complicate treatment of some other disorders, like manic depressive or obsessive-compulsive disorders. Thus, despite the availability of psychopharmacologic agents to treat the disorder, the relearning process that permits more amiable living with others requires an intensive psychotherapeutic effort with the youth and the family (Cantwell, 1985; Gualtieri & Hicks, 1985; Pelham, Walker, Sturges, & Hoza, 1989).

Children who have genetic disorders are often vulnerable to environmental stress. Their prolonged illness may have a debilitating effect on their parents, making it difficult for the parents to collaborate in a treatment program.

CULTURAL FACTORS THAT AFFECT PROGNOSIS

The family's degree of acculturation and the support the family receives from the extended family are important issues to be determined, in treatment planning with Hispanic and American Indian families. An exploration of the family's desire to use native healers and a determination of which family members, both nuclear and extended, can and should be involved in the treatment process will promote a more integrated treatment program.

Among Hispanic families, the usual healers may be either *curanderos* or priests in the local parish. Accepting psychiatric treatment may be very difficult for the family because psychiatric illness is foreign to their thinking. The extended family may also be a factor; disagreement about treatment between the generations in a family may complicate the nuclear family's readiness to be involved in family therapy. The extended family may even make therapy impossible. Some psychiatric disturbances in boys, which may be manifested by acting out and antisocial behavior, are often seen by the family as a natural extension of the male "machismo" and therefore acceptable as normal adolescent behavior.

Because Hispanic families are often closely knit, helping a family to work together on behalf of a daughter who has accused her father of incestuous behavior may be very difficult. The tendency is to protect the father and, thus, maintain the family's denial of the sexual abuse.

In some extended families, the elders may clearly see a child's or adolescent's need for help and may recognize the role of some family members in the young person's illness. In some cases of physical abuse, the elders have committed the family to a treatment program (Casaus, Arciniega, & Castillo, 1982; Martini, 1979).

In American Indian families, the extended family may be dysfunctional; alcoholism may have disrupted its cohesiveness. A search for responsible relatives or other potential reservation foster families is an essential component for family therapy and subsequent discharge planning.

In pueblos and tribes that are matrilineal in the distribution of property, the grandmother is all-powerful and her decision about the need for treatment is often final. The relationship of the hospital staff to members of a tribe or pueblo, but particularly to the medicine men and women, may be a determining factor in how the family views hospital treatment. The staff's relationship with tribal social workers or mental health personnel can also be an important determinant of family cooperation as well as planning for discharge and posthospital treatment.

Any evaluation team working with an American Indian family needs to become aware of the particular traditions and values of the family's community. For example, among the Navajo, speaking about the dead is prohibited. Thus, to try to help a child or adolescent with the process of mourning and depression following the loss of a parent is very difficult. The use of traditional psychotherapy will probably not be effective. Expressive therapies—story telling, art therapy, or play therapy, for example—in which feelings are expressed through metaphor may be more helpful.

The readiness of the staff to support the family's desire for a healing ceremony will often facilitate the treatment alliance and lead to further improvement in overcoming dysfunction. At times, culturally sanctioned healing ceremonies can lead to significant improvement in symptoms.

In some communities, the family's status will often determine whether the parents will be charged by the tribal court with neglect, physical abuse, or sexual abuse of a child. Thus, the victim may be removed from the family for help, but the family will not involve itself in family therapy and the victims return to the home is very difficult. The possibility of enlisting extended family members, especially those who live off the reservation, to become foster parents must then be explored. Or, tribal social services may be able to find other families on the reservation who are willing to become foster parents (Red Horse, 1981; Sander, 1979).

EVALUATION OF THE DEGREE OF PSYCHOPATHOLOGY

To plan treatment effectively, the current degree of psychopathology, its duration, and the past and present contributing environmental factors must all be assessed.

In most severe conduct disorders and in some personality disorders like the borderline or narcissistic personalities, there are data to support early lack of nurturance as well as maternal need to interfere with the developmental process during separation and individuation stages (Kernberg, 1983; Petti & Vela, 1990; Westen, Ludolph, Lerner, Ruffino, & Wiss, 1990). It is certainly clear from the work of pioneer developmentalists, particularly

Spitz and Bowlby, that lack or disruption of bonding or attachment in infancy leads to serious mental illness in the infant and young child (Bowlby, 1973; Spitz, 1965).

The degree of succor or nurturance provided by others in the environment, which may alter the severity of a depression or schizoid withdrawn behavior, must also be evaluated. The willingness of the staff to work with seriously disturbed parents, and their ability to do so without passing judgment on the parents, is an important variable to be considered in treatment planning.

A DEVELOPMENTAL APPROACH TO TREATMENT PLANNING

Effective treatment planning depends on a thorough and accurate biopsychosocial and developmental assessment and formulation. The biopsychosocial model consists of more than just the individual biological, psychological, and sociocultural influences on human health, behavior, and emotions. The model refers to the mutual *interaction* of these influences at all age-stage levels of development, which must be recognized and appreciated to complete a thorough evaluation (Thomas, 1981). In addition, the special and unique characteristics of each individual's psychological evolution must be taken into account.

Biological influences on emotional, cognitive, behavioral, and personality development include such factors as genetic, morphologic, neurochemical, neurointegrative, and temperamental influences; variations in language acquisition; and the occurrence of illness and injury—to name a few. The developing interaction of the infant with his or her environment, especially the primary caretaker, begins the creation of psychological themes that may continually reappear throughout the life cycle. The "goodness of fit" between the child and the environment is an important determinant of subsequent healthy development (Thomas, 1981). Cultural expectations and values also exert considerable influence upon the interaction between the parent and the child (Rosenthal & Bornholt, 1988). Psychosocial developmental models are compared in Table 4.1.

The identification of the developmental level from a biopsychosocial perspective is the first step in creating an effective treatment plan. Areas where the child lags behind can be identified as areas for treatment focus. Realistic goals then can be set for movement along a developmental line, if the treatment planners are familiar with the progression of normal development. This goal-directed treatment planning can be extensive or limited, depending on the degree of disturbance and the projected length of stay.

Goal-directed treatment planning (Nurcomb, 1989) begins with a biopsychosocial formulation, an identification of pivotal problems and potential,

Table 4.1. Developmental Models

Cognitive Development (Piaget)	Moral Development (Kohlberg)	Psychosexual Development (Freud)	Psychosocial Development (Erikson)	Defenses Development (See Table 3.1)
Object Permanence (8–9 months)		Seek immediate pleasure & relief from discomfort (0–18 months)	Trust vs. mistrust (0–1 year)	Early Developmental Defenses Denial Projection Splitting
Stranger Anxiety (2½ years)	Deference to power (2–3 years)	Control of body, self, & others (12–36 months)	Autonomy vs. shame & doubt (1–3 years)	
Egocentric (up to 4 years)		Separation issues (1–3 years)		
Symbolic Activity & Make-Believe Play (2–4 years)		Sexual identity (2–4 years)		Mid-Level Developmental Defenses Acting out Regression Counterphobic behavior Identification Displacement
	Obey to get reward (3–5 years)	Aware of other relationships (3–6 years)	Initiative vs. guilt (3–6 years)	

(continued)

Table 4.1. **Developmental Models** *(continued)*

Cognitive Development (Piaget)	Moral Development (Kohlberg)	Psychosexual Development (Freud)	Psychosocial Development (Erikson)	Defenses Development (See Table 3.1)
Decentration (4–7 years)				
Separate Fantasy From Reality (6–8 years)		Begin to work/compare with others (6–12 years)	Industry vs. inferiority (6–12 years)	
Use of Concrete Logic (7–11 years)	"Good boy or girl" (7–8 years) Authority orientation (8–11 years) Democratic law (11–12 years)			
		Close friendships (12>) Move toward independence (12>)	Identity vs. role confusion (12–20 years)	Later Developmental Defenses Isolation Rationalization Sublimation Humor Altruism
Abstract Thinking (adolescence)	Internal sense of morality (adolescence)		Intimacy vs. isolation (15–30 years)	

and the identification of goals that aim to stabilize the problems that prevent the young person from receiving treatment safely outside the hospital. One or more therapies are then selected, specific objectives and a time line are identified, and a method for evaluation and modification of goals is agreed upon by the staff and the patient's family.

One or more goals may be identified. For short-term hospitalization, one focal problem can be identified and the intervention can be aimed at that problem (Harper, 1989). Another method of treatment planning that identifies one focal problem is the transactional risk model, which aims at improving the "goodness of fit" between the child and his or her interpersonal environment (Woolston, 1989). This model is useful in planning for short- to intermediate-term psychiatric hospitalization.

An essential ingredient in all successful treatment plans is an integrated interdisciplinary team that understands and shares the treatment goal or goals. This team includes all the milieu (staff) workers and school personnel, including allied therapists (speech and language, music, occupational, and recreational therapists). When all treatment team members are working toward integrated objectives, the child's total environment can be directed toward the achievement of the shared treatment goals.

INDIVIDUAL ABILITIES OF MILIEU STAFF AND PSYCHOTHERAPISTS

Some milieu staff and therapists work well with a wide variety of disturbed children. However, individual staff members often have particular therapeutic abilities that allow them to be very effective with regressed and disturbed psychotic children or adolescents but unable to work effectively with those who are angry, aggressive, and manipulative. For other staff, the reverse may be true. Knowledge of the countertransference tendencies of staff may help to identify the therapists and individual milieu staff members who can work effectively with a particular child and family.

The comfort of staff members in working with various minority families and children is an important factor in treatment effectiveness. Some staff find it difficult to work with American Indian children and adolescents and their families because of their tendency to be silent and not very forthcoming about history and family issues and problems.

THE LIMITED GOALS OF INPATIENT TREATMENT

Fostering a Trusting Relationship

A trusting relationship can be fostered quickly in an inpatient setting if some essentials are well-established. The milieu must be structured: the level system and the behavioral expectations at each level must be simply but clearly described. The milieu staff must be adequately prepared for the admission of a new patient, through information on the kinds of problems and behaviors that led to hospital admission and on the probable factors and stresses in the young person's development that contributed to the current disorder. With such preparation, a tentative milieu treatment plan can be created, for testing and later evaluation.

It is important that each patient, on admission, be briefed by two staff members (one is a witness and clarifier in the process) about the milieu rules. Along with a description of the level system and how points are gained and lost, the staff members should give a clear statement about how the kinds of behavior the youth exhibited prior to admission are likely to be handled here. The milieu staff person assigned to the patient should offer to discuss these issues further and should stress his or her willingness to help the patient deal with such behavior when the patient feels it is developing. When working with young children, the milieu staff needs to demonstrate an attentiveness to signs of increased tension and anxiety, to help the children avoid those behaviors that will result in distressing consequences.

The more a patient hears his or her problems and behaviors openly discussed, especially at daily task groups that emphasize the patient's positive behaviors and the staff's interventions to contain disturbing behaviors, the more quickly the child or adolescent will find the milieu a helpful place and the staff a trustworthy ally. Staff members who empathize with the patient's problems promote a sense of the patient's being understood. A feeling of closeness will result, a prerequisite for developing a trusting relationship.

Sharing the Evaluation with the Parents

From the beginning of the evaluation, the parents must be informed that family therapy is an integral part of their child's treatment and that their visits to the unit and their opportunities to talk with milieu staff are important to understanding the treatment program and how treatment is progressing. The evaluation process should focus on the kinds of behavior changes necessary for the patient to be able to return home. Parents may learn from milieu staff how disturbing behaviors can be altered. An explanation should be given as to how various parts of the hospital, such as school and milieu, work together and what is expected of the parents. In family therapy, they need to examine their part in the patient's current problems.

Sharing the Goals of Treatment with the Patient

The young person should be brought to an initial treatment conference, to hear how the staff and therapist view the current problems and what the goals of treatment are. The patient benefits from being aware of the rewards for adaptive and cooperative behavior vs. the consequences for disruptive, hostile, destructive, or self-destructive behavior.

Lorna, age 13, was admitted for a threat to commit suicide, frequent runaways from home, truancy from school, and hostile tirades toward both parents when at home. After admission and instruction about the ward rules, Lorna stonewalled everyone. She retired to her room, came out for all daily events, went to school and to group therapy with peers, but would not speak. A few days after admission, she was brought into the treatment planning meeting. She heard a restatement of her behavior problems, but there was no blaming of Lorna for these problems. The family's and the hospital's goals for Lorna's treatment were outlined. Lorna was asked if she had any comments. She burst into a tirade about how no one could hear her pain and anger in having to deal with a violent, alcoholic father and a defensive, not very effective or caring mother.

She was then asked what *her* goals were for family therapy and her own treatment. Lorna clearly stated the need to have her father stop drinking and cease his violent threats and gestures toward her when she requested to go out or to stay overnight with girlfriends. She also hoped her mother would take a stand, to show she cared for Lorna. Then she stated her need to stop her tirades and runaways and to do her schoolwork and learn to make friends. In response to a question of whether she was ready to begin here to behave as she had described, Lorna replied, "Well, I guess so." She profited from being treated as an adult participant in the planning and felt she had been listened to. Lorna began to work in school and with staff and to state her ideas in family therapy as clearly as she could and without invectives.

Turning School into an Ego-Building Experience

Many of the children and adolescents admitted for inpatient treatment are doing poorly in school; almost 50% of our patients show signs of neurointegrative disturbances that range from ADD with or without hyperactivity to learning problems of various kinds to seizure disorders. These youngsters rarely have had the kind of diagnostic and treatment efforts usually provided by occupational or speech and language therapists and teachers and would benefit from introduction of these specialists' skills.

ESTIMATES OF TREATMENT LENGTH AS USEFUL GOALS

For the child or adolescent, the evaluation may clarify the most dysfunctional behaviors, attitudes, and intrafamilial conflicts. Usually, these are the clearest factors in making hospitalization necessary; their reduction or elimination will make it possible for the young person to return to home and school. Projecting a length of stay, even in general terms, can create a useful goal for treatment and a measure for progress.

Depression

Severe depression in both children and adolescents seriously interferes with learning in school, relating to peers and adults, and being a contributing family member. Sometimes only a suicidal attempt will force adults to view the child's depression as serious and requiring treatment.

Depression can usually be treated by a combination of antidepressant medication, milieu therapy, education, and family and individual psychotherapy. Each treatment method significantly contributes to a reduction of depression, an increased sense of competence and well-being, and a delineation of the family problems that need to be modified. An intermediate-length stay can usually be estimated if outpatient therapy and medication follow-up are available (Alessi & Magen, 1988; McGlashan, 1989; Petti & Law, 1982; Puig-Antich et al., 1987).

Conduct Disorder

Conduct disorder is an admitting diagnosis that, with detailed study after evaluation, may often turn out to be a personality disorder like borderline personality or a depressive reaction to physical abuse or an oppositional disorder (Wishik, Bachman, & Beitch, 1989). Acting-out and acting-up behaviors, disobedience, and breaking of rules at home and at school are frequent symptoms, along with fighting, stealing, and fire setting. The reduction of such behaviors is critical. The milieu and school programs as well as family therapy are usually the essential treatment modalities. Some conduct disorders may turn out to have a comorbid attention deficit disorder or major depressive disorder and are treatable with medication (Alessi & Magen, 1988; McGlashan, 1989). The length of stay is frequently of intermediate length; the borderline personality usually requires long-term treatment (Kernberg, 1983; Pelham et al., 1989; Petti & Vela, 1990).

Psychotic Disorders

Psychotic disorders, including autism and childhood schizophrenia, are serious disorders and often require long-term treatment. Recent onset adolescent schizophrenia has a good prognosis with neuroleptic medication and may be treated by brief hospitalization and follow-up outpatient treatment. While the ultimate goal is restoration of former function in adolescents and young children, some reduction of behaviors that make communication, relationships, and learning very difficult would be essential before discharge from the hospital could be permitted. Neuroleptic medication is most helpful in many adolescent disorders and somewhat helpful in childhood disorders (Campbell, 1977; Campbell, Cohen, & Anderson, 1981; Delga, Heinssen, Fritsch, Goodrich, & Yates, 1989; McDaniel, 1986; Rutter, 1978, 1985; Smalley, Asarnow, & Spense, 1988). The cyclothymic disorders occasionally yield to lithium treatment and to psychotherapy and require an intermediate length of inpatient care (Ballenger, Rieus, & Post, 1982; McDaniel, 1986; Petti & Law 1982; Varanka, Weller, Weller, & Fristad, 1988).

Personality and Panic Disorders

Most child or adolescent psychiatric hospitals are admitting many more borderline and narcissistic personality disorders than in recent years (Westen et al., 1990). These are usually serious disorders of development that require a special milieu treatment program and take a long time to ameliorate. The same can be said of most eating disorders and antisocial personality disorders (Delga et al., 1989; Marchi & Cohen, 1990). In all of these serious psychiatric illnesses, milieu, individual and family therapy, and pharmacotherapy are vital to improvement. These disorders usually require long-term hospitalization.

In recent years, we have also seen an increase in panic disorders in children and adolescents who have been stressed by underlying, long-term problems in socializing with peers, enjoying academic achievement, looking sad, and giving other evidence of depression and who become subjected to stress (Moreau, Weissman, & Warner, 1989).

Physical and Sexual Abuse

The large number of children and adolescents who are hospitalized for severe physical abuse and sexual abuse, usually by family members, is of great concern. In addition to acute symptoms of anxiety, withdrawal, or anger and hostility, they suffer the later symptoms of a posttraumatic syndrome.

In a number of girls, the sexual abuse has led them to develop alter egos as part of a multiple personality disorder. Disorders caused by physical and sexual abuse are now so common that special groups have been designed to facilitate treatment. These disorders require intermediate- to long-term care (Conte & Schuerman, 1987; Dell & Eisenhower, 1990; Thomas, 1989).

Multicultural Influences

From a multicultural viewpoint, psychotic behavior may have a variety of traditional or spiritual meanings which must be understood in order to begin to plan a treatment program.

In traditional Hispanic families, and even in some that have become acculturated, psychotic adolescents who exhibit delusions of persecution and/or hallucinations are often thought to have been bewitched. Believing that someone hostile to the family or the adolescent contacted a witch to cast the spell, the family usually will seek a particularly religious *curandero* to perform rites and prescribe herbs to rid the youth of the spell. If the *curandero* is not successful, then psychiatric care might be sought.

Broken taboos or family misbehavior in different American Indian tribes or pueblos have produced many variations of being "witched" or possessed by evil spirits. In a few tribes, the schizophrenic adolescent's delusions and hallucinations are believed to be signs of the spirits' making the young person a healer. In other tribes, where the same signs are indications of being possessed by evil spirits, the adolescent may be ostracized or cast out of the tribe. In more acculturated tribes, psychotic behavior is quickly referred to the tribe's mental health worker. Sometimes, when such referrals result in evaluation at a psychiatric hospital, it is important to recognize that such a disposition may not have met with the approval of the extended family, especially a matriarch or patriarch who may desire a healing ceremony for the adolescent before hospital care is accepted.

In most minority cultures, schizophrenic behavior is frightening to the family and may be interpreted as a punishment of the family for its misdeeds or evil thoughts. Discovering whether a minority family places a particular meaning on adolescent schizophrenic behavior can be important; the treatment planning can then take into account the meaning of the disorder to the patient and the family (Sander, 1979).

MEDICATION PLANNING

When a young person requires medication for the treatment of depression or other serious disorders, this possibility should be discussed with family members during the evaluation process. The reasons for prescribing the medication should be explained and its anticipated benefits and side effects should be clearly described. Take-home literature, simply stated, and written in the family's native language if possible, can aid the family in making their decision. Families who are reluctant to permit the use of medication can sometimes be given opportunities to discuss the value of the treatment with some of their own healers and with members of the hospital staff who can speak their own language and understand their culture. With some Indian families, a meeting with the extended family, particularly the matriarch of the family or a healer related to the family, may be advisable. Approaching the use of medication as a trial effort, with effectiveness to be assessed by the staff as well as the family, can assuage their anxieties.

Enlisting respected community members to help the family consider the alternatives, if no medication were to be administered to a seriously ill and ineffective family member, can be beneficial. When medication is being considered, the possibility that the family can and will discontinue the medication after discharge must be evaluated. Liaison between the hospital and the community's health workers and mental health workers or professionals may be a critical factor as to whether medications are continued. For example, Navajo social workers will often take an authoritarian, maternal stance and will lecture the mother and aunts of a patient on medication if they seem unable to remember to administer prescribed dosage. The Navajo social worker often commands such status in the community that the family usually agrees to administer the drug as prescribed and to report weekly to the social worker so that the child's or adolescent's progress can be evaluated. Native mental health workers assume similar responsibilities in some communities. In many Hispanic families, the grandmother or a respected male relative will undertake to monitor the medication. These relevant individuals must be identified prior to discharge of any patient who is to remain on medication.

WHEN WILL TREATMENT MILESTONES BE ATTAINED?

From a developmental history, an understanding of the symptoms and the reasons for the evaluation, it should be possible to anticipate the length of time from admission to when the patient begins to trust the staff. Trust is usually developed shortly after the "honeymoon"—the testing period of 1 to 2 weeks. In a setting where the limits are clear and the staff unambivalent, children and adolescents begin to understand that no one is acting in a punitive fashion and that staff members mean what they say. For patients from Hispanic and American Indian cultures, the time required to establish trust is often longer because they need to test the staff's prejudices in various settings. Patients tend to engage quickly in the school setting, which is task-oriented and easier to deal with than the more unstructured milieu setting, and in group or family therapy, where there is a demand that the patients talk about themselves and their feelings, as a way of understanding the reasons for their behavior. Patients from nonverbal, action-oriented family environments have great difficulty with these interactions and avoid them.

Our estimates of how long it will take to engage the family in therapy often depend on our ability to assess the family's degree of caring about the child and their capacity to collaborate with each other rather than use one another as scapegoats in describing the genesis of family problems and the disturbance of the patient.

The parents' capacity to trust milieu staff also depends on the parents' defensiveness about their child's problems and need for hospital care. Trust is derived from the milieu staff's ability to include parents in activities and to begin a mutual sharing of observations; its development often accelerates if the staff's backgrounds are similar to the parents'. Parents often feel blamed and may sense a prejudice among the milieu staff. These issues need to be worked out by staff in staff meetings and supervision. Estimating the time it will take to overcome particular parents' resistances is often more difficult than estimating the end of resistance from their children.

Horace, an 11-year-old American Indian boy from a nearby pueblo, came to the hospital because of repeated attempts to hang himself. He had been quite depressed for about 2 years, since the death of an uncle with whom he was close. His mother managed the pueblo jewelry and pottery store; his father, a road maintenance foreman, was a hard-working and, after work, a hard-drinking man. When he was 5 or 6 years old, Horace developed a strong attachment to his father's younger brother because no other adults spent much time with him. Both parents were nominally traditional (they spoke their native language, but did not involve themselves in clan activities). The uncle to whom Horace became attached had been very active in the clan and the pueblo traditions. He died when his pickup was hit by a drunken pueblo resident. Though the parents were upset by his death, they did not participate in the traditional burial ceremonies. Horace felt his parents did not care about his uncle's death. After his first two suicide attempts, the parents expressed concern but still spent little time with their son. While they asked the medicine man to help Horace and paid his fee, they were the only family members whose work kept them from the healing ceremony.

Subsequent, more serious attempts at hanging, in which Horace came close to killing himself, aroused community concern. The parents had been told by the pueblo mental health worker and one of the social workers that Horace needed to be hospitalized. The parents were responsive to school and court pressure only after Horace's last suicide attempt; they applied for his hospitalization.

During the intake, the pueblo's chief social worker accompanied the family and related some of the family's problems and the parents' efforts to ignore them. A younger daughter was doing poorly in elementary school and a preschool son was an angry, hostile boy who could not get along with peers or teachers. Though both parents understood and were fluent in English, they balked at coming to weekly family therapy, despite the relatively short 50-mile drive from their home to the hospital. Their excuse was their work. The peublo's chief social worker spoke very sharply to them in their native tongue. Both parents began to look upset and concerned. They agreed to come to the weekly sessions. The chief social worker said that she would join the family sessions biweekly to ensure the parents' involvement. Later, she told the child psychiatrist and student social worker conducting the evaluation that she had confronted the parents with their failures as parents and with the concern of teachers, school board, court, and many council members for their children. The fact that each parent had abandoned his or her clan and failed to take part in rituals made everyone wonder whether they belonged in the pueblo, deserved to work at pueblo jobs, and were eligible to live in pueblo-owned housing. Their attitude toward cooperating in their son's treatment would need to be looked at in terms of their other problems.

Horace quickly attached himself to a very warm, young Hispanic woman on the staff who was also working with a boy from another pueblo. Horace was placed on antidepressants. In a week's time, he began to talk about himself to the staff person and could make a few comments in the milieu group therapy sessions.

The parents were suspicious of the staff members and the male psychologist who worked with them in family therapy. They did not want to spend much time on the unit. In the first family therapy session, they would not talk of the events leading to Horace's suicide attempts. Horace also was silent. In the second session, with the pueblo's chief social worker present, they were a little more open. The social worker challenged the parents for not attending ceremonies for the father's dead brother. She expressed anger at their failure to spend time with Horace and to talk with him, despite his obvious depression. Both parents were defensive and, again, gave their jobs as excuses. In the ensuing interchange, the parents were able to admit that they had a troubled marriage, arranged by their families. They found it difficult to care about each other. At a young age, the mother went to school to learn merchandising and bookkeeping so that she could get a job. Both parents used work to escape from each other and from their children, whom they did not enjoy. They had been pleased when Horace and his uncle had become pals.

It took over a month for the parents to trust both milieu staff and therapists. Finally, they were able to feel and express some concern for Horace and begin to look at their difficult marriage.

Our estimate that, under ideal circumstances, Horace would require about 4 to 5 months' hospitalization was close to correct. Horace was very hungry for caring human contact and he related well to his milieu staff person and other staff members whose openness he admired. In school, he like both his teacher and the aide. Under their personal direction, he began to make academic progress. The antidepressant helped him feel more peaceful and relaxed.

The parents began to be more straightforward with each other and could talk of their uneasy desertion of Horace when he was in desperate need of care. Gradually, more honest feelings were expressed and felt on all sides. When treatment ended after 5½ months' hospitalization, the pueblo's chief social worker volunteered to maintain family sessions at the pueblo. The parents agreed that they would bring Horace to the hospital once a week for outpatient therapy, medication regulation, and family therapy with hospital staff. The pueblo's chief social worker related to the treatment staff that she felt it important to help the parents become active members of their clan and begin to spend time with and to enjoy their children. From the parents' reactions to the pueblo's chief social worker, it was clear that she was a committed and powerful person in the community.

In both Hispanic and American Indian families, the inclusion of the extended family may be helpful if these relatives are concerned with the patient's condition and are not interested in minimizing both parental and extended family responsibilities for the child's disorder.

In one Hispanic family, the grandmother often tried to comfort a physically abused patient. In family therapy, she frequently was able to speak for the silent patient until the patient could talk for herself. She was also encouraging to both parents in their efforts to be more direct with each other, more involved with the girl, and more motivated to reduce their drinking. Because the grandmother's role was not initially clear, the estimate for change was off by 2 months. The girl, with outpatient follow-up, was able to be discharged in 4 months rather than 6.

In contrast, the grandmother in an old, prominent Hispanic family was determined that no family secrets would be divulged, despite the sexual assault, by a brother, of her 12-year-old granddaughter. Efforts toward family therapy had to be abandoned and the welfare department was requested to press charges against the brother, who was jailed.

As occurs so frequently, patients may come from chaotic, alcohol-addicted households where the parents are not able to and have no wish to participate in their child's treatment. If the child has been removed from the home and is in long-term foster care, the hospital staff will work with the foster parents. The intention is to help them understand the child's problems and, from their frequent unit visits, learn from milieu staff how certain behaviors are most therapeutically and effectively handled.

When no foster parents have yet been found, the hospital makes clear the need to work with the adults who will be parenting the child. One or another of the alcoholic parents—most often the mother—may begin to visit the child. When that occurs, the therapists try to help the milieu staff make the mother welcome and to talk to her about her child's progress. The mother–child visits are supervised.

The staff will often encourage the child to teach the parents to play "Chutes and Ladders," "Old Maid," or "Dominos." The child may not have played any games prior to admission, which means the parents have not learned to play with their child. If a staff member joins them, to model the pleasure adults can have in playing games with children, the parents may begin to enjoy playing games with their child. In time, some of these parents can be engaged in discussions with the child and staff about the home problems that led to the child's troubles.

DISCHARGE PLANNING

Discharge planning needs to begin with the initial evaluation. It is necessary to be clear about who will take the youngster on discharge so that the planning process can begin at the point of admission. As part of discharge planning, communication must be ongoing with the school that the young person will attend on discharge. Planning and collaboration with the school to determine what problems existed prior to admission and to share the youngster's progress and accomplishments prior to discharge result in a better school experience both in the hospital and on discharge.

A critical discharge planning problem involves working with the responsible welfare department on foster home placement, when the child has been removed from the home. This is especially difficult where the parents have been abusing and alcoholic and no extended family is available or sufficiently functional and concerned with the child to become foster parents. Despite the Indian Child Welfare Act, which grants a tribe the right to keep a child on the reservation if placement can be found, it is often difficult to find suitable foster parents in the tribal community.

One of the authors recently testified at a custody hearing involving alcoholic parents who had had their parental rights abrogated by the tribal court, leaving their young Indian child open for adoption. The Anglo foster parents who had cared for the child since he was 4 months old asked to adopt him. The tribe appealed such an action because they felt the child would become alienated from the tribe. The tribe suggested some extended family members as the adoptive parents, but investigation of them revealed an unstable home with recently alcoholic adults and a very retarded mongoloid natural child who required a great deal of adult attention. Thus, the developmental needs of the to-be-adopted child were the important issues to be dealt with. The boy had bonded well, had been learning rapidly, and was happy in the home of the Anglo foster parents. The court ruled for adoption by the Anglo foster parents with a provision for regular visits to the tribe and the extended family.

Another discharge problem may result from the youngster's lack of attachment to anyone outside the hospital. Stable and caring foster parents are needed, to make attachment possible and to provide a continuing caring experience.

Where extended family is available and sufficiently stable to permit a good relationship, a plan must be developed for working with the foster parents and the youngster to facilitate the discharge planning and postdischarge follow-up.

FOLLOW-UP PLANNING AND RESEARCH

For families who live many miles from the hospital, the social service staff tries to work out a follow-up plan with a local mental health or guidance center. Indigenous mental health workers or social workers at various American Indian reservations and pueblos often will see the child and family on a regular, even though infrequent basis. When families live within a reasonable travel distance, staff may arrange for outpatient follow-up with hospital personnel or at an outpatient clinic of a local child psychiatric agency.

An outreach team from the hospital can follow a few patients to remote areas where there are no mental health services. Usually, the team will travel to the patient's community to help establish contact between the family and the local mental health resources. The team also collaborates with the schools to work out a meaningful academic program for discharged patients.

Outcome data are important to help the hospital refine its treatment techniques, find out what works best, and determine what kinds of young people are most effectively treated and why. Follow-up efforts contribute meaningful data toward outcome research.

CONCLUSION

Effective treatment planning in a child and adolescent psychiatric hospital that serves a multicultural population must follow some clear guidelines and sequences. The evaluation process that has been described is carried out by most psychiatric hospitals serving children and adolescents.

The length of stay is usually determined by the severity of the psychopathology of the patient and the cooperativeness of the parents. The effectiveness of the treatment is often determined by the degree of trust developed among the staff, the patients, and the families.

In a multicultural hospital setting, the sensitivity of all the staff to the traditions of each minority culture represented in the patient population is a determinant of both the effectiveness of treatment and the duration of stay.

With experience, the treatment staff becomes attuned to working effectively with children, adolescents, and families with different psychopathology and from different cultures.

REFERENCES

Adams, P. (1985). The obsessive child: A therapy update. *American Journal of Psychotherapy, 39,* 301–313.

Alessi, N. E., & Magen, J. (1988). Comorbidity of other psychiatric disturbances in depressed psychiatrically hospitalized children. *The American Journal of Psychiatry, 145,* 1582–1584.

Ballenger, J. C., Rieus, J. I., & Post, R. M. (1982). The atypical clinical picture of adolescent mania. *The American Journal of Psychiatry, 139,* 602–606.

Bowlby, G. (1973). *Attachment and loss: Vol. 12. Separation, anxiety, and anger.* London: Hogarth Press.

Campbell, M. (1977). Treatment of childhood and adolescent schizophrenia. In J. M. Wiener (Ed.), *Psychopharmacology in childhood and adolescence.* New York: Basic Books.

Campbell, M., Cohen, I. L., & Anderson, L. T. (1981). Pharmacotherapy for autistic children: A summary of research. *Canadian Journal of Psychiatry, 26,* 265–273.

Cantwell, D. P. (1985). Hyperactive children have grown up: What have we learned about what happens to them? *Archives of General Psychiatry, 42,* 1026–1028.

Casaus, L., Arciniega, M., & Castillo, M. (1982). *Parenting models and Mexican Americans: A process analysis.* Albuquerque, NM: Pajarito Publications.

Conte, J. R., & Schuerman, J. R. (1987). The effects of sexual abuse on children: A multidimensional view. *Journal of Interpersonal Violence, 2,* 380–390.

Delga, I., Heinssen, R. K., Fritsch, R. C., Goodrich, W., & Yates, B. T. (1989). Psychosis, aggression and self-destructive behavior in hospitalized adolescents. *The American Journal of Psychiatry, 146,* 521–525.

Dell, P. R., & Eisenhower, J. W. (1990). Adolescent multiple personality disorder: A preliminary study of eleven cases. *Journal of the American Academy of Child and Adolescent Psychiatry, 29,* 359–567.

Gualtieri, C. T., & Hicks, R. E. (1985). Neuropharmacology of methylphenidate and a neural substrata for childhood hyperactivity. *Psychiatric Clinics of North America, 8,* 875–892.

Harper, G. (1989). Focal inpatient treatment planning. *Journal of the American Academy of Child and Adolescent Psychiatry, 28,* 31–37.

Kernberg, P. F. (1983). Borderline conditions: Childhood and adolescent aspects. In K. S. Robson (Ed.), *The borderline child: Approaches to etiology, diagnosis and treatment* (pp. 101–119). New York: McGraw-Hill.

Marchi, M., & Cohen, P. (1990). Early childhood eating disorders and adolescent eating disorders. *Journal of the American Academy of Child and Adolescent Psychiatry, 29,* 112–117.

Martini, P. P. (1979). *La Frontera Perspective.* Tucson, AZ: Old Pueblo Printers.

Maziade, M., Caron, C., Cote, R., Boutin, P., & Thivierge, J. (1990). Extreme temperament and diagnosis: A study in a psychiatric sample of consecutive children. *Archives of General Psychiatry, 47,* 447–487.

McDaniel, K. D. (1986). Pharmacologic treatment of psychiatric and neurodevelopmental disorders in children and adolescents. *Clinical Pediatrics, 25,* 65–71.

McGlashan, T. H. (1989). Comparison of adolescent and adult onset of unipolar depression. *The American Journal of Psychiatry, 146,* 1208–1211.

Moreau, D. L., Weissman, M., & Warner, V. (1989). Panic disorder in children at high risk for depression. *The American Journal of Psychiatry, 146,* 1059–1060.

Nurcomb, B. (1989). Goal-directed treatment planning and the principles of brief hospitalization. *Journal of the American Academy of Child and Adolescent Psychiatry, 28,* 26–30.

Pelham, W. E., Walker, J. L., Sturges, J., & Hoza, J. A. (1989). Comparative effect of methylphenidate on ADD girls and ADD boys. *Journal of the American Academy of Child and Adolescent Psychiatry, 28,* 773–777.

Petti, T. A., & Law, W. (1982). Imipramine treatment of depressed children: A double-blind pilot study. *Journal of Clinical Psychopharmacology, 2,* 107–110.

Petti, T. A., & Vela, R. M. (1990). Borderline disorders in children on overview. *Journal of the American Academy of Child and Adolescent Psychiatry, 29,* 327–337.

Puig-Antich, J., Perel, J., Lupatkin, W., Chambers, W. J., Tabrizi, A., King, J., Goetz, R., Davies, M., & Stiller, P. (1987). Imipramine in prepubertal major depression. *Archives of General Psychiatry, 44,* 81–89.

Red Horse, J. (1981). *The American Indian family: Strengths and stresses.* Isleta, NM: American Indian Social Research and Development Associates.

Rosenthal, D., & Bornholt, L. (1988). Expectations about development in Greek and Anglo-Australian families. *Journal of Cross-Cultural Psychology, 19,* 19–35.

Rutter, M. (1978). Diagnosis and definition of childhood autism. *Journal of Autism and Childhood Schizophrenia, 8,* 139–161.

Rutter, M. (1985). The treatment of autistic children. *Journal of Child Psychology and Psychiatry, 26,* 193–214.

Sander, D. (1979). *Navajo symbols of healing.* New York: Harcourt.

Smalley, S. L., Asarnow, R. F., & Spense, M. A. (1988). Autism and genetics. *Archives of General Psychiatry, 45,* 953–961.

Spitz, R. A. (1965). *The first year of life.* New York: International Universities Press.

Swedo, S. E., Rappoport, J. L., Leonard, H., Lenane, M., & Cheslow, D. (1989). Obsessive compulsive disorder in children and adolescents. *Archives of General Psychiatry, 46,* 376–380.

Thomas, A. (1981). Current trends in developmental theory. *American Journal of Orthopsychiatry, 51,* 580–608.

Thomas, A., Chess, S., & Birch, H. G. (1968). *Temperament and behavior disorders in children.* New York: University Press.

Thomas, J. N. (1989). Triple jeopardy: Child abuse, drug abuse and the minority client. *Journal of Interpersonal Violence, 4,* 351–355.

Varanka, T. M., Weller, A. A., Weller, E., & Fristad, M. A. (1988). Lithium treatment of manic episodes with psychotic features in prepubertal children. *The American Journal of Psychiatry, 145,* 1557–1559.

Westen, D., Ludolph, P., Lerner, H., Ruffino, S., & Wiss, F. C. (1990). Object relations in borderline adolescents. *Journal of the American Academy of Child and Adolescent Psychiatry, 29,* 338–348.

Wishik, J., Bachman, D. L., & Beitch, L. M. (1989). A neurobehavioral perspective of aggressive behavior: Implications for pharmacological management. *Residential Treatment for Children and Youth, 6,* 101–109.

Woolston, J. L. (1989). Transactional risk model for short and intermediate term psychiatric inpatient treatment of children. *Journal of the American Academy of Child and Adolescent Psychiatry, 28,* 38–41.

Part III

Treatment Modalities
and Issues

The centrality of the treatment team as the body that plans, organizes, and implements treatment is emphasized in this section. The various therapeutic modalities must be integrated, and no decisions on patient or family issues should be made by any treatment person without the team's involvement. In Chapter 5, Kerlinsky stresses that confidentiality in this setting is relative; therapists must keep the team apprised of all information shared by the patient or the family, to promote an integrated treatment effort. Acting-out and violent behaviors are a team responsibility, not that of any single individual.

Stearns emphasizes, in Chapter 6, the importance of group work with children and adolescents as a vital therapeutic process. The group process is able to deal with the group members' need for nurturance and their symptomatic expression in hostility. When accepted and given empathy, each youth's feelings and revelations about previous experiences—especially being depressed, being controlled, and controlling—become an integrative process, especially when acting-out in the group is not permitted.

In Chapter 7, Givler presents the central issues that the milieu staff, therapists, and hospital personnel must work on, to help patients and families from minority cultures feel understood and welcomed in the hospital. Givler also describes the various steps that can be explored by the staff and therapists to further the collaboration throughout the hospitalization process.

In Chapter 8, Porter and Blackwell identify various cultural groups' resistances to hospital care, the use of medication, and family therapy, because of their traditions and the attitudes of staff members toward patients' families. These authors describe in detail and illustrate how these resistances can be recognized and differentiated from cultural and traditional differences about treatment, and they present some ways of dealing with resistances in a sensitive and helpful way.

Cavalluzzo, in Chapter 9, reveals how the educational setting and process can be therapeutic for patients. She emphasizes the need for teachers and aides to be an integral part of the treatment team. She describes how a neutral, task-oriented curriculum that does not press the patient for interaction and self revelation can be especially helpful to some patients. The use of various curriculum elements and specialized instruction by allied therapists combine to enhance the patient's learning.

In Chapter 10, Ponton describes the variations in short-term treatment and the elements of an effective short-term treatment program. She emphasizes the increased need for precise information, to help a skilled staff make the most effective use of the short hospital stay. Cultural consultants who can speak each ethnic group's native language and thus facilitate the information gathering and the treatment process are important contributors to short-term treatment. Ponton also emphasizes the need for continued inservice training on both clinical issues and the attitudes and traditions of various cultures with respect to mental illness.

Anthony, in Chapter 11, provides a contrast; he describes the use of long-term, psychoanalytically oriented inpatient treatment. The division between individual treatment as the most important element and milieu treatment with a separate administrative psychiatrist who decides on the patient's passes, visitors, and so on, stands out as an important contrast to Kerlinsky's view of the team concept of treatment. Traditional, psychoanalytically derived inpatient treatment for adolescents and, where possible, work with their families clearly offers some benefits. The importance of the milieu and of other therapies is vividly described as are the specially oriented analytic principles that guide them. Thus, in contrast to several other chapters, Anthony sustains many convictions about the efficacy of long-term hospital care in which a psychoanalytic model of individual psychotherapy is combined with group and family therapy. Some behavioral principles that are consonant with general psychoanalytic principles are used in the milieu.

In Chapter 12, Critchley focuses on how the milieu staff's childhood and upbringing may lead to countertransference reactions to patients and families from other cultures. A lack of understanding of cultural traditions increases staff prejudices. The need for open discussion of countertransference issues in the staff, as a means of reducing adverse therapeutic effects on patients and families, is emphasized. Continued group or individual supervision, to help reduce countertransference in staff, is very important. These issues are illustrated by vignettes.

Berlin, in Chapter 13, describes how the violence of child and adolescent patients controls the hospital unit. The methods of reducing such control over peers and adults may include temporary restraint, isolation, the quiet room, and so on. The rapidity with which staff can anticipate or react to the first sign of violence begins to reduce the patient's control over others and starts the therapeutic restructuring of some personality characteristics. Several vignettes illustrate the clinical process.

CHAPTER FIVE

Integrating Interdisciplinary Team-Centered Treatment

Daniel Kerlinsky

"Method, Method, what do you want from me? You know I have eaten of the fruit of the subconscious." Jules LaForgue, *Moralités Légendaires* (Bachelard, 1970b)

Although most clinicians utilize several treatment modalities, the integration of treatment models and practices is typically considered "eclectic." Webster defines "eclectic" as drawn from diverse sources, systems, or styles; but eclectic says little about the way these diverse elements are woven together. A systematic integration of interdisciplinary treatment is not developed theoretically or in a short period of time. Therapists in training may search conceptually to enlarge their representations of the worlds of mental illness, but practice often transforms theory and the individuals who hold to it.

Frequently, different therapists are guiding individual, family, group, psychoeducational, and psychopharmacological interventions. Therapists of different training and culture may conceive of problems differently. Each modality of intervention in a multidisciplinary treatment may be carried out in isolation from the others. In outpatient treatment, communication among therapists is often limited and unpaid (the patient may be left alone to integrate diverse approaches). Even in well-staffed inpatient units, it may be easy for a "split" to occur, leading to fragmentation rather than integration of treatment. Little attention may be given to the interfacing of the various therapeutic modalities.

This chapter describes the process of integrating interdisciplinary, multicultural, inpatient treatment of the severely disturbed child and adolescent. The systems that require management are delineated and the rationales that guide our treatment-planning priorities at the critical interfaces of hospital care are explained. The boundary alterations around confidentiality in brief or intermediate-length treatment are related to the advantages of opening up issues from individual therapy for focus in family and milieu therapy. In this context, the developmental use of psychopharmacologic interventions is presented. Careful attention to promote the integration of treatment modalities when working multiculturally multiplies the effectiveness of hospital care.

THE MODALITIES OF INPATIENT CARE

Like the indigenous skill of basketry that gathers, prepares, and weaves fibers into containers, the inpatient team selects from each of the disciplines and treatment modalities. For individual psychotherapy, both cognitive and psychodynamic approaches are helpful. Supportive psychotherapy helps children anticipate consequences of their behavior; psychodynamic work helps unravel the complex, confusing motivational patterns that drive maladaptive behavior. Group therapy promotes relationship development, behavioral control, and exploration of common psychological themes such as abuse and loss. Group work also builds a therapeutic culture, setting limits and expectations for courtesy, confrontation, and exploratory interactions while helping to define the therapists' leadership roles.

Family therapy provides a powerful context that explains relationship patterns and denotes the limits of a particular family member's individual growth. Appreciation of cultural factors also aids in understanding the issues that may limit the range of transition, adjustment, and growth possible to an individual in a given situation. Psychoeducation—the "special education" program—provides not only "structure" for the day but a range of cognitive, expressive, and social skills development. Psychopharmacologic interventions can compensate for developmental deficiencies or "boost" development (Shapiro, 1985), often by improving impulse control and affect modulation. Milieu treatment promotes relationship development and reveals behavior patterns and transferences, while allowing the patient a safe haven in which to develop verbal expression of feelings, new behaviors, and new identifications.

In inpatient, milieu teamwork, especially in a multicultural setting, time for understanding patients and their families, and therapist–staff collaboration are crucial considerations. The team must have a shared view of the patient's problems and progress. Each team member should feel encouraged to wonder about the meaning of the patient's problem behavior. The priorities of intervention need to be clear. In practice, any treatment or family intervention that interferes with the priorities of team treatment needs to be examined, understood, and modified. As much as possible, families should be included in the team, and team splitting should be minimized. The milieu treatment program, dealing with daily behavior problems, takes priority over the individual preference, theory, or practice of team members.

For example, therapist–patient confidentiality must be expanded to include the entire clinical team, to prevent a split that would undermine the therapeutic milieu. A therapist, nurse, teacher, or milieu worker who gives in to the child's or family's wish to keep secrets from the rest of the team usually ends up recreating old pathological family situations. Even the traditional passive stance of the psychotherapist must be modified to permit frank discussion with the patient and staff about the therapist's concerns regarding the consequences of the patient's destructive behavior for himself and others (Berlin, Critchley, & Rossman, 1984).

Special education, milieu, and clinical staff must build relationships with each other, to make their evaluations and program delivery effective and integrated enough to hold a group of emotionally and behaviorally difficult patients who at first resist hospitalization and treatment. This phase of team cohesion requires each discipline to extend into new territory; each member must become familiar with each other's knowledge base, values, and style. Adequate "rounds" time at work and appreciation of each other's professional, cultural, and personal qualities are important. In a hierarchical institution like a hospital, one may need occasional reminders that impulse control, affect modulation under stress, and the ability to handle "feedback" and narcissistic hurt are not conferred by training and professional degrees. The same is true about communication abilities, intuition, comfort with aggression and sexuality, common sense, and many other attributes important to multiculturally sensitive, interdisciplinary treatment.

Each child's own custom-built treatment container is woven from the strands of different disciplines, depending on what external structure and skills are needed for facilitating development (Redl, 1965a, 1965b, 1966). Higher functioning children with good impulse control and the capacity to express feelings in words typically require less external structure than the impulse-ridden, undersocialized, angry, depressed, or abused child (Green, 1978a, 1978b, 1983). One child may require firm, tightly structured and adhered-to behavioral consequences that link the classroom and evening shift milieu; another may require nonverbal, expressive therapy and "safe" hugs while working through family abuse issues. But whenever team members work closely together, the continuity of interventions and the "twist" each individual naturally gives to another's formulation and work creates "tight" treatment. Psychodynamically informed behavioral intervention, for example, is less easily evaded by an oppositional child. Working closely together, each individual's professional experience and personal qualities add to treatment.

Personal and cultural factors often skew the child's, family's, and team members' perception, judgment, meaning, and valuation of events. Cultural ignorance, insensitivity, and derogation are important factors that require constant vigilance from the staff. Distortion that results from amplification (blowing an event out of proportion) or skew (seeing only part of what is going on) requires careful attention and correction for patients, families, and team members.

Team-centered treatment may focus on the same problem from several different perspectives and in several different treatment modalities. The team approach may accelerate treatment by providing numerous opportunities to recognize problems, explore antecedents, and attempt new solutions; it may link progress and rewards in one modality to another where the patient seems stuck. Team-centered treatment helps therapists appreciate and amplify the effects of interventions other than their own. When the therapists help direct the team and the team helps direct the therapists, integration of interdisciplinary treatment is a daily practice.

SPECIAL NEEDS OF MULTICULTURAL CARE

Multicultural treatment adds a number of issues with which the team must work. It requires "goodness of fit" for each problem definition, goal, and modality of intervention. Attention to "fit" is required among therapist, family, team, hospital, and home community. Educational needs include not only familiarity with the world views of a variety of cultures but comfort with the styles and interaction patterns of individuals, families, and social networks. Cultures and individuals are not static, and some assessment of the degree of acculturation or biculturality of the individual, family, and community is helpful. The therapist needs to have some preliminary notions of how he or she will be seen by the patient and client family. How is the therapist's ethnic and professional identity regarded? Are any aspects of the therapist's personality style particularly meaningful or distasteful to the patient or family? Are there elements of "evil influence," "possession," or "transgression" in the family's view of the illness? How are these understood and worked with? Should the family be offered the opportunity to involve native healers in the therapeutic process? Can the therapist carry any of the traditional, cultural expectations that the family has of the "healer"?

Outreach requirements must often be increased to serve "minority" groups. Extra help with arranging child care, elder care, relief from work, and transportation expenses is often required with low-income, distant-dwelling patients and families. Outreach that actively includes important members of the social network who may not be in the "nuclear" family takes time, money, effort, and field trips, especially when these individuals do not have telephones or do not speak English.

Consultation is more frequently required to extend the team's awareness of cultural views, values, and styles that may affect the treatment alliance. Extra consultation may be required when cross-cultural interventions include traditional healing ceremonies or cultural activities in the home community that might be seen as "deviant" by members of the dominant culture. Cultural consultation may be useful when a youth is to be removed from or returned to a traditional community, or when the family values are discordant with the "therapeutic" culture that is being considered. When dramatic changes in culturally supported life plans are being contemplated, cultural consultation can help the individual patient predict the social and psychological consequences of crossing these cultural boundaries. Consultation may also be indicated when cultural beliefs about the etiology of disturbances, such as possession or transgression of a taboo, impact on a family's involvement in treatment.

Each of these additional interventions requires administrative commitment of personnel, time, money, and risk management. Trips to see extended family or community members who may or may not become involved in treatment is often seen as extraneous or unproductive. In the time that it takes a therapist to travel to the home of a patient for a session, several other patients could have been treated and billed. Long-distance phone calls and interpreters cost money. Every pass and alternative treatment intervention carries a risk of medicolegal liability and bad publicity for the hospital, should something go wrong. Despite these costs and issues, clinical administrators can usually be persuaded of the value of these multiculturally sensitive services.

Juan was a 12-year-old with chronic depression, self-mutilation, episodic hallucinations and suicidal ideation, conduct disorder, and explosive, violent aggression. His parents divorced when he was age 7 and his mother lived in another part of the country. He had been sexually abused by his father's girlfriend, whom he hated and had threatened to kill. His father had been known, in the past, in the small Spanish village where he grew up, to have dealt drugs, and he belonged to a motorcycle gang. Juan was in state custody and his father's side of the family opposed hospitalization.

After several months of treatment, just when his relationship with his father was beginning to improve, Juan found out his father had died of a gunshot wound, allegedly self-inflicted. Was a pass to be granted for Juan to attend the rosary and funeral? There were clear risks of suicide, assaultiveness, elopement, and confrontation in the small village where outsiders, including the caseworker, were not welcome. But the psychological costs of denying a son's attendance at his father's funeral seemed high as well. Administrative support was essential to grant a pass in the company of the patient's Spanish-speaking "primary" staff and the team's male nurse, since both Juan's therapist and his mother were out of town.

Multicultural treatment requires that individuals, groups, and institutions work in the same direction. Limits were set with Juan and his family about avoiding issues or conflicts that focused outside of his relation with his father. Juan needed to know that staff was instructed to terminate the pass if impulsive behavior or conflict with his father's girlfriend began. Immediate behavioral consequences were woven in, to support Juan's limited anger modulation. The family needed to hear that whatever the problems had been, and regardless of what might have been better than state custody and hospitalization, Juan needed the chance to say goodbye to his father without getting embroiled in other conflicts. Cross-cultural respect for the family's view of "Anglo" institutions was woven into a strong communication of the team's commitment to Juan's well-being, family relationships, and therapy.

The priest needed to know that Juan was a patient in the hospital's care and possibly would need to be removed from church if agitation developed. The priest was asked whether he would permit that in his church and whether he recommended any other special arrangements. The team's respect for his congregation, authority, and duties encouraged him to assist in determining the seating arrangement that would limit contact between Juan and his father's girlfriend. The hospital administration needed to know the team's assessment: that failure to handle the death adequately with Juan might set up intractable problems for treatment and that Juan's history of clever suicide attempts meant he was not necessarily safer in the hospital. The team wove together therapeutic objectives, risk management, and justification for extra staff. In sharing the responsibility for a difficult clinical decision, administrative members of the team agreed with the plan to send an unstable patient into a cross-cultural home community for a religious service that might lead into untherapeutic acting-out.

Even discussions with the priest and extended family could not remove the elements of uncertainty and risk. But the hospital's willingness to accept some risk and the cost of overtime and extra staffing helped us to not add to this boy's tragedy. As the ordeal of acute grief progressed, Juan was able to describe his ambivalence about the relationship with his father—including his repeated experience of neglect and confusion about having been exposed to drugs, sex, and violence as a child.

PROBLEMS IN INTEGRATING INTERDISCIPLINARY TEAMWORK

Unconscious Processes

Several factors may interfere with integrating treatment modalities; one is the important role of the unconscious. Without appreciating complex motivational factors, cognitive and behavioral treatments can become stymied. Critical history of severe trauma and its aftereffects may be missing from the presenting information. An appreciation of unconscious dynamic factors is not always systematic; different affects, wishes, perceptions, transferences, defenses, and resistances may predominate at any time with a child or adolescent. A child may appear differently to different individuals at different times. The ability to track a theme, repetitive interaction, or problem behavior across settings requires effort by all team members to observe carefully and to share their observations and intuitions.

Having time to discuss a patient's interactional patterns with a variety of individuals promotes a kind of quantitative assessment of transference and defenses that is nearly impossible in individual sessions. The extent to which such patterns interfere with the child's functioning in each setting becomes clearer. The meaning of the maladaptive behavior is seen in relation to the origin of the roles and feelings being re-enacted. Strong countertransference feelings may distract one from understanding the child's misperceptions and motivation. Unconscious cultural biases or prejudices may also interfere with the team's ability to understand behavior or accurately define the priorities and goals of treatment. Destructive behavior may be wrongly considered "normative" for particular minorities and thus ignored.

A multicultural treatment facility promotes team-centered treatment in a variety of ways. Perhaps most important, a multicultural setting entertains alternative world views and treatment models. Holistic world views that accentuate connectedness and interdependency may expand psychiatry's biopsychosocial model to include a full range of traditional, modern, and experimental treatment approaches. In encouraging the consideration of alternative treatment methods, a multicultural setting promotes cross-disciplinary respect and flexibility. This permits the team to reframe the issues from different points of view when the initial treatment interventions fail. The freedom to reframe and try again allows the therapist and child-care worker to support the healthy motives in maladaptive behavior while guiding the child and family.

Team-centered work values the relationships developed by each staff member and gives due respect to the therapeutic, healing effects of child-care workers, the "unsung heroes" of the profession. This respect for what in the United States is considered "nonprofessional" work carries over to cross-cultural respect in a multicultural setting. Each of the child's relationships is important, regardless of the social status of the individual as viewed by the dominant culture.

Biological Limitations

Integrated treatment requires consideration of biological, intrapsychic, interpersonal, group, team, family, community, and cultural factors. Problems occurring in any aspect of functioning can affect each of the others. Central nervous system impairment impacts the delivery of each treatment modality. Biological disturbances typically have profound effects on impulse control, affect modulation, self-esteem, and relationships. Improved impulse control is a typical goal for many hospital treatments (Popper, 1987; Shapiro, 1985).

Luis presented as an out-of-control 12-year-old with seizures, developmental disabilities, poor social relations, low self-esteem, and progressive threatening and aggressive behavior. He had had severe meningitis at age 1 and had been sexually abused by a neighborhood boy in the year prior to hospitalization. His black father had never been able to accept his organic brain limitations and had adopted an approach of pushing Luis to succeed and teasing him when he became discouraged or failed. His Hispanic mother continued to wash and style his hair and pick clothes for him in a protective manner, even as he entered adolescence. Luis and his father blamed the white doctors at the county hospital where he had been treated for meningitis for his severe developmental difficulties.

After Luis's sex abuse victimization, his aggressive behavior escalated and began to include inappropriate sexual behavior. His biological difficulty with impulse control and his deficient anticipation of the consequences of his behavior impacted on all levels of his treatment. Among his peer group, other males challenged and provoked him, then sat back and watched him get in trouble. Female peers, inclined to be more sympathetic, were frightened by his aggressive and somewhat eroticized mannerisms.

The staff felt discouraged about his ever gaining better impulse control. The hospital was concerned about the likelihood that Luis would abuse others in the community, should he be released without control of his problem behavior. The community school that referred him for treatment was having a time-out room built for his special education classroom while he was away. His therapist felt confused, helpless, and overwhelmed, torn between wanting to develop a relationship and wishing somehow to get control of the patient and his unmodulated sexual and aggressive impulses. In rounds, team discussion led to a decision to pursue treatment on several levels at once. Concrete behavior goals were set for the milieu; rehearsal and repetition of what Luis could do when teasing or conflict arose led to Luis's earning points and a higher level. Extensive reaching out to the family and a review of Luis's medical records from the county hospital were arranged. His father was then able to confess that he had trouble stopping himself from pushing Luis, because he felt guilty for sometimes wishing he had not survived such a handicapping illness. His mother agreed to stop bathing Luis now that he was entering puberty and to not try to make up for his father's attitude toward him.

In group therapy, male staff were instructed to sit next to Luis and model other ways—uniquely their own—of "being tough." Luis was given an opportunity to show and teach others his Michael Jackson imitation, and a place was made for him in the talent show. In drawings and play, Luis worked out his rage at being abused and his confusion about being sexually stimulated in the process.

These changes would not have been possible without the improvement in his seizure frequency and impulse control brought about by adding propranolol and low-dose thioridazine to his carbamazepine and diphenytoin regimen. The need for improved impulse control was so great that neuroleptics were used, despite their effect on lowering seizure threshold. Luis's improved impulse control reduced team countertransference pressure and improved his peer relations. It gave his father reason for pride, raising Luis's self-esteem and his willingness to allow the team to rechannel the aggression and sexuality resulting from his sex abuse victimization.

Once Luis passed through the hormonal changes of early adolescence, the thioridazine was discontinued without recurrence of the inappropriate sexual and aggressive behavior. This result often occurs when medication is used as a "developmental booster" (Shapiro, 1985). The medication may no longer be needed as other dimensions of intervention become effective in reducing motivation for dysfunctional behavior, promoting alternative adaptive strategies, and reinforcing newly achieved capacities and compromises.

The treatment here was composed of biological, cognitive, and expressive therapies. An important unconscious factor in perpetuating the disorder turned up in family therapy. With Luis's father, the only clue at first was his reluctance to come to the hospital or participate actively in family therapy sessions. He did not show any hostility to the white male doctor. Only by asking, nonjudgmentally, about his style of "toughening" and "encouraging" his son did the feelings of anger, sadness, and pain emerge. After that, the dynamic of externalizing the blame became evident; Luis's father could see that it had been easier to blame the doctors than to blame himself or accept the loss of what he hoped his son would become. His father became more openly affectionate with Luis and began to notice the angry feelings Luis tried to hide after being teased. His father's "toughening" and demand that Luis had to "take care of himself" diminished, along with Luis's aggressiveness.

The doctor's willingness to review the county hospital records helped to solidify the parent–therapist relationship. There was no evidence of any undue delay or assessment in the emergency room, hospitalization, or treatment, though the therapist was willing to acknowledge that minority patients may often be treated with subtle or blunt discrimination in county hospital settings. Luis's father reported feeling guilty for not taking his son to the emergency room sooner, though there was no reasonable clue that medical help was necessary before the headache and stiff neck developed.

Luis's impulse control was the primary reason for referral and the highest priority for intervention. The referral came originally from the home community school where Luis had disrupted his special education classroom. The parents initially viewed hospitalization as a way to "catch up" on schoolwork. This goal was reframed and incorporated into the treatment plan as an assessment of Luis's school problems and special developmental needs. As in many cases, a mismatch of patient abilities and environmental expectations contributed to difficulties. The reason for the mismatch was probably unconsciously determined.

The cultural factors in this case were interesting. Luis's father came from a large Oklahoma sharecropping family where physical prowess and independence were highly valued. He frequently worked overtime and night shifts as maintenance engineer for a local dairy plant, a highly stressful job because any breakdown of the automated conveyor system or the refrigeration led to spoiling and immediate company losses. Growing up in Oklahoma, in the military, and at work in New Mexico, he had experienced repeated racial discrimination. His son, too, was highly visible in a predominantly Hispanic village.

Luis's mother came from the village; ambition and individual accomplishment were less important there than finding a role in the extended, multigenerational family. Marrying an "outsider" and having a son who did not "fit in" raised a different set of issues for her. The family had become split to the point that the father and mother frequently worked opposite shifts. Luis's father spent time preferentially with the youngest son, who was athletically gifted; his mother took care of the two older boys, trying to get Luis's clever, socially adept younger brother to take Luis along with him and "look out" for him. Although many family issues were evident, the family cultural split became the treatment priority. It became clear that Luis, because of his developmental disabilities, would not do well except in his extended family. There he would find a more culturally adaptive and sustaining setting.

Milieu Safety Issues

Open sexual and aggressive behavior can disrupt not only families and schools but treatment objectives and milieu team functioning as well. There is never enough individual supervision time for staff to deal with their reactions to a week of 8-hour onslaughts. At crisis times, the team leaders, including the therapists, must make unit safety and the team's functioning their highest priorities, at least for the time being. Once patient safety and teamwork are assured, setting limits on disruptive behavior by the patient group often helps reduce "inappropriate" sexual, aggressive, and abusive behavior. At the same time, the team works to increase its ability to handle the feelings and impulses that the patients stir up in other patients and in staff members.

In addition to effective limit setting that promotes external support for impulse control, increased patient supervision and milieu structure reduce team and patient group anxiety. Soon, free time more closely resembles a schoolday; activities are scheduled and individuals' participation in group and recreational functions is determined by staff. When there is contagious acting-out in the milieu, optional entertainment and outings are typically suspended. Safety issues of both patients and staff get highest priority. Patient groups are typically reduced in size and the rules of group interactions are reinforced; courtesy, patience, focusing on reduced teasing, and challenging by group members are buttressed by immediate behavioral consequences. Increased attention to the patient group and the team process during these periods of "slowdown" or "shutdown" helps reestablish a therapeutic atmosphere.

The children repeatedly tell the team that "therapeutic" coping strategies will not work in the "real" world. In the real world, no one cares about your feelings. In the real world, they will never be safe. At this point, the multicultural resources of the team are important, to be able to put the child's experience of abuse in context. The team needs to assess with the child the allies he or she may need to call on, in each particular cultural setting, for protection from abuse. The "therapeutic culture's" belief in the patient's autonomy and the child's capacity to develop his or her own identity and friendships is important (Aichhorn, 1967). So are the therapists' belief in the patient's potential for learning to problem-solve and their continuous help in promoting the good judgment to avoid potentially dangerous situations.

In a multicultural treatment process, the consideration of how a particular patient's behavior would be received outside of the hospital often provides a reality base for the therapeutic work to be done. Typically, a multicultural team that values a plurality of views and lives "day in and day out" with a patient is oriented toward that patient's changing reality and adaptive functioning. In our rapidly changing world, many cultural adaptations may be possible.

Typically, staff and family attempt to control bothersome behavior or adapt to it in other ways. Only when a bothersome pattern is aversive enough or repeated enough do people stop to problem-solve or discuss it (Bion, 1961). A team-centered therapist who follows charting on the unit and meets regularly with milieu staff can pick up the beginning elements of a pattern outside the regular therapeutic sessions.

The ability of the team to describe not only patient behavior but the entire interaction—the feelings evoked in them as well as those displayed by the patient—provides the therapist with a wealth of transference–countertransference material. The therapist's ability to rethink the issues, using psychodynamic principles, at times of crisis may be crucial in understanding the meaning of the patient's behavior and finding a variety of interventions to promote reduction of psychopathology.

Team Limitations

Each new advance in any particular aspect of treatment alters the current state of clinical art by requiring changed relationships among all of the treatment modalities. A team-centered "multimodal" therapist should have a sense of what a variety of treatment disciplines can offer to deal with particular child or adolescent problems. For example, a psychologist who is unaware of the beneficial effects of stimulant medication for ADHD (Attention Deficit Hyperactivity Disorder) cannot provide what is currently considered optimal treatment. Similarly, a child psychiatrist who is unaware of behavioral intervention options will not provide state-of-the-art treatment.

A psychiatrist who does not believe in seeing the family, a social worker who does not believe in genetics or the brain, a behaviorist who does not believe in unconscious motivation, or a nurse who does not believe in limit setting would each deny some therapeutic interventions that are available, should they as individuals be in charge of treatment. A team-centered, multicultural treatment model, however, allows for a variety of views and approaches, if each team member can accept feedback and overcome his or her limitations.

When these approaches can be woven together, each modality can augment the others. Whenever family therapy, group therapy, milieu, behavior therapy, psychoeducation programs, and psychopharmacology are effective, clearly much more goes into treatment than what happens in an individual therapy hour—the "old" child therapy model. For example, progress in family work facilitates individual work by creating credibility for the therapist, freeing the patient from undue projections, confronting unresolved separation and oedipal issues, providing for some appropriate dependency gratifications, and reducing the dominance of hostile and control fantasies.

Kurt presented for admission because of repeated vandalism, provocative oppositionality, excessive preoccupation with knives and violence, fire setting, and school suspension. His biological parents were Eskimo and Navajo, but he and his brothers were adopted at an early age by two white VISTA volunteers who had previously been foster parents for his mother. His adopted parents were now a teacher and a guidance counselor at the school where he was getting into trouble. In fact, his behavior seemed designed specifically to embarrass them.

In family therapy, his mother insisted that Kurt remain at the hospital for the two years of treatment she had been advised he would require. When informed that that length of treatment would not be possible, the mother angrily wished to appeal to the hospital's medical director. What gradually emerged was that his mother was convinced that Kurt was planning to kill her, and that he had "bad blood."

Kurt was torn between wanting to win his mother's love and wishing to revenge himself on her for what he perceived as her cold, rejecting ways. Each of his attempts to do well in the hospital program was met with minimization, scorn, and disbelief from his mother. He obtained support for his view of his mother's rejection from his psychiatry resident therapist and then reported to his mother a provocative version of what his therapist had said. In the uproar that followed, it became clear that his father had adopted a conciliatory, protective role with his wife, frequently "giving in" to her demands, as perceived by Kurt. Kurt seemed to be trying to model, for his father, the image of the adult male that Kurt needed to identify with.

In doing so, however, his manipulative, splitting, demanding, callous, haughty behavior made him resemble his mother. When it was suggested that he was acting like her, Kurt looked shaken, confused, and embarrassed. If Kurt really saw his mother as cold and rejecting, why had he not given up long ago on trying to get love from her? With this, the delayed separation and the beginning of a grieving process for the mother he never had began to evolve.

Kurt's provocative, derogatory treatment of women created profound stress for the milieu staff, especially his sensitive, recently hired "cottage primary," who just happened to be a woman. The intensity of humiliation, hopelessness, confusion, and anger he induced in others suggested that he himself had been subject to an onslaught of projective identification. Identifying this dynamic with Kurt's primary staff helped her to understand where these feelings were coming from and what they stirred up in her; identifying it in individual therapy helped Kurt realize that he had accepted his mother's view of him and had been acting in a way to "prove" that she was "right" about him.

An important issue needed to be moved from milieu to individual therapy—Kurt's discourteous, callous, demeaning attitude toward women. His male psychiatric resident therapist had engaged him in competitive board games like "Risk," which revealed Kurt's intelligence and grandiosity but did little to remedy his denial of problems and his provocative behavior outside of sessions. With supervision, the resident was encouraged to follow Kurt's milieu behavior problems more closely and to raise them for discussion, if Kurt did not.

Although this method spoiled the "friendly" atmosphere of the sessions and stopped the therapist from providing the narcissistic "mirroring" he believed Kurt needed, it began the process of approaching Kurt's problems with his mother, which he studiously avoided.

The emotional distress Kurt and his mother created provided a natural focus and priority for intervention. Following the "heat," the natural, distressing emotional problems and priorities led to the central dynamic for hospitalization: Kurt's inability to separate himself from his mother and his drive to get revenge. Revenge dynamics typically require immediate identification, confrontation, and discouragement. Even more so than "blaming," revenge motives lead to a cycle of aggression and disrupt therapeutic work. Revengeful attitudes destroy the goodwill of potential helpers, create long-term aversive consequences, and set up the fear of retaliation.

Kurt's case also required the shifting of issues back and forth between individual and family therapy. Because it was a "safety issue" that Kurt's parents needed to know about, in order to responsibly parent him and his siblings, Kurt was pressured to tell his parents the secret locations of knives he had hidden around the house. When he made sufficient progress to begin to feel guilty for hurting his mother, Kurt was encouraged to apologize in letters and in family therapy. Although his mother never fully accepted his apology and considered him to be attempting to manipulate, Kurt's father felt him to be sincere and their relationship began to develop. Finally, when his mother was unable to accept or enjoy any of Kurt's progress, Kurt was pushed, in individual sessions, to confront the fact that what he wished for from his mother was unlikely to happen; as a matter of fact, the sessions focused on what was stopping Kurt from pursuing other, more age-appropriate relationships to get his needs for intimacy met.

In guiding the back-and-forth flow between individual and family therapy, a few rules about defining boundary conditions may be helpful. As mentioned in Kurt's case, parents have a right to know anything that is necessary for family safety or for responsible parenting of their child. How to raise other issues that come up in the child's therapy and that the therapist deems important for family work must be worked through with the child in individual sessions first, whenever possible. Issues can be raised generally, with the therapist prompting the patient to present issues in a nonhostile way. Children and adolescents need to know that they cannot put off working on important family issues because they feel uncomfortable or would have to tell their parents things that would lead them to be more closely supervised.

As Kurt began to do well in school and to succeed in his behavior therapy program, further leverage against his introjection of and identification with the "bad blood" appeared. He became interested in his Eskimo heritage and presented a unit of his own design to the class. A decision was made to use paradoxical technique, since Kurt was improved and had understood much of why he behaved as he did. Kurt was then informed that he would be unable to control himself in the face of his mother's pessimism. The family was informed, that, as they predicted, Kurt would require long-term, out-of-home placement.

Although emotionally exhausted, the team was gratified when the family decided to refuse the recommendation and take Kurt home. After hurried good-byes, Kurt never called or wrote, but "proved us wrong" by doing well despite his mother's beliefs.

UNDERSTANDING CHANGE

In addition to differences in interpersonal experience between therapist and team, a clinician must be prepared for variability of a child's function, particularly in group as compared to individual sessions, or structured versus unstructured situations. Peculiarities of history and setting, such as unusual difficulties with mealtime, bathroom functions, bedtime, wake-up, and school may lead to markedly different levels of function within a single day. Thus, the team arrives at a series of images of a particular child's functioning in a variety of settings which, taken together, creates a profile against which to measure growth, regression, and change.

Each new dynamic or developmental change that then emerges unfolds into potential growth in a variety of areas of functioning. Providing careful linkages across modalities of therapeutic work for each individual helps the treatment plan to become continuously more effective. This reflects the value of integrated treatment.

The term "integration" is defined by the dictionary as organization into a whole. One way of integrating interdisciplinary treatment would be to consider the changes in impulse control, affect modulation, relationship capacity, problem solving, and other functions developed in each of the treatment modalities. As noted above, pharmacotherapy, behavior therapy, cognitive therapy, group therapy, family therapy, psychoeducation, and milieu work can all improve such functions as impulse control and expression of feelings.

Another way of looking at integration would consider the development not only of specific capacities but of the general capacity to undergo change and participate in a broader range of experience (Mindell, 1985). This general capacity is related to entropy (Prigogine & Nocolis, 1989; Prigogine & Stengers, 1984), defined scientifically as the capacity of a system to undergo spontaneous change. Entropy is also proportional to the number of configurations a system can realize. Applied to clinical situations this means that interventions that disrupt maladaptive behavior and promote new experiences increase entropy and are helpful. Viewed in this way, cultural factors can promote or inhibit change.

Jean, a 13-year-old Hispanic/native American girl, displayed episodic oppositionality that proceeded into power struggles, crying, hiding, self-aggressive and assaultive behavior with paranoid ideation, and accusations that no one cared and that the staff wanted to hurt her. Direct limit setting, consequences, time-outs, and extensive discussion all failed to end the episodes, which continued for several hours at a time. Staff and therapist felt extremely angry and frustrated that the patient could do very well for several weeks and then be so completely unresponsive. Jean's family culture seemed to support nondisclosure and passivity between her episodes of acute disturbance.

The feelings of helplessness and anger Jean stirred up in others and her pattern of unremitting unresponsiveness reminded the therapist of a report that Jean had been repeatedly raped by a group of males. Rather than struggle to control her, the team decided to allow Jean to go to one of several preselected "safe" hiding places in subsequent episodes. This "joining in" resulted in Jean's being able to disclose a full range of post-traumatic experiences, including flashbacks and nightmares that were triggered by her feeling out-of-control.

Once a psychodynamic formulation is worked out, trial interventions can be designed to alter a defense or go directly to one side or the other of a conflict. So-called paradoxical intervention often encourages acting-out of an undesired behavior. Acting-out under instruction, as Milton Erickson pointed out (Rossi, 1980), takes away some of the gratification of defiant omnipotence; it forces increased awareness on the patient and it decreases tension between patient and staff. Acting-out under instruction may confuse and unbalance a patient's defenses, calling forth a spontaneous, compensatory increase in more adaptive ego defenses. Paradoxical techniques disrupt the behavior pattern by introducing a new element—novelty (Dolan, 1985). In Jean's case, support for her need to hide disrupted the therapeutic impasse.

CONCLUSION

Integrated, multimodal treatment of the severely disturbed and disturbing child requires a flexible approach. As we repeatedly talk over the problems that recur time and again, we build up a data base of problems, progress, intervention options, strategies, tactics, and results. In our repeated discussions of problems, especially repeated symptomatic behaviors, we uncover hidden relationships and meanings that contribute to the tenacity of overdetermined, maladaptive, pathological, and often partially gratifying behaviors.

Structuring the environment to reduce the reward of destructive behavior and to gradually find effective methods of reducing such behavior is often a painstaking process. When biological factors limit a patient's impulse control, anticipation of consequences, and reward from relationships, pharmacological treatment helps to control these behaviors and facilitates the other treatment efforts. Only when better impulse control is established will the psychological factors in the disorder emerge.

Sometimes behavioral change precedes a child's ability to consciously look back, acknowledge, or understand troubling issues. In our understanding of systems theory, interactions and identity are codetermined (Spencer-Brown, 1972; Varela, 1979). Thus, exploration of identity issues has no intrinsic priority over behavioral techniques, to promote changed interactions. Identity changes lead to new interactions just as new patterns of interaction lead to identity development. Behavior change can lead to insight and vice versa. We therefore are alert to change wherever it first appears and we attempt to maximize the ramifications of change (Berlin, 1979; Berlin & Critchley, 1982).

In general, we have found that many traditional cultures have more in common with each other than most traditional cultures have with the dominant culture. Almost any traditional cultural value—respect for elders, concern for maintaining values, ceremony and identity across generations, willingness to share and work with an extended social group, understanding of natural consequences for transgression—can be helpful in the therapeutic process. With a little patience, respect, and reframing (Bandler & Grinder, 1975), a therapist can explain the special circumstances that lead him or her to request the temporary setting aside of a particular custom or belief for the sake of the patient's recovery. In some indigenous cultures, such requests may be expected of the community healer.

With severely disturbed children whose maladaptations may be deeply entrenched and whose trust and relationships have been significantly limited, we often search out the possible dimensions of change, no matter where they may be. Verbal interactions, behavior, cognitive changes, altered peer relations, shifts in family relations, and behavior shifts due to the use of pharmacotherapy all help in the attempt to interrupt behavior disruptive to treatment. We support and reinforce the possibilities of socially adaptive growth.

Multicultural treatment depends on interdisciplinary interventions that disrupt maladaptive behavior and foster growth. These results do not occur without discomfort and pain to both the patient and staff. Accepting the possibility of defeat often has a liberating effect for the team and patient. Many of our patients have been defeated in their attempts to protect their healthy development or reform abusive others. Admitting feelings of helplessness helps severely abused children feel understood (Schact, Kerlinsky, & Carlson, 1990). Hidden identifications with abusive others then emerge. Helping abused children relinquish distorted relationships with their abusers requires cross-cultural respect for the positive aspects of those relationships that the child experienced or imagined. Only then can the loss of the wished-for and needed good parent be appreciated and mourned.

"I always come then to the same conclusion," Gaston Bachelard (1970a), the French philosopher of science, psychoanalysis, and imagination, wrote in *The Poetics of Space*. "The essential newness of the poetic image poses the problem. . . ." This newness, the capacity for spontaneous change, delights the artist and gives the child therapist some small measure of progress and satisfaction.

REFERENCES

Aichhorn, A. (1967). *Delinquency and child guidance: Selected papers of August Aichhorn.* Menninger Foundation Monograph Series. Independence, MO: International Universities Press.

Bachelard, G. (1970a). *The poetics of space.* Boston: Beacon Press.

Bachelard, G. (1970b). *The poetics of reverie: Childhood, language, and the cosmos.* Boston: Beacon Press.

Bandler, R. & Grinder, J. (1975). *Patterns of the hypnotic techniques of Milton H. Erickson, M.D.* Cupertino, CA: Meta Publications.

Berlin, I. N. (1979). A developmental approach to work with disorganized families. *Journal of the American Academy of Child and Adolescent Psychiatry, 18;* 354–365.

Berlin, I. N. & Critchley, D. L. (1982). Fostering normal development in abused children—work with child and group home parents. In A. Kazdin (Ed.), *The child and his family.* (International yearbook.) New York: Wiley.

Berlin, I. N., Critchley, D. L., & Rossman, P. G. (1984). Current concepts in milieu treatment of seriously disturbed children and adolescents. *Psychotherapy, 21,* 118–130.

Bion, W. (1961). *Experiences in groups and other papers.* New York: Basic Books.

Dolan, Y. M. (1985). *A path with a heart: Ericksonian utilization.* New York: Brunner/ Mazel.

Green, A. (1978a). Psychopathology of abused children. *Journal of the American Academy of Child and Adolescent Psychiatry, 17,* 92–103.

Green, A. (1978b). Psychiatric treatment of abused children. *Journal of the American Academy of Child and Adolescent Psychiatry, 17,* 356–371.

Green, A. (1983). Dimension of psychological trauma in abused children. *Journal of the American Academy of Child and Adolescent Psychiatry, 22,* 231–237.

Mindell, A. (1985). *River's way.* Boston: Routledge & Kegan Paul.

Popper, C. (1987). *Psychiatric pharmacosciences of children and adolescents.* Washington, DC: American Psychiatric Press.

Prigogine, I. & Stengers, I. (1984). *Order out of chaos: Man's new dialogue with nature.* New York: Bantam Books.

Prigogine, I. & Nocolis, G. (1989). *Exploring complexity.* San Francisco: Freeman.

Redl, F. (1965a). *Children who hate: The disorganization and breakdown of behavior controls.* New York: Macmillan.

Redl, F. (1965b). *Controls from within: Techniques for the treatment of the aggressive child.* New York: Free Press.

Redl, F. (1966). *When we deal with children: Selected writings.* New York: Free Press.

Rossi, E. L. (Ed.). (1980). *The collected papers of Milton H. Erickson.* New York: Irvington.

Schact, A. J., Kerlinsky, D., & Carlson, C. (1990). Group therapy with sexually abused boys: Leadership, projective identification and countertransference issues. *International Journal of Group Psychotherapy, 10,* pp. 401–417.

Shapiro, T. (1985). Developmental considerations in psychopharmacology: The interaction of drugs and development. In J. Wiener (Ed.), *Diagnosis and psychopharmacology of childhood and adolescent disorders.* New York: Wiley.

Spencer-Brown, G. (1972). *Laws of form.* New York: Dutton.

Varela, F. J. (1979). *Principles of biological autonomy.* New York: Elsevier.

CHAPTER SIX

Inpatient Group Treatment of Children and Adolescents

Frederick A. Stearns

Although most of the children admitted to psychiatric hospitals generally need an intermediate length of stay (2 to 6 months), some children's conditions may warrant short-term assessment/stabilization or long-term treatment. Most of the children have severe emotional disorders and a few have a mixture of emotional and conduct disorders. The use of group treatment has grown in importance as lengths of stay have been shortened and treatment goals have become more focused. Generic groups, once intended for psychodynamically oriented insight or group behavior management on the unit, have become more directed toward presenting problems, social skills/problem solving, and time-limited objectives. Along with dynamic group therapy, inpatients may receive group treatment for sexual abuse, drug abuse, satanic involvement, or social skills deficits.

Children admitted for inpatient psychiatric treatment typically have a history of neglect and rejection in their early experiences and relationships. Interpersonal events with family, caretakers, peers, neighborhoods, and schools have been largely disappointing and frequently traumatic. Consequently, many of these children have difficulty developing trust in adults. Latency age children and early adolescents may have a developmentally appropriate reticence in talking with adults about distressing inner feelings or family problems. Group therapy with peers tends to complement the growth tasks associated with normal social maturation during latency, pre-puberty, and early adolescence. For children with serious developmental pathology, the use of developmentally appropriate group treatment approaches can facilitate the engagement of the young people in other modalities of hospital treatment. Dependency needs, which are often experienced as overwhelming, can be met in group treatment without the intensity, intimacy, or demands of individual therapy. For children of different cultural backgrounds, the group serves as a learning experience for both majority and minority cultures. This is achieved by the patients' learning that they can safety share differing values, meanings, and beliefs without stereotyping, blaming, denying, or humiliating one another.

GUIDELINES FOR GROUP WORK: A REVIEW OF THE LITERATURE

As early as 1943, Slavson persuasively reported that young children can and do exert a corrective influence on one another. The nondirective play group or activity group therapies described at that time introduced arts and crafts materials that could be used to promote regressive play in the service of the ego or to promote mastery (Axline, 1947; Slavson, 1943). However, the "permissive," "nondirective," and "neutral" process of these early activity therapies could evoke so much fantasy material and regressive play that children at a preoedipal level of development were traditionally considered inappropriate for group treatment. Many of the children requiring inpatient treatment are so deficient in ego equipment and in verbal and social skills that greatly increased group structure, therapist activity, and understanding and interpretation of nonverbal communication are essential.

The degree of group structure should be carefully established to address the areas of ego functioning that are objectively defined to enhance the emotional, cognitive, and social development of the patients. A differential treatment approach based on the recognition of underlying dynamics is as crucial in group therapy as it is in individual treatment (Schamess, 1976). Modifications in activity group therapy with severely deprived children clarify the very active facilitation required with the patient population (Scheidlinger, 1960). When the therapist sets a tone of neutrality and permissiveness by minimal verbalizations, few behavioral expectations, and failure to interfere with threatening group interactions, children's anxieties increase and acting-out soon follows. Group members do not perceive the therapist's lack of activity as warm, protective, or helpful. Lifton and Smolen (1966), through their group work with schizophrenic children, suggested that limits and structure alleviate anxiety in the ego-damaged child. Verbal and physical restraint are at times crucial to set limits, institute boundaries, establish controls, and substantiate feelings of protection.

Setting limits as protection and not punishment requires firm, nonretaliatory intervention (Frank, 1976). Children feel safe and better about themselves when their own impulsivity is not left uncontrolled. Children are more likely to try out and learn new, more adaptive behaviors when they do not have to be preoccupied with protecting themselves from the aggressive or sexual impulses of peers. Cohesiveness and trust result when group members feel accepted and supported by one another.

Therapists impose external controls in which listening, sharing of materials, interacting in activities, and verbalizing can safely occur. Therapists act as gatekeepers in preventing children from aggressively acting-out or leaving the room. They take planned positions in the room, maintain eye contact, and deescalate aggression by recognizing early warning signs and thus stopping the spread of group contagion. Play and art materials are carefully selected to focus expression of feelings for eventual emotional and cognitive mastery over impulses. Scapegoating, sarcasm, and sexist or racist gestures or verbalizations require immediate limit setting.

Within an active limit-setting environment, the young people can safely talk about any maladaptive interpersonal patterns in the course of the group session (Yalom, 1975). Trafimow and Pattak (1982) enumerated three elements of group process which enhance the child's capacity for progressive ego development. First, children are often less anxious with peers than with adults. They are more likely to express their developmental needs in the company of other children and to identify with the more adaptive characteristics and coping strategies of the group members. Interacting with the other children provides a range of "objectal alternatives." Second, the cotherapy leadership team members function as auxiliary group egos. They aid and support ego functioning through clarification of distorted perceptions, reality testing, and interventions needed to prevent abusive interactions. Third, the group as a therapeutic entity is perceived as positive and larger than the individuals in it or the member groups of children or therapists. Others have related this last phenomenon to the concepts of "mother-group" (Scheidlinger, 1974) or the group as transitional object (Kauff, 1977). Trafimow and Pattak (1981) suggested "the group-as-a-whole" may substitute for the therapist by serving the maternal function and defining the self, just as the inanimate object may represent self and mother for the developing infant (Winnicott, 1948/1958).

Frank (1983) suggested that these ego-impoverished children need not only the safety of protective limits, but also active teaching to facilitate ego capacities. Group members need to be shown various strategies for handling painful feelings or frightening impulses. Many of these young people act only on the basis of their feelings. They cannot discriminate between their feelings and actions and they have a limited ability to perceive how their actions might affect how others feel. Role playing is an active modality that offers emotional distance and a less charged opportunity to learn about themselves. Role playing facilitated by the therapist models and teaches the acceptance of feelings, but not necessarily actions, and begins a problem-solving process.

Yalom (1975) recommended that the therapist distinguish between content and process, when observing and facilitating group interaction. By reviewing the process of the interaction, group members learn to pay attention to the message about the relationship of the people involved in the interaction. The young people learn that it is often crucial to look beyond the context of the words to discern a subtly exploitive interaction.

Other group techniques include various forms of ego support. Talking about feelings and impulses diminishes acting-out, enhances reality testing, and decreases magical thinking. Skillful confrontations help the observing part of the ego look at the experiencing part and confront itself intrasystemically. The patient is less likely to refute and reject internally perceived insight (Blank & Blank, 1974). Interpretations are made not only to make historical connections for the individual, but also to promote awareness of underlying feelings such as sadness or anger. Interpretations are also directed toward interpersonal consequences of behavior and toward painful feelings that negative peer interactions evoke in the individual. The group process is also designed to help its members problem-solve various situations that previously would have resulted in a rapid, critical response. Thus, they begin in the groups to understand the need to delay immediate action and to be able to examine the issues involved in any course of behavior. Schamess (1976) reminded us of the limitations of interpretation with characterologically disturbed children:

> *These children tend to view interpretation in one of three ways: at best it is seen as an expression of the therapist's interest, positive feelings, and wish to be helpful; at worst it is experienced as a criticism or humiliation and an expression of the therapist's dislike; usually it is simply ignored because the child (defensively) feels it is irrelevant and uninteresting.* (p. 43)

THE HOSPITAL AND THE PATIENT POPULATION: AN EXAMPLE

The University of New Mexico Children's Psychiatric Hospital (CPH) provides inpatient treatment for children requiring various lengths of hospitalization. The patients admitted may come from anywhere in the state, range in age from 5 to 14 years, and are from Anglo, Hispanic, Afro-American, or native American cultural backgrounds. New Mexico is geographically the fifth largest state, has one of the lowest per-capita incomes, and is primarily rural outside of the Albuquerque area. There are 28 very different Indian tribes throughout the state. Hispanics settled the region before there were settlements by the English on the East Coast. Much of the Anglo population arrived after World War II. It is normative for the patient groups to be a mixture of very divergent cultural backgrounds, family configurations, and socioeconomic circumstances.

At CPH, boys and girls are assigned to one of six separate units or cottages, according to their chronological and developmental ages. Nine young people reside in each cottage and interact in a wide variety of group settings throughout the milieu, including school.

Many of the children have suffered multiple losses, separations, or abandonments from primary caretakers. Severe deprivation and abuse, extended family history of major psychiatric disorders, and family multi-substance abuse are part of these patients' histories. The children present with low frustration tolerance, impulsivity, aggressive outbursts, and poor peer relationships. They are needy, are unable to feel positively about themselves, and have poor self-esteem. They also have a profound distrust of adults. They can be anxious and preoccupied with primitive fears of punishment and bodily injury. Most have major deficits in ego functions; behavior, rather than speech, is the primary means of communication. These children have little capacity to talk meaningfully about painful internal experiences or interpersonal relationships. Typically, these children lack an intact "observing ego" and initially do not benefit from insight-oriented interventions.

ASSESSMENT OF CULTURAL FACTORS IN INPATIENT GROUP TREATMENT

To facilitate corrective group interaction, it is critical to assess how the minority child and his or her family are able to respond to an inpatient setting that reflects the cultural orientation of the majority culture. For example, tremendous differences may exist among cultural groups regarding the value of expressing feelings in a group setting. A comprehensive psychiatric evaluation should include consideration of the cultural context of a disturbance. Time should be spent exploring with the family their beliefs about the identified problem areas and "mental illness" in general. Their thoughts about the cause of the disturbance, what might help, and what they have tried previously are essential to any treatment formulation. Information should be gathered on how the family communicates emotional pain or how presenting symptoms are understood. Attitudes toward helpers and expectations of treatment provide information as to how the patient will interact with others in the various hospital group activities.

Confusion may arise when treatment recommendations are formulated without careful consideration of cultural variables. An example recently occurred in what was initially labeled as "resistance." An 11-year-old Pueblo boy was referred for molesting two younger boys in foster care. The boy's mother, an alcoholic, had abandoned him and the state's Human Services Department had taken custody for the purpose of placement. A maternal aunt who was unable to care for the child became understandably alarmed by the molestation incident, which had occurred while the boy was in state custody. The aunt was further concerned when hospitalization was recommended and group treatment was described as part of the boy's therapy. She attempted to prevent his hospitalization. Outreach contacts to the tribal authorities and the aunt's residence, and pre-admission discussions at the hospital revealed the extent of secrecy and shame felt by the tribe and the aunt with regard to the sexual abuse. An exchange of ideas as to what would be helpful to the boy resulted in integral involvement of the aunt and tribe in the treatment plan and their agreement to hospitalization. The patient initially denied being sexually abused himself. Yet, a month after hospitalization, during a sexual issues group session, he disclosed extensive sexual abuse. What aided the group therapists in facilitating the disclosure was their knowledge that, for this particular patient, the extent of shame, secrecy, and humiliation had a cultural context and went beyond the typical shame and secrecy encountered in their clinical experience or described in the sexual abuse literature.

Gathering information about the cultural context of a patient and family requires assessment of the community systems in which the patient lives. Knowledge of the patient's peer group at school and at home is essential. Outreach teams composed of social service workers and clinicians can be of enormous value, especially if they travel to geographically or socially isolated areas and learn the unique cultural framework of some children's disturbances. Outreach contacts to the family and the community's helping agencies are helpful before, during, and after hospitalization. These outreach efforts prevent stereotypical assumptions about the cultural or socioeconomic background of patients. They provide clues as to how patients will express themselves to others, whether they will share or be interdependent, confront or support, and form a therapeutic alliance or withdraw.

For Roberto, an 11-year-old, depressed Hispanic boy from a small town in north-central New Mexico, an outreach visit to the home early in treatment proved indispensable. One month into treatment, family history remained inadequate, the mother had not attended family therapy, and the patient was especially reluctant to participate in group therapies. An outreach visit to the school, home, and social service agency significantly furthered the assessment. Interviews at school confirmed the impression that Roberto only marginally interacted with his peer group and classmates because of intense shyness and limited social skills, and also revealed his tremendous proficiency and interest in New Mexico history. During the home visit, Roberto's mother disclosed two family secrets: her mother's suicide and her divorced husband's sexual deviancy. Both secrets had a crippling effect on the family's adjustment and consequently its acceptance in the community. The mother did not feel accepted by her church or her neighborhood and had rejected both, out of fear. Discussion at the social service agency revealed that this family was economically deprived, yet the mother would not accept reimbursement for bus fare to attend family therapy. The treatment plan needed to be radically changed, to reflect this information. Instead of resistance, the family was without transportation and had too much pride to accept reimbursement for attendance at family therapy. Roberto's proficiency in New Mexico history was used to foster a treatment alliance and facilitate his acceptance in his peer group. Once Roberto's mother felt relief, following her disclosure of her family's secrets, she recognized some potential benefit from treatment and accepted state reimbursement to attend family therapy. When Roberto's mother accepted treatment, she also gave Roberto permission to engage in treatment. When Roberto's mother began to look at her relationships in her neighborhood and church, Roberto started to interact with friends and classmates.

INPATIENT GROUP THERAPIES

The Task Group

The basic group structure for the patients at CPH is created among the nine children who live in the same cottage and attend school together. Child-care workers maintain a benign, family-like setting where a safe, consistent, predictable, and gratifying environment is maintained. Task groups focus on "here and now" interactions that occur during the daily routine of personal hygiene, chores, mealtimes, school, recreation or games, team sports, and less structured "quiet times." Because the child-care workers provide concrete gratifications (food, assistance with hygiene, school projects, play or leisure activities), the patients may be very available to the corrective interactions and modeling of social skills that are facilitated in task groups.

Safety, acceptance, and nurturance are vigorously maintained in the 24-hour milieu. The one-to-three staff-to-patient ratio provides adequate supervision and invites the children into relationships with adults and peers. Because the children are clustered by developmental and chronological age, schoolwork and activities can be compatible with their developmental levels and abilities, thereby preventing some acting-out and regression among patients. Before too long, the patients begin to recapitulate the family dynamics of their home environment and provide multiple opportunities for corrective intervention.

Child-care workers are aware that most of the patients communicate through behavior rather than language and consequently intervene in more concrete behavioral and nonverbal expressive modalities. Helping the children appropriately express feelings and develop social skills is approached through games, pictures of feelings, cooperative play with toys, and sports activities. Children learn to delay impulses in order to listen, share, support each other, label feelings, and confront each other in a caring manner. Many spontaneous disclosures of physical and sexual abuse occur during task groups focusing on distressing "here and now" behaviors of daily living.

A striking example of almost "accidental" disclosure took place within a task group, after a cooperative game. A group of eight boys, ages 8 to 10 years, had been involved in a cooperative game of moving from a sitting position on the ground to a standing position, by locking arms. A staff member suggested they all count to three, lock arms, and stand together. As the boys began to count in unison they became agitated, yelled at each other, and began striking out. While verbally processing the activity later, one boy stated how uncomfortable he became when counting because he had had to count aloud the "swats" he received from a caretaker when he was being physically disciplined. Oddly, all but one of the boys had received the same form of corporal punishment, but had not wanted to talk about it until this group activity.

The Dynamic Group Therapy

The nine boys and girls who live in the same cottage and attend school together also participate twice a week in a dynamic group therapy led by a child psychologist or psychiatrist and a senior child-care staff member.

The clinicians integrate knowledge of the patients' family and individual therapies into the dynamics of the group interactions. Information about the patients' caretakers, extended relatives, and particular family constellations helps the therapists to understand what they observe in group interactions. Typical family dynamics include multiple separations from and losses of caretakers, parent and child role reversals, lack of generational boundaries, and poor impulse-control modulation. Across age groups, the safe expression of feelings among group members is the broad goal of group therapy. The children often are confused over the expression of feelings because they lead to a distressing sense of vulnerability. Some patients carry the conviction that expressing anger inevitably results in hurt and eventually loss of significant caretakers. Other patients distort needs for nurturance with eroticism and sexuality. Still other patients fuse sexual impulses with violent impulses. Many hospitalized children tend toward aggressive acting-out as a useful defense against the formation of desired but previously unreliable close relationships. Corrective group interactions encourage healthy identifications with others and better ways of positively regulating self-esteem.

For the youngest children (ages 5 to 9), the use of dyads (Crawford-Brobyn & White, 1986; Fuller, 1977) or subgroups has proven useful. Many of these children have not learned to play, much less to participate in cooperative play. In a group with many new admissions and little group cohesion, playing a favorite board game in subgroups facilitates learning group rules—sharing of materials; delaying of impulses to always win, in favor of the group pleasures and camaraderie of playing together—and thus acquiring rudimentary social skills. The youngest children relate best to nonverbal expressive therapies, which may include storytelling, puppetry, drawing of pictures, modeling of clay, and games that focus on labeling and mastering feelings. For older children who have some rudimentary social skills and capacity for verbal interaction, the group focuses more on verbal expression of feelings, anger management, problem-solving skills, and conflict resolution. Even the more ego-damaged early adolescents will enjoy role playing of stressful scenarios with peers, teachers, and parents.

Learning tolerance of racial and cultural differences among group members is one of the most frightening and potentially healing factors in dynamic group therapy. Children with out-of-control behaviors warranting inpatient hospitalization frequently have negative identifications with caretakers who have severely abused or exploited them. Some patients have learned to overidealize their abuser and internalize aspects of the abuser. They identify with the aggressor to feel powerful, in control, and seemingly less anxious about themselves. Unfortunately, this sense of power is usually accompanied by feelings of self-hatred. Racial and cultural scapegoating can be challenged, interrupted, and worked through. Tolerance for cultural differences can facilitate the development of empathy in interpersonal relationships. The following clinical vignette provides an example of a young Hispanic male working through an intolerance of cultural differences and intense self-hatred. The group process enabled him to develop a tolerance for interpersonal differences, better regulation of his self-esteem, and a more positive ethnic identity.

Juan, a 10-year-old Hispanic boy, was hospitalized for extremely aggressive outbursts at school, at home with younger siblings, and toward younger children in his neighborhood. His academic performance deteriorated and school officials became concerned about sexual behaviors with male and female peers. His past history included multiple abandonments by caretakers, prolonged custody struggles between his divorced parents, and physical abuse by his father, requiring intermittent investigations by the state's social services agency. The patient on two occasions had been placed in an emergency shelter during these investigations.

After two months of hospitalization, Juan disclosed the occurrence of anal rape by a male caretaker who was a friend of Juan's mother. He also disclosed that he had been anally penetrated by an older boy while placed at the emergency shelter. After the disclosures, Juan was able to discuss in group therapy his fears of being permanently physically damaged and therefore less strong or able to take care of himself. He also was preoccupied with the possibility that he had been "changed into a homosexual." As the patient began to talk guardedly about these feelings and attitudes, he suggested to the group that his name be changed from Juan to John, apparently in an effort to cope with his changed sense of self. It seemed that he associated his vulnerability to rape with his Hispanic heritage and hoped to make himself less vulnerable in the future by Anglicizing his name.

In family therapy, the patient's biological father was asked to describe the intergenerational significance of the name Juan. Juan learned for the first time many positive attributes of his deceased paternal grandfather. He heard and began to identify with the positive expectations his father had for him in naming him after this important family member. Nonetheless, Juan continued to insist with peers that they refer to him as John.

The boy's therapy group became the pivotal modality for working on issues of ethnic identity. They were encouraged to share the different ways their families celebrated holidays, fixed meals, and expressed feelings. The boys were from Anglo, native American, black, and Hispanic backgrounds and immediately recognized enormous differences in their family backgrounds. Tolerance was supported by actively setting limits on ridiculing, stereotyping, denying, or withdrawing from the discussions. Eventually, the boys themselves began to challenge Juan's need to change his name to be more accepted or to feel better about himself. Most of these boys also had abuse issues and had tended to bully or exploit others. Gradually, they were able to take responsibility for ways in which they colluded to reinforce one another's feelings of helplessness. Sensing that

Juan's desire to change his name to John implied vulnerability and uncertainty about himself, the boys went along with the name change because of the sense of power they felt over Juan. Eventually, some discomfort was expressed over taking advantage of Juan's confusion, and all agreed they did not feel better about themselves by taking advantage of Juan. Another Hispanic group member confronted Juan's confusion and in a caring way supported their shared ethnic identity through talking about pleasurable ways in which Hispanics celebrated holidays. Ultimately, Juan used what he learned in the group to announce proudly to his father in family therapy that he no longer wished to change his name and was glad his father had given him his grandfather's name.

Pinderhughes (1979, 1983) suggested that any issue in group treatment can be used to define values, meanings, and beliefs unique to an individual's background. In Juan's case, the group process helped members understand and respect the differences they discussed. Tolerance for differences facilitates the ability to manage conflicts, negotiate, and compromise. Group therapists can help develop such tolerance by encouraging the sharing of differing perceptions in a protected atmosphere. This requires active limit setting, clarifying, challenging, and support. Allowing group members to blame, deny, withdraw, or scapegoat when other members express differences creates an unsafe group environment.

The Sexual Issues Group

In response to the enormous increase in reported victims and perpetrators of sexual abuse, the hospital has developed specialty groups referred to as sexual issues groups. Shortly after these groups were formed, the rate of disclosure of sexual abuse increased across all age groups in the hospital. Clinicians reported their individual and family therapies were more productive as children became more available to work through their abuse dynamics.

These groups are best formed by clustering same-sex children with close chronological and developmental ages. Using group therapists of both sexes has proven most helpful for observation of group dynamics as well as balanced interventions. Separating perpetrators from victims is optimal for initial development of trust and group cohesion, although mixing the groups in later stages can be helpful.

There are many indications for group treatment of sexually abused young people. The group provides acceptance and sympathetic understanding of disclosure and increases the feeling of being believed. In the group experience, the sexual abuse becomes easier to discuss because the group member learns to listen and empathically respond to another's abuse. Dependency needs are met without the intensity, demands, or intimacy of individual therapy. Individual therapy with an adult therapist may be inhibited by a fear of recapitulation of abuse dynamics. The one-to-one relationship evokes concerns about secrecy or increases fears that the patient's homosexual anxieties may not be understood. Group therapy facilitates learning to depend on peers rather than adults. The group can diminish feelings of isolation and secrecy and can enhance social skills. A group of peers can effectively confront denial and minimization around painful affects such as anger, guilt, sadness, shame, and fear. A group provides a safer atmosphere in which to ventilate anger toward the perpetrator or caretaker who did not adequately protect the young person, or toward relatives who did not believe him or her. Suppression of painful effects associated with the abuse can be challenged with repetitive ventilation and expression of feelings. The repeated sharing of painful emotions helps the young person to gain a sense of cognitive and affective mastery over the abusive events. Group discussions can also prepare the child or adolescent for the legal processes that will be experienced. Interviews with detectives, investigators, and attorneys, and experiences in court can be shared and clarified. Alternatives to exploiting others are generated by the group. Concepts of responsibility and interdependence are rehearsed in an effort to promote autonomy.

Repeated opportunities arise within the group context to provide education that will correct distorted perceptions of sexuality. Frequently, abused children's lack of anatomic and sexual knowledge reinforces their perception of damage.

An important component of the group treatment approach, therefore, is sex education, including anatomy and physiology. Although abused children have precocious sexual knowledge, their impressions include very distorted and inaccurate information. Learning of social skills and street safety is especially important for younger children. They quickly recognize the difference between "good touch" and "bad touch" and can rehearse how to safely enlist the help of adults who can be trusted. Behavioral interactions and consequences are employed to keep verbalizations, gestures, and interactions nonabusive and supportive. Psychodynamic development of empathic group support encourages individual disclosure of abusive incidents and the consequent painful feelings associated with the abuse. Art therapy and metaphorical storytelling can be especially useful with latency age children. For children suffering from Post-Traumatic Stress Disorder, the use of certain words can evoke intrusive, painful memories or flashbacks that are not helpful; accessing painful effects indirectly through expressive therapies and metaphors can be more beneficial than direct expression of feelings. Finally, experimental therapy, such as wilderness or outdoor stress initiatives, has been found to be empowering for some victims of sexual abuse. Use of rope or rock climbing with perpetrators of sexual abuse has helped interrupt and challenge their omnipotent, narcissistic, and exploitive interactions because of the efforts needed to master these difficult and fearful experiences.

At the start of a sexual issues group, roommates Craig and Mathew appeared to have supportive verbal interchanges. Upon closer scrutiny, it became evident that although Craig made helpful comments to Mathew, he actually controlled when Mathew spoke and how and what Mathew said. This dominance was achieved through visual glances, subtle gestures, and a slightly sarcastic tone of voice. As Mathew was coached to become more assertive and to complete his statements of his feelings, Craig became more agitated. Eventually, Craig was escorted out of the group for his rudeness toward the entire group. This setting of limits prompted Mathew to disclose the extent of verbal intimidation, including threats of sexual abuse, he had received from his roommate when they were alone. By distinguishing between the content and process of Craig's group interaction, group members uncovered a very exploitive relationship and took pride in keeping Mathew and themselves safer.

The Substance Abuse Group

Many of the children admitted as psychiatric inpatients are from families directly affected by chemical dependency and substance abuse. It is widely recognized that chemical dependency must be addressed if other problem areas are to be dealt with effectively within individual and family therapies. A drug education and substance abuse group was formed at CPH to meet this need. As in the sexual issues group, these children form a cohesive group working on common issues of secrecy, denial, minimization, guilt, and shame.

The substance abuse group quickly identifies the level of drug involvement and the risk factors for each child. Through peer questioning and group discussion, the patients, ages 12 to 14, learn to take responsibility for how they became involved with mood-altering substances and why they continued to use them. They learn how substance abuse interfered with the development of positive self-esteem, choice of friends, family relationships, and school performance. Group members learn to confront denial and look at painful feelings rather than glamorize drug use through "war stories." The group establishes positive peer pressure to increase their refusal skills, improve their peer selection, and increase their level of assertiveness and problem-solving abilities. Education is provided to correct misinformation, to answer questions regarding chemical dependency, and to learn the effects of drugs and alcohol on the body, the mind, and the realization of future plans.

Many nonverbal modalities may be helpful with this specialty group. Discussion can be improved through the use of art therapy, cooperative games, individual journals, group role playing, outdoor cooperative play activities, and videotaped sessions. Increasing each child's repertoire of leisure activities, including the pursuit of certain interests, hobbies, or sports, has been enormously helpful. Knowing how to have fun with others without abusing substances is often a new experience for these children. As they experience an increase in drug-free activities, their self-esteem is enhanced.

Finally, attendance at Narcotics Anonymous, Alcoholics Anonymous, or a related, appropriate self-help group exposes young people to a support group who value being chemical-free. Establishment of this connection to an outside support group may be extremely valuable in the transition to a new peer group outside the hospital.

CONCLUSION

Guidelines for inpatient group work with ego-damaged, impulse-ridden, acting-out children have been described. The level of group structure must be carefully monitored to address areas of ego functioning that are available to group interventions to enhance the emotional, cognitive, and social development of patients. Within the safety of protective limit setting, children try out new interpersonal strategies and learn to better regulate their self-esteem. Tolerance of cultural and racial differences is learned through sharing different perceptions of values, meanings, and beliefs. Tolerance is a learning experience for both majority and minority cultures and is a powerful tool for the development of empathy. Group therapies demonstrate that young people can and do exert a corrective influence on one another.

The intensity of having to live cooperatively with other young people who are ethnically and racially different becomes most evident in the group treatment modalities. Instead of such intensity evoking fear and distrust, group treatment provides the opportunity to safely explore and affirm those differences. The young person experiences the interpersonal rewards of being cared for through confrontations, and a feeling of being understood through support by other young people.

REFERENCES

Axline, V. (1947). *Play therapy.* Boston: Houghton Mifflin.

Blank, G., & Blank, R. (1974). *Ego psychology: Theory and practice.* New York: Columbia University Press.

Crawford-Brobyn, J., & White, A. (1986). A two-stage model for group therapy with impulse ridden latency age children. In A. Riester & I. Kraft (Eds.), *Child group psychotherapy future tense* (pp. 123–135). Madison, WI: International Universities Press.

Frank, M. (1976). Modifications of activity group therapy: Response to ego-impoverished children. *Clinical Social Work Journal,* 4, 102–109.

Frank, M. (1983). Modified activity group therapy with ego impoverished children. In E. S. Buchholz & M. J. Mishne (Eds.), *Ego and self psychology* (pp. 145–156). New York: Jason Aronson.

Fuller, J. S. (1977). Duotherapy: A potential treatment of choice for latency children. *Journal of the American Academy of Child and Adolescent Psychiatry,* 16, 469–477.

Kauff, P. (1977). The termination process: Its relationship to the separation–individuation phase of development. *International Journal of Group Psychotherapy,* 27, 3–18.

Lifton, N., & Smolen, E. (1966). Group psychotherapy with schizophrenic children. *International Journal of Group Psychotherapy,* 27, 85–96.

Pinderhughes, E. (1979). Teaching empathy in cross-cultural social work. *Social Work,* 24, 312–316.

Pinderhughes, E. (1983). Empowerment for our clients and for ourselves. *Social Casework,* 64, 331–338.

Schamess, G. (1976). Group treatment modalities for latency-age children. *International Journal of Group Psychotherapy,* 26, 455–473.

Scheidlinger, S. (1960). Experiential group treatment of severely deprived latency-aged children. *American Journal of Orthopsychiatry,* 30, 356–368.

Scheidlinger, S. (1974). On the concept of the "mother-group." *International Journal of Group Psychotherapy,* 24, 417–428.

Slavson, S. R. (1943). *An introduction to group therapy.* New York: International Universities Press.

Trafimow, E., & Pattak, S. (1982). Group treatment of primitively fixated children. *International Journal of Group Psychotherapy,* 32, 445–452.

Yalom, I. D. (1975). *The theory and practice of group psychotherapy.* New York: Basic Books.

Winnicott, D. (1958). Pediatrics and psychiatry. In *Collected papers* (pp. 157–173). New York: Basic Books. (Original work published 1948)

CHAPTER SEVEN

Working Therapeutically with Parents of Hispanic and American Indian Children and Adolescents in the Hospital

Thomas L. Givler

The effectiveness of hospital treatment of children and adolescents depends in large part on the capacity of the patient's family to engage cooperatively in the treatment effort. The quality of the relationship between the hospital team and the family is critical to the success of the hospital's intervention. Establishing and maintaining a constructive relationship is a difficult process under the best of circumstances, given the staff expectation that family members look at themselves, their past and present behavior and its effects on the child, their hopes and projections directed at the child, and their expectations of themselves. The difficulty of the process is compounded when severely emotionally disturbed children are involved. Therapeutic work with disturbed, noncommunicative children who are very angry, hostile, withdrawn, depressed, suicidal, or psychotic may arouse a variety of angry, hopeless, uneasy feelings among the staff. These feelings can lead the staff to blame parents for their children's condition and can delay or even negate the formation of a constructive relationship between the hospital team and the parents. Successful negotiation of such a relationship requires considerable trust on the part of parents and empathy on the part of the professionals working with the family.

This bond of trust and empathy is established most easily when the professionals and the family share a similar cultural background. The family feels understood and more readily trusts the professionals. The professionals feel empathy for the family, seeing in the family's past and present circumstances enough similarity to their own past and present situations to enable them to imagine being in the parents' shoes. The greater the degree of cultural difference between the parents and the professionals, the more difficult it is for the parents to feel that the professionals have sufficient potential for understanding the family's past experiences, goals, values, and aspirations. Parents often feel ambivalent about the efforts to help their child grow within a culturally different context and about whether they will ever develop trust in the hospital team. The family's concern may be well founded. When the professional perceives as callous or pathological behavior that is expected in the family's culture, the professional may see the family as "not caring" and lose the capacity to feel empathy for their circumstances.

This chapter discusses the process of working effectively with the parents of children and adolescents in the psychiatric hospital, particularly when the process of cooperation is complicated by major cultural differences between the family and the hospital team. Obstacles to the development of a respectful, trusting, working relationship that stem from cultural differences between the professional team and families from minority cultures are discussed. Special issues related to work with Hispanic and Indian families in New Mexico are used as illustrations.

THE WORKING ALLIANCE WITH PARENTS OF HOSPITALIZED CHILDREN

If the therapeutic team in the hospital is to work effectively with children and their families, care must be taken to build a working alliance with the children's parents. The concept of the working alliance was developed to describe a critical aspect of the relationship between the analyst and the patient in psychoanalysis (Greenson, 1967). It is used here in a broader sense, not just to refer to one aspect of the relationship between the family therapist and the family, but to include the interrelationship among all members of the therapeutic team. The working alliance is between the hospital as an institution and the family (Stewart, 1981).

The character of the relationship between the family and the hospital begins to take shape from the first moment of the family's contact with the hospital. Family therapy does not begin until some time after the child has been admitted. By then, the family's contacts with hospital personnel will have begun to shape the nature of the family's alliance with the hospital therapeutic team. If the policies, program, and personnel of the hospital are sensitive to the needs of parents and supportive of their parental functions through the hospitalization, the parents are likely to have formed a positive working alliance with the hospital and to be open to forming a therapeutic alliance with the family therapist and other members of the therapeutic team (Stewart, 1981).

Establishing this working alliance is complicated when there are cultural differences between the family and the hospital staff. Usually the Anglo culture is identified among Indian, Hispanic, or black people as having taken their lands, freedoms, and, through prejudice, their equality of opportunity in employment and education. The sensitivities developed in response to racism frequently lead culturally different parents to be guarded with hospital staff until the hospital's commitment to working with them to strengthen the functioning of the family has been demonstrated. Special efforts on the part of the hospital staff are needed, to reach out to the child and parents, and to develop and exhibit an understanding based on appreciation of their unique experience.

In work with American Indian families, outreach activity should begin prior to the child's first visit to the hospital for evaluation. The long, unhappy history of adoption of Indian children by non-Indians (Green, 1983) has left a legacy of suspiciousness toward Anglo social agencies. A referral from a school or even from an Indian social agency, describing symptoms that would usually alarm a parent may not be enough to overcome previous experiences with uncaring and indifferent Anglo agencies.

The first step in setting the stage for an evaluation at the hospital is frequently a visit by a team member, accompanied by a native mental health worker, to the family in their home, to discuss the family's view of the child's problems, the family's efforts to get help, and the services the hospital offers. In exploring the family's previous efforts to get help, the mental health worker should be requested to discover whether native healers have been used and to what effect. Raising the question in a respectful way can communicate the hospital staff's commitment to working in a culturally sensitive fashion with the family. Involving Indian social agencies in support of the hospital evaluation is often important in making it possible for the family to come for the evaluation. Assistance with transportation may be needed, but, the implicit sanctioning of the hospital's program by tribal social services, health, or mental health workers may make engagement in the evaluation possible.

Some families need active outreach services before they can work with the hospital team. Miguel was a 12-year-old, Hispanic child who had a long history of incorrigible behavior at school and uncontrolled anger at home. He was referred for evaluation following an episode in which he fondled a girl in his classroom. He was found on evaluation to have a Major Depression with psychotic features. The biggest problem facing the team appeared to be how to engage Miguel's mother as an ally in the hospital treatment. This 30-year-old mother from a small, isolated community had a long history of involvement with social service agencies because of her neglect of Miguel and his two younger siblings. She experienced the agencies (and all institutions of social authority) as the enemy. Her job in relation to them was, she felt, to comply with as few of their regulations as she could, while still mollifying them. Indeed, a part of her seemed to relish the challenge of getting away with as much as she could before the agency intervened. It became clear soon after Miguel entered the hospital that she had transferred this relating style to her interactions with the hospital staff.

One of the hospital's social workers visited her in her home with the goals of dispelling her fears of the hospital and engaging her in the work with the treatment team. On his first visit, he spoke reassuringly about the staff's commitment to helping her son so that he could come home. He told her that the team needed her help in figuring out how to help her son because she was the one who knew him best. Miguel's mother responded by talking about her own unhappiness. The social worker said that her feelings were terribly important, too, and offered to arrange an appointment for her at the branch of the community mental health center in her town. She agreed to go but said that she would have major difficulties finding reliable transportation to the hospital to participate in therapy. The worker offered to talk to an agency that could assist her with transportation. By the end of this visit, Miguel's mother was looking differently at the worker—as if she had begun to consider the possibility that the worker might be able to help her. The worker called her three times in the next week to confirm the details of the appointment he had set up for her at the mental health center and the transportation he had helped to arrange. By the end of this series of contacts, she sounded happy to hear from him when he called and she came to the hospital as arranged, to visit her child and begin work with the team.

This social worker's contacts with Miguel's mother set the stage for her involvement with the hospital in several ways. First, he surprised her by responding to her resistance and distrust calmly and without showing evidence of hostility or discounting her concerns. When services were arranged for her own needs, she began to hope that, by working with the hospital staff, she could get some help with her many other problems. Feeling that the hospital staff was interested in helping her enabled her to consider that they might be interested in helping her son rather than in controlling and manipulating the family, motives that she had experienced during previous contacts with courts and social agencies.

Impediments to a Constructive Working Alliance

Powerful transference and countertransference feelings involving the child, the parents, and the hospital staff are stimulated when a child enters a psychiatric hospital (Palmer, Harper, & Rivinus, 1983). Working with vulnerable children stimulates a range of protective wishes in the staff. Some are appropriate to the staff's caretaking role, and some are not, such as fantasies that if only the staff member were the child's parent, the child's psychopathology would disappear. The fairy-tale theme in which the child hero, who has been secretly left by a royal parent in the care of humble or evil surrogate parents, finds happiness when restored to his rightful home is a common fantasy among children of European background. The combination of the child's separation from the parents, the orientation of the hospital program to the child's needs, and the child's psychopathology creates a fertile environment for the flowering of these fantasies in some children during their hospitalization. Known as the "family romance" (Freud, 1909/1961), these fantasies often lead Anglo children to act toward staff in subtle ways, as if to say that all of the child's internal tensions would disappear if the staff were their parents.

Feelings of responsibility for the child's distress usually stimulate a sense of failure in the parents, which may lead them to join the child in the fantasy that the child's problems would be solved if only he or she had a better parent. Parents' responses to these feelings of failure include avoidance of or defensive hostility toward staff or a guilt-based presentation of themselves as incompetent parents. The combination of the child's and the parents' feelings, along with the staff's own wish to care for and protect the child, creates subtle but powerful feelings in all the participants in the child's treatment—child, parents, and staff—that the staff should "adopt" the child and replace the parents. When these subtle feelings are not dealt with by the staff, a constructive working relationship between the hospital and the parents is not possible.

Parents of Hispanic children and parents of Indian children from various reservations often are given the feeling by Anglo social service agencies that they are incompetent. When, in addition, they are alcoholic, abusive, or helpless in dealing with their children because of their own chaotic life-style or their economic inability to provide for their children, they are particularly vulnerable to the agencies' attitudes. In any case situation, it may be the treatment team's duty to assess the viability of the family to care for the child. This assessment can be done ethically only if it is based on a realistic evaluation of the child's and the family's strengths and weaknesses and of the alternatives open for foster care. It must not be based on unconscious or unrealistic reasons stemming from the treatment situation.

Strengthening the Parental Function of the Family

Family systems theory, mainly based on work with Anglo families, maintains that the family is an interacting system that has several subsystems, such as the sibling subsystem and the marital subsystem. The parental subsystem is the most important subsystem for nurturing the growth of the children in the family. When a child develops psychopathology sufficiently severe to require inpatient treatment, it suggests that the parental subsystem is not performing adequately. Therefore, in addition to treating the individual psychopathology of the child, a significant part of the hospital's intervention should be directed toward strengthening the parental function of the family. Hospitalization will benefit the child and the family when it strengthens the parental function. Finding parental strengths to work on in minority families is often difficult, unless the family therapist personally understands how the particular minority family functions and what other persons, besides the nuclear family, are vital to the process of working through family problems.

Recent literature on work with the parents of children in psychiatric hospitals describes efforts to reformulate the relationship between the clinical team and the parents. Central to this literature is a concern with strengthening the parents' role in the treatment of their child. These strategies all have the effect of supporting the parents in their parental function and thereby helping to contain the powerful transference/ countertransference feelings in parents and staff that are stimulated by the child's hospitalization and consequent interactions with staff.

The most frequently described strategy is to involve the parents actively in the child's treatment; in some cultures, the extended family must be included. Williams (1988) made parents members of the interdisciplinary team by involving them in each step of treatment planning and progress assessment and by having them attend the regular case conferences.

Woolston (1989), in addition to including the parents in the child's team, required that parents spend time on the hospital unit, not in the role of visitor but in carrying out activities usually performed by staff—doing the child's laundry, observing and discussing staff interactions with the child, and implementing behavioral protocols. This level of participation requires that a mental health professional who is familiar with a particular culture translate treatment-planning progress reports, to make sure they are meaningful.

Miguel's mother, who was initially resistant to engagement, as described above, became involved in a collaborative way with the team. After comprehending that working with the hospital team could be concretely helpful to her, she quickly began to see the hospital as a potential source of nurturance for her children as well as herself. She began to discuss with the team her concerns about Miguel's younger sister. On evaluation, it turned out that Miguel's sister had been sexually abused by the mother's ex-husband and was suffering from posttraumatic symptoms. The mother supported a period of hospital treatment for the second child. She continued to participate weekly in both of her children's treatments, despite a three-and-a-half-hour trip each way to the hospital. Toward the end of Miguel's hospital stay, she became concerned about her capacity to manage his continuing aggression toward two younger siblings in the home. She worked cooperatively with the staff to arrange a foster home placement for him.

Some writers have proposed rethinking the role of the clinical staff and the way they regard the family. Palmer et al. (1983) suggested that, in addition to clinical responsibilities, the staff should see themselves as "consultants to the child's parents" (p. 292). Hanrahan (1986) proposed that the first task in family therapy with parents of children in psychiatric hospital is to "reframe the whole family as competent" (p. 394). This may be challenging when parents are alcoholic or abusing or have permitted others to abuse their children. Their guilt and sense of being blamed by others may make Hanrahan's approaches difficult to implement. Harper (1989) took this a step further. He proposed developing a succinct problem statement as the focus of treatment; the team and the parents share this problem statement as the goal they are working toward. Harper emphasized the importance of framing the problem involving the interaction between the child and the family in "language that views the patient and the family sympathetically . . . , strengthens the alliance between the patient, parents, and staff, [and] strengthen(s) the alliance with, and foster(s) empathy (among the clinical team) toward patient and parent(s)" (p. 32).

Levy, Joyce, and List (1987) viewed severe estrangement from parents in adolescence as an impediment to separation/individuation tasks rather than an appropriate response to parental inadequacy. They proposed that reconciliation between the parents and the adolescent is often facilitative of the adolescent's progress toward separation/individuation and that such reconciliation should be viewed by the team as an appropriate treatment goal. They cited the case of a 14-year-old suicidal black girl whose angry stalemate with her single mother had its roots in early attachment problems between mother and child. These were related in turn to the mother's tenuous attachment with her own mother. Focusing the clinical work on the goal of helping mother and daughter find a way to make peace between them led to exploration of feelings of hurt and fear of rejection, which lay behind the dominant affect of anger. Exploring these feelings in individual and family sessions enabled the parent and patient to begin relating as mother and daughter, an experience that had been impossible for both, prior to the hospitalization. Both the mother and the daughter began to move toward age-appropriate separation/individuation and toward distancing themselves from their disappointment in the experience of being mothered, which had been the basis of their angry stalemate (Levy et al., 1987).

In American Indian and traditional Hispanic families in New Mexico, the separation/individuation process described in Anglo psychological literature may not pertain. In many Indian tribes, the adolescent and young adult offspring remain in the family and their duties are prescribed by the family matriarch or patriarch, depending on the tribe. Separation occurs only when they move out of the family home to form their own household. The young adults, however, remain obedient to the dictates of the family elders. In Hispanic families, a similar situation pertains. The grandfather or grandmother often still exercises control over adult children and their spouses in making major decisions of living—a change in jobs, a move away from the family to obtain work, the education and marriage of their children's children, and so on. Consultation with these family elders may continue until the grandparents' death. Thus, the vicissitudes of separation/individuation in childhood and adolescence may be different for minority cultures than they are for middle-class Anglo culture (Attneave, 1979).

Team Attitudes Conducive to the Family–Hospital Alliance

The attitude conveyed by the hospital staff to parents is critical to the formation of an alliance between the hospital and the family. If all members of the hospital staff are seen as having an open, curious, and exploratory attitude toward understanding the child and his or her relationship to the parents, in time the parents usually respond cooperatively. If the hospital staff's response to parents is perceived as blaming, the guilt and anger that interfere with the development of a working alliance will be increased (Berlin & Szurek, 1973). Thus, while it is important to understand the interaction between the child's psychopathology and the parents' conduct of their parenting function, and while limitations in the parents' conduct of their role often contribute to the problems of psychotic, personality-disordered, hospitalized children, only rarely has it been the parents' intent to harm the child. Usually, these parents have been doing their best to cope with a bewildering situation that they have found themselves helpless to control. At times, what they have found difficult to control is an aspect of development, usually in adolescence, as manifested in the child's behavior. At other times, the child's uncontrollable behavior is related to impulsive behaviors or feelings in the parents. In either case, parents respond to an approach that demonstrates empathy for the parents' struggle, acknowledges their efforts to cope, and supports their attempts to master the situation.

Reluctance of both American Indian and Hispanic parents to discuss their child's psychological and behavioral symptoms may be traceable to a belief that the child or adolescent was "witched." If symptoms persist despite the efforts of native healers, the parents believe (usually correctly) that Anglos will not understand such an explanation for the symptoms. Psychiatric symptoms are often viewed as a disharmony between various spirits or a lack of the patient's faith in the healing power of "the gods." The staff member's ability to express his or her awareness that there may be specific cultural factors that could be looked to as causes for the problems helps the parents to feel understood and more optimistic about the outcome of the hospital's treatment.

Parents who have abused their children are the most difficult to work with in this regard. Central to assessing the parents' capacity to change abusive behavior is an assessment of the parents' potential to feel empathy for the child, particularly the child's experience of the abuse, and to appreciate the impact of the abuse on the child's development. Abusing parents who have been abused themselves and who have the capacity to recover the effect associated with the abuse have a good prognosis (Fraiberg, Edelson, & Shapiro, 1975). Making this assessment requires engaging the parents in a working relationship with the hospital staff, to explore what has happened and the parents' capacity to acknowledge their part in it. The staff must relate to parents as whole, multidimensional people and must contain any countertransference pressure to treat these parents as terrible human beings. Countertransference feelings are increased when the parents are alcoholic and are likely to be most powerful toward parents who have nearly killed or severely sexually abused the child. The child's best interest, however, will be served best by a thorough evaluation of the child's and the parents' capacity to change. Only through forming a working relationship with the parents while the child is in a safe place such as a hospital can that evaluation be properly obtained.

Parents respond to an approach that demonstrates empathy for the burdens they have shouldered in parenting the child. Systems theory has helped us to appreciate the family as a dynamic system in which several subsystems and role relationships interact with a variety of forces. The relative impact of those forces, however, cannot be known in advance of knowing the specifics of a particular family's situation. For example, the stresses in the family do not all flow from parent to child. Parenting a seriously disturbed child can pose significant additional stresses on parents. Palfery, Walker, Butler, and Singer (1989) found that the parents of emotionally disturbed children reported that their children's difficulty created particular problems in the areas of child care, the parents' job situation, and family friends. The authors concluded, "Practitioners may have to reach out more to some families to understand the full impact on their lives of a disturbed child and to promote increased involvement and an increased sense of effectiveness" (p. 103).

Building a sense of trust, then, provides the foundation for the alliance. Drawing attention to the parents' strengths—their efforts enlist remedial help beyond the spiritual or indigenous methods, and their willingness to try to find help for their child's problems through the hospital—enhances their parental function and thereby strengthens it. This approach also communicates to the parents that the work to be undertaken is to be based on an appreciation of their strengths as parents and will be directed toward working cooperatively to reinforce their parental functioning, not to replace them. For example, many parents have gone to great prior lengths to get help for their child and, even though the child's hospitalization indicates that those efforts were not completely successful, the parents' strength in seeking help should not be overlooked. Other parents may have tried to find local healers to work with their child's problems independently. These parents should also be supported in their parental role by acknowledgment of their earlier efforts and of their strength in deciding to seek professional assistance at this point.

The team's initiative in sharing information with the parents demonstrates the hospital's trustworthiness. The contact with the parents on the day following the child's admission to the hospital and the parents' involvement in the Initial Planning Meeting (IPM) are critical to laying the groundwork for a working alliance. The team must take the initiative, to ensure that these contacts happen. Many parents are demoralized about their parenting and may doubt their capacity to provide the kind of parenting their child needs. This is a frequent reaction among most parents, but those from oppressed cultural groups are more likely to approach majority institutions passively, with the expectation that they will be replaced as parents. Their demoralization may lead them to fear secretly that they should be replaced. The staff's initiative in informing the parents on how the child is adjusting and ensuring that they will attend the IPM communicates two powerful messages: The hospital and the team believe in the parents' potential to be appropriate parental partners to the team, and the staff is committed to working cooperatively with the parents to strengthen their parental functioning. The staff's commitment to including the parents may require scheduling some IPMs outside of the regular workday, to accommodate the reality of parents' employment.

Special efforts, beyond choosing a nonworkday time, may be necessary to convince parents of the importance of their participation in the IPM. The meeting is an important opportunity for the team to initiate the desired respectful working relationship by explaining their role in the child's treatment, sharing their observations, and soliciting the parents' response. Not all parents begin as cooperative, objective participants in this process. Some parents respond provocatively as a way of testing the team. An important step toward trust will be taken if the team remains unprovoked and responds with an effort to understand the underlying concern. When parents' visits and participation in the program are limited by their living at some distance from the hospital, such contacts are vital. However, even parents who participate regularly in the program need to be kept informed frequently about their child's daily life.

Minority parents may never openly acknowledge their role in their child's problems. If the family matriarch scolds them for their drinking or other failures as parents, they may mask their feelings of anger or shame. Their loss of face when such scolding is done in front of staff may be offset by the staff's continued contacts with the nuclear and extended family. If the parents feel that the hospital views them as being important to the child, they may be encouraged to form a new attitude toward their child.

STRATEGIES IN WORK WITH MULTICULTURAL PARENTS

Earning Trust

Similar cultural heritage certainly does not guarantee mutual understanding and empathy, but the task of earning trust becomes complicated when the therapist and family do not share a common cultural background. Earning trust becomes still more complicated when the family comes from a culture with a history of racist oppression, because the barriers of unfamiliarity are reinforced by expectations of exploitation. Thus, black, Hispanic, and native American parents tend to approach majority institutions psychologically armed. The consequences of our nation's history of racism have ranged from misunderstanding, the most benign level, to distorted perception, to frank racist exploitation of the vulnerable. They come prepared for the possibility that their wish to find help will be frustrated. The overrepresentation of children from oppressed minority backgrounds in foster care and other out-of-home placements is an example of the impact of institutional racism on child welfare policies.

For example, Adam, a 12-year-old black child, was referred to the hospital after six years of continuous residential treatment, much of it in a respected psychiatric hospital in another state, the remainder in a residential treatment center of high quality. The welfare department had taken custody of Adam and his sister because of their drug-addicted mother's neglect of them. Adam responded with curses and physical attack to foster parents' and welfare workers' attempts to parent him. He was admitted to the first hospital shortly thereafter, because of his violent behavior. His treatment had continued for all of this time, as had his verbal abusiveness, oppositionality, physical attacks, and attempts to run away. He foiled attempts to sustain him in a residential treatment center; he remained unrelentingly determined to use the less restrictive structure as an opportunity to run away. Adam had occasional and inconsistent visits from his mother and her siblings, who had significant problems with drugs as well. During these visits, Adam became a different child—warm, responsive to limits, and eager to please.

Although Adam had severe learning disabilities and an IQ in the 70-to-90 range, his behavior seemed articulate. He appeared to see himself as a political prisoner; the staff, even those who were black, appeared to him as the enemy. He would take no comfort from them, responded with verbal abuse or physical attack to efforts to lure him into friendly relations, and used any opportunity for escape. His destination was always his family. The well-intended efforts of the hospital and welfare department staff to reunite him with his family failed. Family members who lived near the hospital were not capable of following through with plans to visit on a reliable basis.

His maternal grandmother wanted to try her hand at raising him. She was raising Adam's sister and several other grandchildren successfully. Unfortunately, she lived in another state. The welfare department in that state found her home lacking the amenities required of a proper foster home, despite the obvious developmental successes of the children under her care. It seemed likely that the officials in her state were reluctant to take responsibility for a child who might again need expensive hospital care. Our hospital became involved as the result of the initiative of a particularly resourceful social worker to have Adam transferred from the hospital in his state to our hospital, in the grandmother's state, to test his capacity to function with his grandmother. We were struck by her efforts over the previous six years to have Adam live with her and the apparently insurmountable barriers she had encountered. It was hard to believe that a white grandmother would have found the bureaucracy so unyielding for such a long time.

Although they frequently appear cooperative, parents from minorities that have experienced discrimination usually approach exchanges with Anglo institutions with a certain reserve. They watch the representatives of the institution carefully, to assess both their trustworthiness and that of the institution. Their familiarity with the hypocrisy of Anglo culture usually leads them to base trust on actions rather than words. Thus, the first stages of trust are more likely to be earned by actions taken to demonstrate respect for their parental role rather than by exhibitions of psychological sensitivity. Special attention, therefore, needs to be paid to outreach activities, especially those that provide the family with information. Parents usually understand the importance of information, and the hospital team's initiative in sharing information with the parents demonstrates the hospital's trustworthiness. Sharing with the family the information from the initial evaluation, the treatment plan, and the course of treatment provides a new experience of continued evidence of the staff's respect and its desire for collaboration.

Adam's grandmother was polite and cooperative in her contacts with the hospital team. However, she made it clear that she saw the plan to have Adam at our hospital to test how he would do with her as just another hoop the bureaucracy required her and her grandson to jump through before he could be reunited with his family. Her feeling seemed justified by Adam's behavior. Although he continued to be verbally abusive of staff and physically aggressive with staff and peers in the hospital, he did well when he was on pass with his grandmother. He appeared willing to accept his grandmother's authority, whereas staff's efforts to exercise authority compelled him to resist. His grandmother remained skeptical about the staff throughout most of Adam's hospitalization. Only at the end of Adam's stay, when the hospital staff joined her in negotiations with the Department of Human Services to ensure that Adam was returned to her care, did she begin to trust the staff.

One of the recurrent problems for staff is the fact that American Indian and Hispanic families who are not acculturated have a different time frame than staff. Linear time is primarily an Anglo invention. These families may forget the time of an appointment, come on a different day, or come late and still expect their full appointment time. These behaviors are not deliberate tests of the staff. In some minority cultures, time is not accounted for by looking at a clock, but by a feeling of timeliness or readiness to partake of an event. Unless we can relax our Anglo worship of the appointment time, we may, in our early involvement with the family, lose them. We must understand patients' families' attitudes toward time, spiritual harmony, and life forces or we will be included with other Anglo institutions that can tolerate only behavior that conforms to Anglo ways of living and doing business. We need to be cautious that we are not seen as manipulative and rigid.

To work effectively with culturally different families, the team must develop the capacity to remain curious about the meaning of any behavior that seems alien to the team. It is useful to maintain the idea that the parents have the best interest of the child in mind; the task of the team is to figure out in what way the parents' behavior makes sense and expresses the parents' effort to carry out their parenting responsibilities. Understanding the behavior from this perspective will enable the team to respond most effectively to the real issues that cause the team concern.

Coppolillo (1987) related a vignette that illustrates this process. After the first of a series of painful operations, a 6-year-old Apache boy packed his bag and announced that he was going home from the hospital. Much to the distress of the staff, his mother refused to coerce him to stay. Only the absence of transportation back to the reservation prevented him from leaving that day and allowed time for a psychiatric consultation with the boy and his mother. Coppolillo observed:

> *In the course of listening to the shy, but very candid and devoted mother, I became aware that the notion of forcing children to do something simply did not exist in her mental repertoire. I must admit that I had, at first, felt irritation at the mother's passivity. With a bit of reflection, however, I realized that my frustration had more to do with my ignorance of that Apache culture and the rigidity of my own value system. As I realized this and indicated to the mother that I was willing to listen instead of recommend, she herself suggested a solution. There were several people on the reservation that her son admired, and had chosen as his mentors. She was sure that if any one of them were to be brought to the hospital and were to indicate to the boy that it was a desirable and manly thing to be operated on and cured, he would permit treatment. (p. 37)*

This procedure was followed and the medical treatment was successful.

The point is not that parents from different cultural backgrounds always engage in growth-promoting behavior, if only we could understand the family's cultural context. The point is that most of us understand the behavior of parents and children in the context of the culture in which *we* were raised and, therefore, cultural difference tends to breed misunderstanding unless vigorous efforts are made to counteract it. An effort to ward off a rush to judgment about behavior or ideas that do not appear to make sense usually leads to a more respectful relationship between family and team and to more effective intervention. Both the team and the family are likely to begin stereotyping each other if the team prematurely judges behavior that is culturally syntonic to the parents. When this happens, the possibility of a cooperative working alliance is lost.

CONCLUSION

Working with parents from different cultures places increased burdens on inpatient staff. Unless some staff members belong to one of the minorities or, from working for a long time with them, have learned to respect them and to understand their views of life, illness, and death, work with the family is likely to be wrecked on the shoals of misunderstanding. The role of the extended family and the powerful people in a particular family must be understood, and these individuals might be included in family conferences. We must be sure that our communications are correctly translated. Continuous attitudes of respect for the ways, ideas, and holistic approach to life and illness of each minority are essential for maximal family involvement and effective therapeutic work with the child or adolescent and the family.

REFERENCES

Attneave, C. L. (1979). The American Indian child. In J. B. Noshpitz (Ed.), *Basic handbook of child psychiatry* (pp. 239–248). New York: Basic Books.

Berlin, I. N., & Szurek, S. A. (1973). Parental blame: An obstacle in psychotherapeutic work with schizophrenic children and their families. In S. A. Szurek & I. N. Berlin (Eds.), *Clinical studies in childhood psychoses* (pp. 115–126). New York: Brunner/Mazel.

Coppolillo, H. P. (1987). *Psychodynamic psychotherapy of children: An introduction to the art and the techniques.* Madison, CT: International Universities Press.

Fraiberg, S., Edelson, M., & Shapiro, V. (1975). Ghosts in the nursery. *Journal of the American Academy of Child Psychiatry, 14,* 387–421.

Freud, S. (1961). Family romances. In J. Strackey (Ed. and Trans.). *The standard edition of the complete psychological works of Sigmund Freud* (Vol. 9, pp. 237–241). London: Hogarth Press. (Original work published 1909)

Green, H. J. (1983). Risks and attitudes associated with extracultural placement of American Indian children: A critical review. *Journal of the American Academy of Child Psychiatry, 22,* 63–67.

Greenson, R. (1967). *The technique and practice of psychoanalysis.* New York: International Universities Press.

Hanrahan, G. (1986). Beginning work with families of hospitalized adolescents. *Family Process, 25,* 391–405.

Harper, G. (1989). Focal inpatient treatment planning. *Journal of the American Academy of Child and Adolescent Psychiatry, 28,* 31–37.

Levy, L. P., Joyce, P. A., & List, J. A. (1987). Reconciliation with parents as a treatment goal for adolescents in an acute care psychiatric hospital. *Social Work in Health Care, 13,* 1–22.

Palfrey, J. S., Walker, D. K., Butler, J. A., & Singer, J. D. (1989). Patterns of response in families of chronically disabled children. *American Journal of Orthopsychiatry, 59,* 94–104.

Palmer, A. J., Harper, G., & Rivinus, T. M. (1983). The "adoption process" in the inpatient treatment of children and adolescents. *Journal of the American Academy of Child Psychiatry, 22,* 286–293.

Stewart, R. (1981). Building an alliance between families of patients and the hospital: Model and process. *Journal of the National Association of Private Psychiatric Hospitals, 12,* 63–68.

Williams, B. E. (1988, Spring). Parents and patients: Members of an interdisciplinary team on an adolescent inpatient unit. *Clinical Social Work Journal, 16,* 78–91.

Woolston, J. L. (1989). Transactional risk model for short and intermediate term psychiatric inpatient treatment of children. *Journal of the American Academy of Child and Adolescent Psychiatry, 28,* 38–41.

CHAPTER EIGHT

Working with Resistance in Families: A Cross-Cultural Perspective

Natalie Porter
Scott Blackwell

The literature focusing on the delivery of mental health services to various ethnic and racial minority groups has been clear: These groups often experience therapy negatively, are underrepresented in receiving services, and are overrepresented in early terminations (La Fromboise, 1988; Sue, 1977; Sue & Zane, 1987). For example, Sue (1977) reported that 55% of American Indians seen in Seattle mental health clinics said they were highly unlikely to return. The President's Commission on Mental Health (1978) reported that ethnic minority clients were underserved, were not receiving services relevant to their needs, and felt abused by the mental health system.

Resistance is a primary way in which clients may register their discomfort or dissatisfaction with the psychotherapy process. McGoldrick (1982) argued that the medical model of viewing psychiatric problems is inadequate for understanding illnesses and help-seeking behaviors of various ethnic groups because it ignores the clients' cultural frame of reference. This model is blamed for increasing noncompliance, dissatisfaction with treatment, and failure. Studies have demonstrated that the differences in ethnic groups are manifested in "how they communicate about their pain or symptoms, their beliefs about the cause of their illness, their attitudes toward helpers, and what treatment they desire or expect" (McGoldrick, 1982, p. 6).

Resistance is by no means limited to minority populations nor reserved as an expression of displeasure with therapy. Historically, resistance has been assigned a central role in psychotherapy. Freud (1952) described its purpose as being similar to the role of defense mechanisms: to protect the individual from experiencing the anxiety associated with unresolved conflict. Maintaining symptoms maintains equilibrium in the patient by keeping unacceptable and unresolved conflicts, thoughts, or impulses at bay. Analyzing resistance became a major task of analysis.

Psychotherapy's definition of resistance has contributed significantly to effective treatment through the understanding of the role of a client's resistance. However, it assigns all of the responsibility for resistance to the client, permitting the ways in which a therapist may foster resistance to go unexamined. This view of resistance is particularly flawed, and perhaps dangerous, when working with minority clients because the therapist's own assumptions, values, and biases may be responsible for initiating or exacerbating resistance in the therapy hour.

Family therapists have embraced resistance as a key concept in treatment, but have elaborated on the definition to encompass the entire therapeutic system. Anderson and Stewart (1983) included the family, the therapist, and the setting in their definition of resistance:

> *Those behaviors in the therapeutic system which interact to prevent the therapeutic system from achieving the family's goals for therapy. The therapeutic system includes*

family members, the therapist, and the context in which the therapy takes place. . . . Resistance is most likely to be successful, that is, to result in the termination or failure of family therapy, when resistances are present and interacting synergistically in all three components of the therapeutic system. (p. 24)

This chapter discusses resistance in all three areas, as it is experienced in working with families in inpatient, cross-cultural settings. We differentiate resistance caused by therapist or contextual (institutional) factors from the classically defined resistance emanating from the family. We also discuss behaviors that are often defined as resistance in the family but may actually reflect social, racial, or economic barriers. Finally, we present some cultural variations in the ways therapeutic resistance may be manifested.

THERAPIST COMPONENT

Therapists involved in cross-cultural treatment may contribute to therapeutic resistance in several ways:

1. They may simply represent a poor ethnic or cultural match with a family;
2. They may be unwilling or may lack the necessary knowledge to adapt their perspective to that of the family, and therefore fail to provide culturally relevant therapy;
3. They may insist on their own cultural values or definitions of mentally healthy functioning, disregarding the family's perspective;
4. They may ignore factors they consider tangential to psychotherapy which are highly salient to the family, for example, how a family's history of acculturation or oppression impacts its functioning and its relationship to the therapist.

The Ethnic-Validity model of cross-cultural counseling (Tyler, Sussewell, & Williams-McCoy, 1985) proposed a way of understanding the benefits and costs of therapist–client cultural matches or mismatches. These authors described three types of ethnic validity that can occur in the relationship between a client and therapist:

Convergent validity—both individuals share beliefs about what constitutes psychological well-being, for example, a therapist and a client with Northern European roots who both value autonomy and individuation;

Divergent ethnic validity—beliefs about what is acceptable or psychologically healthy differ as a function of culture, for example, a therapist with Northern European roots working with a client with Asian roots; filial piety is valued in one culture and independence in the other;

Conflicting ethnic validity—what is considered healthy in one culture is seen as unhealthy in another, for example, an Asian who believes that one never speaks of one's problems, is considered unhealthy by a therapist from Northern European origins.

Divergent ethnic validity offers no particular difficulty for therapy, provided the therapist is aware and supportive of the client–therapist differences. Frequently, however, the therapist values his or her own dominant-culture perspective and devalues that of the clients.

Two Navaho girls, ages 5 and 7, were living in foster care after being sexually abused. Their caseworker was planning their return to their grandmother, whom the girls visited on weekends. The grandmother complained angrily to the caseworker after the foster mother cut the girls' hair. The caseworker did not intervene, considering the complaints symptomatic of a control battle between foster mother and biological grandmother. When the foster mother cut the girl's hair again several months later, the grandmother became irate. At this point she was in family therapy, and explained to the therapists that the girls could not participate in a Navaho healing ceremony until their hair had grown back. The therapist intervened and prevented further disregard of the grandmother's wishes (Berman, 1989).

Falicov (1982) underscored the divergent validity between Anglo therapists and Latin families. She cited the cultural values of most mainstream therapists as "individualism, egalitarianism, self-determination, self-fulfillment, future orientation, achievement and optimism" (p. 145). Clients should "keep appointments, and be on time, take responsibility for their own actions, . . . solve problems, . . . plan for the future, and . . . express verbally all of their concerns" (p. 145). She contrasted these expectations with those of Latin American families, who wanted the therapist "to be casual about keeping appointments, to take the initiative for change, and to give advice or educate them as a solution to their problems. . . ." The expectations stemmed from Latin American values of "family interdependence and loyalty, age and sex hierarchies, collectivism and continuity, affiliation and cooperation" (p. 146).

Conflicting ethnic validity usually represents the biggest problem for minority clients, because the values and definitions of the dominant culture typically preempt those of other cultures. La Fromboise (1988) cited fear of acculturation as a source of mistrust among American Indian clients, who believe that therapists from the dominant Euro-American culture consider their life-style and values more valid than those of the various American Indian cultures. La Fromboise wrote that American

Indian communities are characterized by strong social ties and group cohesion. Highly individualistic behavior, which is generally associated with conceptions of Western psychiatry, is viewed as contrary to the goals in American Indian culture. Concepts such as "self," "personality," and "mental health" are seen either as lacking a focus on naturalistic or holistic health or as a breach of cultural and community values. American Indian writers uniformly express the concern that Western psychiatry interprets the mental health problems of American Indian clients from a Western bias and therefore influences the client to behave in ways that conflict with their cultural origins (Jilek-Aall, 1976; Trimble, 1982; Trimble & La Fromboise, 1985). La Fromboise (1988) argued that the Euro-American perspective emphasizes the individual, intrapsychic processes, and weakened community ties, whereas the American Indian tradition emphasizes the transcending of self for the greater good of the community and the social causes of illness.

Bradshaw (1988) also described this bind. Japanese clients are viewed by Anglo therapists as pathologically dependent because their culture, which values interdependence and familial and community loyalty, conflicts with the Western European ideals of independence and autonomy. She cited Masterson (1985), who in essence labeled all Japanese as pathological by diagnosing them as either narcissistic or borderline because of their early childhood rearing which emphasizes parental indulgence and dependency more than North American culture does.

Tyler et al. (1985) concluded that, in order to work cross-culturally, therapists must learn to accept the validity of their clients' values and perspectives, to validate their clients' goals even when they differ from those of the therapist, and to understand when their beliefs can be harmful to a client who has a different cultural perspective.

A Navaho adolescent girl was hospitalized after her mother killed a sister and then herself. The staff encouraged this girl to express her grief openly in order to resolve her loss. This form of expression, considered by dominant-culture therapists to be *the* way to resolve loss, contradicts the Navaho way: Death is not discussed. At the mother's funeral, the girl was vehemently reprimanded by her grandmother for shedding a tear, which fell on the mother in her casket. "Now your mother will never be able to find peace."

Sue (1988) argued that outcome studies on cross-cultural therapy have been conceptualized too simplistically. Often, the only dimension considered is whether the therapist and client share an ethnic or racial heritage. Sue argued that an ethnic match may or may not represent a cultural match; for example, a Chicano therapist who values Mexican American traditions may be working with a highly assimilated Mexican American family that values Anglo traditions. He stated that ethnicity *per se* is too distal a factor to the psychotherapy process to account for outcome. More proximal factors, such as the translation of one's knowledge about a cultural or ethnic group into specific therapeutic interventions, must be developed.

Sue and Zane (1987) considered two basic processes, credibility and giving, as the proximal factors necessary for effective treatment. *Credibility* refers to the family's perception of the therapist as an effective and trustworthy helper. *Giving* is the therapist's ability to provide something real to the client and culminates in the client's perception that something was gained from the therapy contact. Resistance occurs when either credibility or giving is absent, particularly when the client and the therapist view the problem differently, develop different treatment goals, and believe the problem should be solved in different ways. The therapist may also set up resistance by failing to establish credibility in several other ways, as described in the following sections.

Treating All Minorities as Being Alike

There are in the United States 511 federally recognized native groups and an additional 365 American Indian tribes with widely varying cultures (La Fromboise, 1988). Yet we speak of "American Indian culture." There are persons from Mexico, Puerto Rico, the Philippines, El Salvador, and Argentina who share a language but not a culture and who may represent different racial groups. They are all called "Hispanics." We often respond to West Indians, Jamaicans, Haitians, and African Americans as if they possess a common culture. Most members of minority cultural groups report that they are often expected to speak for all members of their racial group. What therapists may consider resistance may be the therapist's own failing to differentiate among groups.

Overstereotyping and overgeneralizing may happen in several ways. One way is to view all members of a particular ethnic background as similar and rationalize providing the same form of therapy to all; for example, all Mexican Americans respond better to directives and to authoritarian therapists in family therapy. When lack of success should serve as a cue that the therapist's interventions are missing the mark, it is seen only as resistance, and the therapist escalates the directives rather than changing course (Vargas, 1989).

Another form of overstereotyping is to overattribute symptoms to culture and miss signs of emotional disturbances (Lopez & Hernandez, 1987). For example, to attribute Caribbean clients' hearing of voices of a spiritual nature only to cultural beliefs would be an underdiagnosis of psychosis. To view rigid marital roles in Mexican American families as normative would ignore the empirical evidence to the contrary (Cromwell & Ruiz, 1979; Lopez & Hernandez, 1987; Zinn, 1980).

A third way to overgeneralize is to not take into account the interaction of ethnicity with acculturation. Family issues will differ, depending on the family's identification with the dominant cultural group or their own ethnic origins, the extent of the identification, and whether they aspire to move closer to or away from their own background. These factors may influence a preference to work with a therapist from their own background or one from the dominant culture, as well as the therapeutic issues they will consider important. For example, when the young child of an American Indian family was hospitalized, the father, who held traditional Pueblo beliefs and worked on the reservation, sought a therapist who would support his values. The mother, who commuted 60 miles to a city to work as a professional and identified more closely with the upwardly mobile mainstream culture, did not ascribe to traditional ways for women in the Pueblo culture and wanted a less traditional therapist.

Ignoring Class Issues

Therapists frequently confound status in an ethnic or racial group with socioeconomic class. Characteristics that often result from poverty are stereotypically attributed to all members of a minority group. Late arrival to appointments may be a function of using the bus system or not being able to leave hourly wage jobs rather than the domain of a particular ethnic group.

Ignoring the History of Oppression

Traditional therapy practice says to let clients initiate discussion about important issues. Therapists, in adhering to this dictate, usually fail to raise questions regarding racial issues. Families may be acutely aware of them but fear to initiate this discussion, especially not knowing whether there will be reprisals. The more racial or ethnic tension in a community, the less likely that clients will share their concerns. Because their feelings of discomfort will influence their ability to develop an effective therapeutic alliance, the therapist must initiate this discussion. His or her openness and willingness to discuss the issues help the family feel easier about contributing their views. Even if the family chooses not to disclose their concerns at that moment, they will feel free to raise them later. The therapist's demonstration of concern and sensitivity will also permit the family to trust at a deeper level.

Ignoring a Family's Strengths

All too frequently in inpatient treatment, deficits overshadow strengths. By the time a child or adolescent is hospitalized, family functioning may have deteriorated under stress so that family strengths may seem minimal. Therapists may not even be aware of the resilience that is being demonstrated. To focus on deficits and ignore strengths may sabotage treatment with any family; to focus on weaknesses in minority families, who may be more aware of the negative judgments of Anglo-Americans, may jeopardize any forward motion. Minority families feel the daily scrutiny of a hostile society; replication of this behavior by a therapist or hospital staff may prove intolerable.

Ignoring a Family's History of or Fears About Assimilation

Falicov (1982) suggested that family structures change to meet the presses of acculturation. These transitional changes, often necessary to cope with immigration, may be viewed as pathological by therapists. For example, the loss of extended family and friends through immigration may increase the cohesiveness of the nuclear family. This may be labeled enmeshment by the family therapist—and it well might be a valid label. However, the cohesiveness may reflect a healthier state than the alternative of social isolation. Outside attempts to diminish the closeness of family members would certainly encounter resistance. Effective intervention would require decreasing this isolation before diluting the family bonds.

In New Mexico, this issue is encountered in American Indian and Hispanic families. The Hispanics, although newcomers by Indian standards, were established in New Mexico before the Pilgrims landed in Massachusetts. They have maintained their traditional cultures as firmly as have the Navaho, Pueblo, and Apache groups. Currently, the pressures for them to assimilate have multiplied dramatically as outside developers seek to devour their land and tourists invade their culture. In the hospital, they fear a further onslaught to their values and culture.

A native American adolescent who was experiencing disturbing psychotic symptoms refused to take medication even at the urging of his parents. However, after a meeting with his medicine man, who prescribed tossing sacred corn toward the rising sun each morning, the young man was willing to take his medication because it was not replacing his religious beliefs.

A northern New Mexico family refused to meet in the therapist's office for family therapy sessions even when transportation and lodging were offered. A home visit was then arranged. The therapist wisely discarded his own agenda and let the family take the lead; his objective was to participate fully in the family's agenda for the day. The therapist met three generations of family members and was taken out to the forest to pick piñon nuts. There the father demonstrated his dexterity and skill at piñon nut picking. The therapist offered respectful praises. During lunch, the family began to openly discuss the recent difficulties in the family and their concern for their son.

As these examples suggest, adapting cultural aspects to the therapeutic process can help mollify minority families, concern that they will have to sacrifice their beliefs and values. Working within the cultural milieu may result in a greater likelihood that changes will be maintained following treatment. For example, a Navaho girl who became quite proficient at identifying and discussing her feelings became viewed as a "counselor" for other troubled youths on the reservation.

INSTITUTIONAL COMPONENT

The setting influences a family's resistance in a number of ways. Inpatient treatment presents special hurdles to all family treatment and may increase resistance in all families. However, it may pose an even greater problem to minority families, who may already feel more powerless and disenfranchised than mainstream families.

Sue and Zane's (1987) factors—credibility and giving—refer to the institutional context as much as the therapist factors. The particular ethnic or racial group must view the institution as responsive to its needs and sensitive to maintaining its cultural integrity. Barriers inhibiting the use of comfort by minority families must be reduced. Increasing the number of bilingual staff at all levels, having materials available in representative languages, having the racial makeup of the staff similar to that of the clientele, celebrating special events and holidays with traditions borrowed from a variety of cultures—all these measures increase the feeling that the institution provides valuable services to families.

Family therapy is altered by virtue of placing one family member, typically a powerless one, away from the family and in a setting that has several layers of caretakers. If the family's inclination is to push the ill child or adolescent out of the family, hospitalization facilitates that goal. The family's resistance serves the function of maintaining the child outside of the family, for improvement in the family will mean reunification with the child or adolescent. Motivation to change may be reduced once the "problem" is out of the home. The family can organize around the hospitalized child or adolescent while avoiding the family conflicts or issues that generated the problem (Haley, 1976). This tendency may be the greatest in centrifugal or disengaged families (Beavers, 1982). Once the child is hospitalized and other caregivers are involved, the family no longer has to parent. They may feel vindicated by the hospitalization, which "proves" that the child is the "sick" family member. The rest of the family then feels no need to change; they are not the problem. Frequently, families with these dynamics will offer support to the identified patient and articulate their deep desire to help in any way possible. However, their energy is usually turned toward maintaining the child in the sick role and in the hospital.

A 13-year-old boy was referred for hospitalization for suicidal ideation and a variety of conduct problems, including stealing and lying. Following admission, the father and stepmother offered their total support in helping their "mentally ill" child. However, the father opposed all exploration of family history or of the family's role in his son's problem. When the son received privileges for behaving well in the hospital, the father would argue that any changes were temporary and were only the boy's successful manipulations of a gullible staff. After a great deal of frustration of both sides, the father admitted his concerns: he was fearful that if the therapist exposed his failings as a father, his current wife (this was his sixth marriage) would leave him.

Hospital and milieu staffs may collude with the family's lack of improvement by considering themselves as better able to parent the child or adolescent or viewing the family as too flawed to improve. The greater the economic or cultural disparity between the family and the staff, the greater the blame that may be projected on the family. If the staff attributes positive changes only to their actions, the family is left in an uncomfortable bind. Either the family must credit the staff for success or they must resist change in order to prove that the staff is no more competent than they are. In this struggle, the minority child may be rewarded for increased acculturation and rejection of nonmainstream values and traditions. The staff may be inadvertently linking improved mental health with acceptance of mainstream values and beliefs. The family may experience the hospital staff as literally stealing their child or adolescent from them by condoning the young person's rejection of the family's cultural manifestations. Adoption of Anglo ways may also serve to isolate a child who returns to a traditional culture. Understanding the risk that the acculturation will make the child an outcast, the family may resist the change. The staff will only see the family's lack of cooperation.

The family may also feel undermined by the child-centered environment of an inpatient unit. Alliances will be strong between the staff and the child or adolescent, and the parents may feel their own power has been diminished while that of their child has been augmented. The family may feel threatened by the lack of support they experience relative to their child.

If the family has strong ties, they may interpret hospitalization as their personal failure. Their resistance serves to reduce the humiliation of accepting that other caregivers succeeded where they have failed with their child or adolescent. Resistance becomes a matter of saving face. Families with a strong sense of control may feel that they have lost control over their child or adolescent and, therefore, over their family. Issues that may impact their cooperation or resistance include: whether they were self-referred; whether they wanted the hospitalization; whether they perceive they had choices regarding alternatives to the hospitalization; whether they feel they are able to maintain some control over the treatment; whether the removal of one family member impacts the family's self-definition or roles.

Ironically, the skills that assist a family in functioning positively outside the hospital setting are frequently viewed as maladaptive and resistant within the hospital. For example, staff may label families as trouble makers or as overly controlling when they serve as advocates for their children, want to be part of the treatment team and participate in decision making regarding care, or disagree with the treatment team. Involving parents as active members of the treatment team, providing frequent feedback, and involving the family in the initial assessment and planning diminish these resistances (Pearson, 1987).

Voluntary versus involuntary commitments are significant in a family's ability to cooperate. In New Mexico, for example, all children must be involuntarily committed for inpatient treatment via a court hearing at which they are represented by an attorney. This procedure occurs regardless of the family's, the child's, or the professional's opinions regarding the child's need for inpatient treatment. Thus, the parents are thrust into an adversary relationship with their child even when both may agree on the need for treatment. For many families, this process highlights their sense of loss of control over their hospitalized child. In addition, many families overtly or unconsciously perceive the commitment process as a loss of their custody of their child. The family then may seek ways to reestablish control, and power issues may get played out in the hospital. For example, the family's availability for visits, passes, or family therapy may be tied to their attempts to reassert their importance in the child's therapy. Parents may offer gifts to the child to "win" him or her back.

Financial need may increase the family's humiliation and loss of control. In many states the Human Services Department, or its equivalent, may provide financial backup when the family can no longer support the hospitalization. However, the state may require that the parents relinquish voluntary custody to the state during this period. The parents automatically lose control of the child in doing so. Furthermore, the parent may only be able to relinquish custody by signing a statement that directly states or indirectly implies a neglect of or an inability to care for the child. Thus, even parents willing to turn over custody must swallow the bitter pill of an imposed "confession" in order to do so. This may be particularly painful for families that are unsure whether they can trust the system to return custody of their children. American Indian families may recall the number of their children adopted by Anglo families prior to the Indian Children's Welfare Act.

Resistance in families may also be increased by their lack of faith in caregivers. The need for hospitalization may represent a failure of previous therapeutic attempts. The family may experience a greater sense of helplessness and hopelessness, because treatment has moved to a more restrictive and intensive alternative. Furthermore, the family's experience in previous settings with other systems will influence their motivation and trust in the inpatient setting. Families who felt regarded, respected, and listened to in previous settings are more likely to feel initially positive toward an inpatient setting than families who felt misunderstood, discounted, or blamed by former agencies.

The circumstances described above represent ways in which resistance is an interaction between institution and family. Although the parents are typically labeled as resistant, the behavior of the staff can ameliorate resistance in most of these situations. Some inpatient facilities, for example, have incorporated family nights or similar opportunities for the child and family to interact with milieu staff in a nonthreatening activity in order to support the privacy of the family, and for milieu staff to develop relationships with parents, thereby decreasing the likelihood of splitting.

FAMILY COMPONENT

Clark, Zalis, and Sacco (1982), in describing low-income, chronically deprived families, listed three types of resistance frequently encountered— situationally based, reality-based, and pathologically based resistances. They described *situationally based* resistances as including lack of transportation and a telephone, and entrance into therapy because of someone else's referral. *Reality-based* resistances consist of fears related to bureaucratic entities—fear of having children removed or fear of losing some portion of public assistance. *Pathologically based* resistances include fear of exposure of their own problem behavior to others, for example, fear of exposure of abuse without feeling guilt or conflict over the abuse.

With racial or ethnic minority families who also experience poverty, many of these resistances will be manifested in an inpatient setting. Reality-based resistances such as loss of control over their own and their children's destinies have previously been partially discussed. This section examines:

1. The economic hardships of poor families which interfere with treatment but may not reflect an unwillingness to go along with treatment;
2. Further ways in which families protect themselves from boundary intrusions;
3. The threat acculturation may represent;
4. Parental psychopathology issues.

Economic Realities

The harshness of poverty may manifest in therapy in many ways. A father may be labeled as peripheral or as resisting treatment because of his lack of involvement in therapy. However, the father's absence may reflect the economic survival needs of the family and his "resistance" may reflect a breadwinner who must work several jobs to make ends meet (Hines & Boyd-Franklin, 1982). Some therapists may halt treatment until all family members participate, a dictum that may place impossible demands on the family.

A father who was working two jobs as a mechanic was viewed by treatment staff and school personnel as neglectful for his unavailability for meetings. Arranging appointment times in the early morning or evening, at the home, allowed the father to participate in his daughter's treatment while not sacrificing the need to provide financial stability.

Many authors report that various ethnic groups do not arrive for appointments on time. Hines and Boyd-Franklin (1982) pointed out that poor people who experience long waits and are given no set appointment times in medical clinics expect similar treatment in mental health settings. Similarly, the therapist may label a family that has no phone or experienced a car breakdown as resistant when the fact that the family came in at all may represent an impressive commitment on their part.

Structural differences in families may occur out of economic necessity and must be approached with flexibility. For example, many family therapists work to remove all children from "parentified" roles in families, believing that no older siblings should have ongoing responsibilities for younger children. However, it is impossible generally for a working single parent not to rely on her older children to provide child care and perform household tasks. The goals are not to remove these responsibilities but to ensure that the child or adolescent has authority and privileges commensurate with responsibility and to meet the adolescent's developmental needs.

Furthermore, because low-income families may be involved with many agencies and individuals, they may receive advice on the same problem from a variety of sources. Failure to follow through with one particular set of recommendations may be a function of confusion over having received contradictory advice rather than of resistance (Pinderhughes, 1983). Solicitation of advice from many sources may also be viewed as resistance and the families may be accused of "splitting" professionals. However, the training the larger social system imposes on poor families, to listen to all professionals as the experts and to not trust their own views, needs to be considered.

Boundary Intrusions

Families may resist change because of the level of intrusiveness the intervention represents. Minority families may be particularly vulnerable to these boundary violations. Wynne (1980) theorized that families must maintain a "dynamic equilibrium" between continuous change and stagnation. Too much change could lead to chaos, whereas too little could imply role rigidity. The Timberlawn Study (Lewis, Beavers, Gossett, & Phillips,

1976) found that healthy families balance their need for solidarity and identity with influence from the environment. The researchers described families who fail to achieve this balance as *centrifugal* (they have overly permeable boundaries that make them susceptible to accommodation of external pressure, even when negative) and *centripetal* (they possess rigid boundaries and are unyielding to outside influence even when desirable or necessary). Pinderhughes (1983) pointed out that black families protect themselves from a hostile, often dangerous environment by developing rigid family boundaries. Pinderhughes's description of boundary formation is similar to Wynne's premise that boundaries prevent chaos. The more chaotic, alien, or dangerous the environment, the greater the need for tight, impermeable boundaries. Thus, a family style that may appear inflexible and may make therapist intervention difficult may have originated as an adaptation to environmental demands. Furthermore, many minority families recall negative experiences at the hands of social service agencies. They may feel that providing detailed family information to a therapist or hospital makes them vulnerable to further loss of control of their family (Clark et al., 1982). If they perceive a great disparity (which may exist) in power between themselves and the hospital staff or in the extent to which they are out of the mainstream culture, their fear of loss of control and the hospital staff's actual animosity toward them may increase.

Acculturation Pressures

Resistance is part and parcel of change. Family theorists have a range of definitions of resistance: the family's way to avoid psychic conflict, even for several generations (Boszormeny-Nagy & Ulrich, 1981); a mechanism to maintain homeostasis (Bowen, 1978); a normal part of the therapy process (Haley, 1976). The Strategic school theorizes that families seek help only when they have reached an impasse in their own coping and adaptive patterns. Anderson and Stewart (1983) pointed out that families seek therapy not out of a desire for change but because of a failure to accommodate to changes that have already occurred.

The process of acculturation can be seen as this type of family developmental crisis. The family may perceive the assimilation of the younger generation as a threat to their survival, as well as a loss of a relationship. Parents who may not feel comfortable with the new language or new way of life may feel dependent on their children. This sense of a threat may propel families to distrust the schools, the churches, the children's friends, and any mental health professionals who enter the scene. The parents may deny the consequences of their isolation; for example, they may label the child's depression a result of the pressure of acculturation rather than of the imposed isolation. They may view their behavior solely as protective.

The therapist must walk a tightrope between opening up possibilities for the child and respecting the parents' concerns. Montalvo and Gutierrez (1989) emphasized that therapists must understand that individual members of the same family will represent many levels of acculturation.

Psychopathologically Based Resistance

Some forms of resistance represent a level of psychopathology on the part of the parent. One form of resistance derives from the parent's need to maintain contact with the therapist or therapeutic community, but to feel able to do so only if the child is in the "sick" role. The self-esteem of the parent, often a single parent, appears tied to her or his ability to work with the hospital staff. However, as the child improves, the future loss of the hospital staff's support threatens the parent, who must covertly sabotage the treatment so that the child can remain in care. Another common pattern of parents is to offer a second sibling for inpatient care as the hospitalized child improves. This behavior may not be expressly linked to ethnic minority clients, but it is linked to clients who have few social or economic supports.

Another form of resistance is the parents' extreme alliance with the child against the hospital. Although this may occur for reasons discussed previously, such as the hospital's insensitivity to the role of the parents, it may also occur because of parental projections. Parents who are enraged at their child may project their own unacceptable, punitive fantasies onto the hospital staff. The parents then overcompensate for their own anger by allying with the child against the harsh, arbitrary hospital system and supporting the child's acting-out against the system (Rinsley, 1980). This resistance may be manifested more frequently by parents who have their own history of authority problems or of abuse and neglect. In dealing with minority families, it will become crucial to differentiate legitimate expressions of concern against a hospital that represents mainstream culture from uses of cultural differentness as *raisons d'être* for their rage.

Similarly, a family may resist change because of the feelings triggered by the care provided to their child. Depending on their own family histories, they may feel angry and jealous that their child is receiving attention and nurturance they never experienced as children. Their own fears of abandonment may be further triggered by watching their children attach to "strangers."

A 7-year-old girl was placed in foster care after allegations of sexual abuse by her father. The father was incarcerated, and the girl was eventually hospitalized. After a period of hospitalization, the therapist began working to reunite the girl with her mother. The mother, who had been working diligently in therapy, dropped out of her own incest survivors' group and missed family therapy. She insisted that the abuse could not have occurred because her daughter primarily lived with the maternal grand-parents on a reservation away from the rest of the family. After extended exploration, the mother became aware of her rage at her daughter. She had originally placed the child with her parents because she was jealous of her husband's affection toward the infant. The grandparents' obvious affection for the child contrasted with the neglect and abandonment the mother experienced with them, mostly living in boarding schools. Finally, the ther-apist's and the state's concern for her daughter's victimization infuriated her, an ignored victim. Once these issues surfaced, the mother resolved much of her ambivalence and warmed up to her daughter.

Decreasing parental resistance by joining with the parents in their con-cern for their child and in their anger regarding the problem behavior of their child may permit an exploration of all of the fears and concerns of the parents. Decreasing or carefully supervising the child–family contact while increasing parent–therapist contact may be helpful in joining the family and may provide an opportunity for evaluation of mental disorders in the parent.

CONCLUSION

Suggestions have been given throughout this chapter for reducing resist-ance. We conclude with some general comments.

With minority families, a family orientation serves to reduce resistance because it better matches their cultural values. Family therapy fits their priority of community and family cohesiveness over individualistic goals. However, the therapist must recognize that important family members may extend beyond the nuclear family. In a Navaho family, for example, the grandmother is often the pivotal decision maker. She must be included, for therapy to advance. In Hispanic and black families, the extended family must be involved even though some of the important extended family mem-bers may not be biologically related. In Hopi families, the maternal aunts and uncles are responsible for discipline and the biological parents are re-sponsible for nurturance. As in many other American Indian groups, all are called "mother" and "father" by the children. To misunderstand family ties, limit who is involved, or pathologize these relationships would set up a therapeutic failure. However, the tendency of the therapist might be to attribute the failure to the family's resistance rather than to the therapist's not working with the appropriate family members.

Therapists must validate their clients' values, perceptions, and goals (Tyler et al., 1985). They must learn to translate knowledge about a culture into actual interventions (Sue, 1988). They must remain aware of tendencies to overgeneralize and stereotype and must remain open to guidance from the family (Montalvo & Gutierrez, 1989). Lastly, in the words of Tyler et al. (1985), cultural pluralism must be respected. Therapy must respect diversity, build on an ethnic group's strengths, neither systematically advantage or disadvantage any group, and provide for individual and social change.

REFERENCES

Anderson, C. M., & Stewart, S. (1983). *Mastering resistance: A practical guide to family therapy.* New York: Guilford.

Beavers, W. R. (1982). Healthy, mid-range, and severely dysfunctional families. In F. Walsh (Ed.), *Normal family processes* (pp. 45–66). New York: Guilford.

Berman, J. R. S. (1989). A view from rainbow bridge: Feminist therapist meets changing woman. *Women & Therapy, 8,* 65–78.

Boszormeny-Nagy, I., & Ulrich, D. (1981). Contextual family therapy. In A. S. Gurman and D. P. Kniskern (Eds.), *Handbook of family therapy* (pp. 159–186). New York: Brunner/Mazel.

Bowen, M. (1978). *Family therapy in clinical practice.* New York: Jason Aronson.

Bradshaw, C. (1988). *A Japanese view of dependency: What can it contribute to feminist theory and therapy?* Paper presented at the Advanced Feminist Therapy Institute, Seattle, WA.

Clark, T., Zalis, T., & Sacco, F. C. (1982). *Outreach family therapy.* New York: Jason Aronson.

Cromwell, R. E., & Ruiz, R. A. (1979). The myth of macho dominance in decision-making within Mexican and Chicano families. *Hispanic Journal of Behavioral Sciences, 1,* 355–373.

Falicov, C. J. (1982). Mexican families. In M. McGoldrick, J. K. Pearce, & J. Giordano (Eds.), *Ethnicity and family therapy* (pp. 134–163). New York: Guilford.

Freud, S. (1952). *A general introduction to psychoanalysis.* New York: Washington Square Press. (Original work published 1900)

Haley, J. (1976). *Problem solving therapy.* San Francisco: Jossey-Bass.

Hines, P. M., & Boyd-Franklin, N. (1982). Black families. In M. McGoldrick, J. K. Pearce, & J. Giordano (Eds.), *Ethnicity and family therapy* (pp. 84–107). New York: Guilford.

Jilek-Aall, L. (1976). The western psychiatrist and his non-western clientele. *Canadian Psychiatric Association Journal, 21,* 353–359.

La Fromboise, T. (1988). American Indian mental health policy. *American Psychologist, 43,* 388–397.

Lewis, J. M., Beavers, W. R., Gossett, J. T., & Phillips, V. A. (1976). *No single thread: Psychological health in family systems.* New York: Brunner/Mazel.

Lopez, S., & Hernandez, P. (1987). When culture is considered in the evaluation and treatment of Hispanic patients. *Psychotherapy, 24,* 120–126.

Masterson, J. F. (1985). *The real self: A developmental, self, and objects relations approach.* New York: Brunner/Mazel.

McGoldrick, M. (1982). Ethnicity and family therapy: An overview. In M. McGoldrick, J. K. Pearce, & J. Giordano (Eds.), *Ethnicity and family therapy* (pp. 3–30). New York: Guilford.

Montalvo, B., & Gutierrez, M. J. (1989). Nine assumptions for work with ethnic minority families. In G. W. Saba, B. M. Karrer, & K. V. Hardy (Eds.), *Minorities and family therapy* (pp. 35–52). Binghamton, NY: Haworth.

Pearson, G. (1987). Long-term treatment needs of hospitalized adolescents. *Adolescent Psychiatry, 14,* 342–357.

Pinderhughes, E. (1983). Afro-American families and the victim system. In M. McGoldrick, J. K. Pearce, & J. Giordano (Eds.), *Ethnicity and family therapy* (pp. 108–122). New York: Guilford.

President's Commission on Mental Health. (1978). *Report to the President.* Washington, DC: U. S. Government Printing Office.

Rinsley, D. B. (1980). *Treatment of the severely disturbed adolescent.* New York: Jason Aronson.

Sue, S. (1977). Community mental health services to minority groups: Some optimism, some pessimism. *American Psychologist, 32,* 616–624.

Sue, S. (1988). Psychotherapeutic services for ethnic minorities: Two decades of research findings. *American Psychologist, 43,* 301–308.

Sue, S., & Zane, N. (1987). The role of culture and cultural techniques in psychotherapy: A critique and reformulation. *American Psychologist, 42,* 37–45.

Trimble, J. E. (1982). American Indian mental health and the role of training for prevention. In S. M. Manson (Ed.), *New directions in prevention among American Indian and Alaska native communities* (pp. 147–168). Portland, OR: Health Sciences University.

Trimble, J. E., & La Fromboise, T. (1985). American Indians and the counseling process: Culture, adaptation, and style. In P. Pederson (Ed.), *Handbook of cross-cultural mental health services* (pp. 127–134). Beverly Hills, CA: Sage Press.

Tyler, F. B., Sussewell, D. R., & Williams-McCoy, J. (1985). Ethnic validity in psychotherapy. *Psychotherapy, 22,* 311–320.

Vargas, L. A. (1989). *Providing culturally responsive supervision.* Paper presented at the American Academy of Child and Adolescent Psychiatry, New York.

Wynne, L. C. (1980). Paradoxical interventions: Leverage for therapeutic change in individual and family systems. In J. S. Strauss, M. Bowen, T. W. Downey, S. Fleck, S. Jackson, and I. Levine (Eds.), *The psychotherapy of schizophrenia* (pp. 191–202). New York: Plenum Medical.

Zinn, M. B. (1980). Employment and education of Mexican-American women: The interplay of modernity and ethnicity in eight families. *Harvard Educational Review, 50,* 47–62.

CHAPTER NINE

The Educational Process as Ego Enhancement in Inpatient Settings

Virginia A. Cavalluzzo

Teaching children who are from various cultures is a complex process. The teaching–learning relationship is dynamic and constantly changing. Significant differences exist in how each culture expresses its values, customs, and beliefs; what is considered successful in one culture may be a taboo in another. Yet, across cultures, two common qualities of life are essential: feeling valued and feeling competent about the things that one does. Both qualities are often missing in child and adolescent patients, whether they are Hispanic, American Indian, black, or Anglo. Many of these children suffer from severe trauma caused by experiences such as abandonment and neglect (especially in the early years of their lives), physical and sexual abuse, and neurological anomalies due to fetal alcohol syndrome.

Children from different cultural backgrounds also experience a sense of not being valued if they are members of a minority culture whose value systems are different from those of the dominant culture in which they are trying to function. This is especially true for Hispanic and native American children, for whom the extended family may play a vital part in their upbringing and may create an interdependence not valued in Anglo society. When the Hispanic or native American family unit becomes dysfunctional or is reduced to that of a poorly functioning single-parent family, the child is less likely to feel cared about.

The role of any psychiatric hospital for children and adolescents is to use its various modalities, including the school, to work in a culturally sensitive way with these disturbed patients. This chapter describes the educational goals, curricula, activities, administrative procedures, and interactive approach at the University of New Mexico Children's Psychiatric Hospital (CPH). These data on the hospital population known best to the author are offered to exemplify some successful results of a comprehensive therapeutic educational program and to communicate with other professionals who, in parallel endeavors, may have recommendations for continued progress.

ADMISSIONS DATA AND STAFFING

As an intermediate-care hospital, CPH serves children aged 5 through 14 from throughout the state of New Mexico. A multicultural state, New Mexico has three major cultures: Anglo, Hispanic, and native American. Child residents aged 5 through 14, according to the 1980 Census, are made up of 54.5% Anglos, 34.5% Hispanics, and 8.85% native Americans. Blacks are 1.6% of the child population, and all other cultural groups together make up .35%. Children are admitted into the hospital under the New Mexico Mental Health Code and reflect a cultural diversity of 62.13% Anglo, 28.16% Hispanic, 5.83% native American, and 3.88% black.*

* CPH Annual Statistical Report, June 1989.

Diagnoses on admission to the hospital include major depression, attention deficit disorder, conduct disorder, posttraumatic stress syndrome resulting from severe physical and/or sexual abuse, and a range of personality disorders. In addition, the children often are learning disabled or mildly retarded, or have chronic physical illnesses such as seizure disorders, juvenile diabetes, and severe hearing impairment.

At the time of admission to CPH, each child is assigned to a cottage/classroom unit according to his or her age and treatment needs. Each unit has a treatment team whose regular membership is composed of the child's clinician, cottage program manager, child-care workers, nurse, social worker, teacher, educational diagnostician, and therapeutic recreation therapists. Other treatment team members are included when their special skills are required to respond to a child's unique treatment needs. Referred to as allied therapists, these other treatment team members are the occupational therapist, speech/language therapist, adaptive physical education teacher, art therapist, music teacher, and children's librarian.

As psychiatric inpatient treatment for children has evolved over the past 30 years, so has the role of the in-hospital school. CPH's Mimbres School program, with its psychodynamic conceptualization, has drawn upon the work of those who pioneered the development of educational programs for severely emotionally disturbed children and adolescents. Influenced by psychoanalytic theory, Bettelheim (1974), Redl and Wineman (1954), and Fenichel (1971) were leaders who developed successful approaches to educating severely emotionally disturbed children in specialized settings. Their approaches were based on an understanding of children's psychopathology and the kinds of relationships with teachers and other staff that facilitated conflict reduction and new learning. Through the years, other work by Hobbs (1966), Haring and Phillips (1962), and Hewett and Taylor (1980) developed approaches that drew heavily on behavioral theory. Their work stressed the importance of operant conditioning, environmental design, and applied behavioral analysis in creating a successful educational program for emotionally disturbed children.

THE MIMBRES SCHOOL

The Mimbres School, an accredited New Mexico public school on the CPH campus, is an integral part of the CPH treatment program. Its status as an accredited public school assures the children and their parents that a legitimate educational program will be provided during hospitalization. The school can both receive and transmit educational information and credits from the hospital school are guaranteed to be honored by other schools. Accreditation also makes the school eligible to receive a wide range of public education funds to support programs in basic skills, science, the arts, special education services, and other special program and research grants.

Upon admission to CPH, each child is automatically enrolled in the Mimbres School and attends each weekday, beginning with the first schoolday following admission. CPH patients have such severe and complex psychiatric problems that they are designated, under the 1989 Educational Standards for New Mexico Schools, as eligible for special education services.

Public schools in the United States, with few exceptions, operate on a 10-month, 180-day school year with a 6-hour workday for teachers and support staff. This traditional school-year organization is not compatible with the needs of an inpatient hospital school. The Mimbres School operates on a 12-month, 252-day school year with an 8-hour workday for teachers and support staff. Thus, the teachers and allied therapists are able to actively continue as members of the clinical treatment teams.

The School's Operational Methods

The Mimbres School has merged behavioral and psychodynamic concepts in creating a therapeutic school environment that supports each child's clinical treatment goals and enhances his or her sense of competence. Throughout the school day, as a continuation of milieu therapy, significant emphasis is placed on providing the children with immediate feedback about their social behavior with their peers, teachers, child-care workers, and other adult staff. The classroom provides a stable, consistent, and predictable environment in which the teachers and child-care workers are able to teach various subjects. In addition, their personalities enable them to be sensitive to and empathic with such issues as the children's feelings, fears, pain, needs for contact, and control of aggression. With the help of task oriented, concerned teachers and child-care workers, children are helped to take risks, make decisions, establish positive interpersonal relationships, and enhance their ability to communicate effectively and to attain new knowledge and skills.

The staff help all children to feel comfortable in the classroom by focusing attention on their competencies. Respect for each Hispanic and native American child is demonstrated by using culturally relevant activities in the educational process, particularly the preparation of indigenous foods with each child's help. For one Zuni child, storytelling became the medium through which he could comfortably express his feelings and ambivalence about being "different" from the other children. As he recognized that others liked his stories, he acknowledged his Zuni heritage by telling the stories of the Shalakos (annual religious ceremonies performed during the winter solstice) that he had heard so many times. He was able to help other children to share stories and dances from their cultural backgrounds and in the classroom he began to take pride in learning academic skills. A Hispanic female adolescent who was very withdrawn and unable to express herself in individual and family therapy was equally noncommunicative in the classroom. The skillful teacher did not pressure the girl to speak, but maintained a consistent, matter-of-fact, nonjudgmental manner in teaching her basic academic skills. Gradually, a rapport was established; as this girl became a more effective learner, she was able to trust the teacher enough to begin sharing her pain and fears, the effects of many years of abuse suffered from family members. The teacher's therapeutic, instructional approach was the catalyst that enabled the girl to communicate her painful experiences to her clinician.

Inherent to the Mimbres methods are the beliefs that every child, no matter what his or her previous experiences have been, can learn and that the process of learning makes the child feel better about himself or herself. As each child's knowledge and skills increase so do his or her self-confidence and self-importance.

Educational Diagnostic Procedures

A recent study by Tramontana, Hooper, Curley, and Nardolillo (1990) affirmed the importance of considering neuropsychological factors that may influence the learning achievement of children with severe emotional disturbance. The educational assessments can be particularly effective in identifying underlying elements of a learning disability. This leads to a consideration of the most effective method to reduce the learning problems.

The Mimbres School's program emcompasses all the usual diagnostic procedures leading to a comprehensive assessment and develops an individual educational plan (IEP) for each child. The IEP details how skills will be taught and is shared by the teacher in a meeting with the parent(s) and the child.

The School's Role in the Treatment Process

A child is able to achieve healthy emotional growth when the goals and experiences provided for the child in the home and school environments are reasonably compatible. When a child lives in a chaotic home and is a member of a dysfunctional family, the school's role in socializing the child, particularly in an inpatient hospital, is of great importance. When a child's norms and rules of socialization are from a different culture, these differences must be kept in mind to facilitate the slow acquisition of new relationships as socialization opportunities are provided.

When children have experienced serious emotional trauma and are hospitalized for treatment, participating in a treatment milieu that incudes a therapeutic school environment is a crucial aspect of the total effort to promote their healing and their continuing growth. Integration of the educational program into the treatment milieu is a task that requires constant attention. It can begin to occur only after trust and respect are established among staff across all the professional disciplines that are involved in developing and implementing the treatment program. Once this trust level has been established, ongoing staff training and clinical supervision across and within disciplines are important, in order for the staff members to obtain a common base of knowledge about the children's pathologies and milieu treatment modalities.

Each cottage/classroom unit has a core team: the cottage clinician, teacher, program manager, evening supervisor, social worker, and nurse. This team, in a group meeting, examines the treatment issues for each child and his or her family. Skillful leadership from the cottage clinician and the program manager enable all members of the team to examine their own feelings and attitudes about the treatment issues, to recognize the subtleties of the child's and parents' behaviors, and to develop a unified approach that will be used by all staff. Issues of transference and countertransference are examined repeatedly in the core team meetings. In this supportive and nonthreatening atmosphere, the kinds of behaviors that elicit difficult countertransference issues are clarified. Strategies are suggested by the team or identified during supervision to assist team members in addressing their own feelings, attitudes, and interactions with each other, the child, and the family.

THE MIMBRES PROGRAM

Instructional strategies are varied, to enable children from different cultural backgrounds and in different developmental stages to participate in meaningful learning experiences, both independently and in groups. Teachers structure the daily schedule to include opportunities for children to participate in cooperative learning activities.

Hewett's "engineered classroom" (Hewett & Taylor, 1980) is one model. Based on behavioral theory, the engineered classroom emphasizes a hierarchy of educational tasks, token reinforcement principles, and a physical arrangement of the classroom that creates individual and group learning centers. This model can be adapted and combined with strategies from the psychoeducational model to meet successfully the needs of an in-hospital classroom. Both behavioral and psychoeducational concepts, when combined, provide the most functional classroom model for teaching seriously emotionally disturbed children.

Each classroom at the Mimbres School has the capacity for the furnishings to be arranged to create spaces for both individual and shared activities in the classroom and on an adjoining patio. Instructional materials such as maps, bulletin board displays, computers, and games are among the items available to the children during the course of the day. With staff guidance, the children determine the "rules" for acceptable classroom behavior. Behavior management strategies in which children receive positive rewards (e.g., stickers, points, tokens, popcorn, praise) are used throughout the day. Each classroom also has a "time-out room," which is used as one consequence when a child is out of control.

A teacher and two child-care workers regularly assigned to each classroom unit comprise the teaching team. The classroom structure, the daily schedule, and the individualized instructional program are organized, under the leadership of the teacher, to provide the essential stability, consistency, and predictability needed. Attention is given also to the overall ambience of the room, to ensure that the classroom atmosphere is inviting and comfortable and reflects an environment in which the children feel safe. The children assist in creating the desired classroom atmosphere by participating in the decisions concerning the arrangement of furniture, preparation of bulletin board exhibits (especially the artwork created by the children), and the varied uses of classroom space.

The cottage/classroom teams at CPH have developed a behavior management system that is built on staff agreement on acceptable and unacceptable behavior for both school and cottage life. Behaviors are clustered and prioritized into a "levels" system. At the lowest level, the children have the least control of their independence; at the highest level, they have most control over their independence. A reward system used in conjunction with the levels program is agreed upon by the staff and ranges from tokens to a "special" activity with a favorite staff member. The staff team reviews the reward system regularly as new children are admitted to the hospital. In this way, the staff is able to assess which rewards have been and will be most effective.

Students' Need for a Known and Predictable Environment

The staff was reminded, quite dramatically, of the importance of having a stable and predictable environment when the hospital underwent a major refurbishing. Although the staff and children had discussed the process of replacing carpets, window blinds, and some furniture, and painting all the rooms, the preparation was not sufficient to allay the children's fears of losing a safe milieu when they saw everything being moved out of the school so that the new carpet could be installed. Interior furnishings remained outside, clustered near the building, for several days. Plans had been made for the staff to take the children on trips to the zoo and museums on days when they were unable to occupy the school building. All of the plans relevant to the refurbishing had been discussed with the children and adolescents prior to its beginning, and they all had seemed to feel comfortable about what was going to happen. However, as some of the younger children watched the school being emptied, they began to cry and became exceedingly anxious. They were convinced that they were being abandoned. The older children and adolescents didn't cry but were equally anxious about what was happening. The departure time for the field trips was delayed, to enable the staff to help the children with their feelings and to reassure them that they were not being abandoned. Upon their return from the field trips, some of the children, accompanied by staff, were allowed to stand in the doorway of the school to see what progress had been made with the carpet installation. Everyone, children and staff alike, was relieved when everything was back in the building and normal routines were reestablished. It became clear that fears of being abandoned and not cared for are very difficult to alter.

The Teacher's Role

The teacher, serving as facilitator, takes primary responsibility in arriving at a good balance and consistency in scheduling psychotherapy, allied therapies, and the classroom instructional program. This task requires careful planning and continued monitoring by the treatment team. The teacher is able to alert the other members of the child's treatment team if the child appears to be becoming overwhelmed or fragmented by the schedule and/or the range of program activities.

It is not essential for each member of the teaching team to have the same teaching style. It is essential, however, for the teaching team members to have a common philosophy, a unified commitment to implement the treatment plan, and an agreed-upon standard regarding each child's behavior in school. The team also develops behavior management strategies specific to the different pathologies of the children. For example, a hyperactive child who must learn to deal with the hyperactivity in constructive ways is rewarded each time he or she does not interrupt someone and is ignored when he or she is disruptive. Rewards also are given for increasing "on-task" behavior. Children are taught to use the time-out room when they need to regain self-control and are encouraged, again through the use of rewards, to go there voluntarily when they begin to feel a loss of control. The teachers are empathic toward the depressed children, encouraging them to discuss their concerns with their clinicians, redirecting their attention to the school task at hand, and in general providing encouragement and rewards for their efforts to participate in the immediate task.

Based on each child's pathology, the teacher modifies the school program on an individual basis. This is done by simultaneously varying the amount and level of the subject content that the child receives, adjusting the pace at which the child participates in the instructional activities, and choosing instructional strategies that emphasize using visual, auditory, and/or kinesthetic materials to introduce and reinforce concepts according to the child's particular major sensory intake modality, his or her main avenue for learning. When these essential requirements have been met, the diversity of teaching and personal styles of the staff enhances the educational experience for the children.

Curricula Development and Implementation

A multidisciplinary approach to curricula development is used. Several subjects such as language arts, science, music, and art are integrated through the development of a common set of goals and skills to be learned. Through coordinated planning, these goals are addressed simultaneously when each subject area is taught (Quattrone, 1989).

At CPH, one way in which this has occurred has been through the implementation of the Stress/Challenge Outdoor Adventure Program (SCOAP). Overcoming fears and learning to trust others as well as oneself are addressed through participation in the "ropes" course, backpacking, and camping activities. Activities that involve the children in cooperative learning, role playing, and building of models of their cities, towns, or communities are very successful.

Whether using a multidisciplinary, thematic, or unit structure to develop the curricula, the concepts to be learned must be organized along a developmental and cultural framework. Activities that stir a child's curiosity, provide opportunities to explore his or her world, and offer involvement with problem solving are crucial for a child's gaining of a sense of competence (Taba, 1962).

Expressive arts projects enable children to access and express their feelings creatively through drawings, storytelling, dancing, and so forth. As children increase their capacity to problem-solve and to express themselves creatively, they gain a sense of competence and self-worth (Berlin, 1980).

Some of the expressive arts activities at CPH that are most successful in enhancing the children's language and ego development are implemented through the Chapter I Language Enrichment through the Arts Program (LEAP) and the Artist-in-Residence programs. Instructional modules from LEAP which encourage creativity focus on activities such as mime, puppetry, dance, music, storytelling, and photography. These and other expressive arts activities serve as vehicles for involving children in nonthreatening, guided learning experiences with the facilitating activities of adults who by their skills can engage most children and thus reduce their cultural and emotional barriers to communication. Children gain a powerful new view of themselves as they interpret their personal experiences through an expressive arts format. The diversity of the arts experiences enables each child to gain a greater awareness of self and sensitivity toward others.

Following a visit to a museum where they were permitted to examine musical instruments from many parts of the world, the children were asked to speculate as to how the instruments were constructed and to create stories about why the instruments were used in a particular culture. A study of the music of the people of West Africa was the cultural context from which generalizations were drawn. The decision to study about the West African people was made to help one black girl in the group develop a sense of pride in her black heritage. Comparisons with Hispanic and native American music were interwoven throughout the project.

Using folk tales, the children learned how ideas and beliefs are transmitted from one group of people to another and from one generation to another. Listening to selections of international folk music, the children learned how feelings are expressed differently in different cultures and some of the common elements of musical expression of happiness, sadness, and playfulness. As a culminating activity, the children presented an interpretive musical performance at a West African folk story, *Why Mosquitoes Buzz in People's Ears: A West African Tale* (Aardema, 1975). The children made their own instruments and costumes for the performance.

The black girl, who had very low self-esteem, believed that she didn't fit into any group. Her usual behavior was to become so disruptive that she would be isolated from the group. She initially refused to participate in the performance, but changed her mind when she learned that everyone would create another image of himself or herself by designing a mask to wear as part of the costume. She created a beautiful mask for which she received many compliments from her peers. The clinician was able to use this experience to help the child deal with her feelings about her identity.

In addition to the expressive arts projects provided for all children at CPH, some children receive art therapy. The program provides these children with a unique avenue for self-expression and self-exploration when verbal communication may be very difficult for the child because of a psychological status or cultural background. In one instance, a native American, teenage girl who refused to discuss her abuse (physical and sexual) was referred to the art therapist. When clay was introduced as a medium for expression, the girl worked with the clay much like bread dough and was able to relate experiences in which her grandmother showed her how to make bread. She created a small *horno* (clay oven) and, through a discussion about making a fire and releasing heat, the repeated activity allowed her to eventually be able to talk about her anger. The art therapy sessions helped the girl to reconnect with her cultural heritage and marked the beginning of a series of images, created using beadwork and masks, through which she could express her feelings of anger, sorrow, and, eventually, hope for her future.

In another situation, a highly verbal Hispanic teenage boy who had a long history of physical abuse defended against any affect around these issues. In art therapy, he told his story through a diorama depicting a village where a tyrannical god ruled and punished innocent people for crimes committed "before they were born." The village people had to learn to "live underground" to avoid this god's wrath. This was the beginning of the exploration, in both individual and group therapy, of the fear of punishment and the hatred brought about by keeping feelings hidden ("living underground"). The boy began to see, in the treatment setting and later in his extended family, allies who were rescuing him from his having to live underground. Leisure-time skills are taught through scouting and recreational activities such as playing games and working on craft projects. Through group discussions in the cottage, the recreation therapists help the children to understand what leisure-time activities are offered and to guide them as they try several activities until they find one they enjoy.

As one group art therapy project, the adolescents created images of their "life's road" and where they were on their journey. One girl, a survivor of sexual abuse and rape, painted herself ". . . out in the open with wild flowers. I just came from my journey through the dark canyon between the mountains. My path was black, but now it is new. There aren't even any tracks on it yet." She related this image of her own life, her past, and her new feeling of self-confidence and hope for her future.

Because many adolescents at CPH have a history of sexual abuse, guiding them toward development of healthy attitudes about human sexuality is an emotionally-laden task that demands the participation of the entire treatment team in a unified effort. Each treatment team determines when and how the instructional module on human sexuality will be presented to its cottage/classroom unit. The instructional module is developed by the teacher only after the treatment team establishes the goals, defines the role for each team member during the project, and determines a schedule for implementation. The clinician provides the primary leadership in guiding the team members to examine their own attitudes about sexuality and to develop skills that will adequately respond to the children and adolescents. This project always opens a floodgate of emotions for everyone. The ways in which the treatment team members respond to the children and adolescents and to themselves are crucial to the healing process.

The children's initial reactions to the human sexuality unit are embarrassment, curiosity, feigned interest, or pretended casual interest. As lessons progress, some children become very agitated and anxious as they recall their own encounters with sexual abuse. Other children react by becoming sexually provocative.

One child turned her back on the teacher throughout the first two lessons, as a signal that she did not want to participate in the discussion any more. The teacher acknowledged the child's feelings and told her that she needed to talk with her clinician and other staff so that she could be helped to cope with feelings such as embarrassment, guilt, fear, and anger. When verbal communication is too painful, art therapy, play therapy, and role-playing techniques are used. Attitudes and feelings about human

Table 9.1.   An Integration of Services Model for Speech/Language and Occupational Therapies

1. Go outside of the classroom for individual therapy one-on-one with the therapist.

2. Go outside of the classroom for small group therapy with the occupational therapist or the speech/language therapist.

3. Go outside of the classroom for small group therapy; use a therapy room, with the speech/language therapist and the occupational therapist doing team teaching.

4. Use team teaching in the classroom with the classroom teacher and either the speech/language therapist or the occupational therapist.

5. Stay in the classroom for modified speech/language or occupational therapy programs when the speech/language therapist or occupational therapist is providing the specialized therapy.

6. Hold weekly collaborative consultation for speech/language and occupational therapists and the classroom teacher, to develop ideas, identify instructional strategies, and select materials through which the teacher can implement the program in the classroom. Modify the program as needed.

7. Identify specific levels of task mastery through diagnostic/prescriptive teaching done with individual children by the classroom teacher, the speech/language therapist, and the occupational therapist.

sexuality are revealed also in role-playing activities such as how to be a good baby sitter.

For students who have difficulty communicating, computers provide a new avenue for expressing themselves. Word processing and advanced desktop publishing programs are ideal for those who have difficulty with handwriting, spelling, and sequencing of ideas. The computer is nonjudgmental. Errors are easily corrected and the finished product always looks "professional," thus enabling the student to feel a sense of accomplishment for having achieved a new level of competence in communicating with others.

Pairing a nonverbal child with a verbal child to play problem-solving computer games provides them with a highly interactive process of communication in which they help one another and communicate successfully with one another.

Computer technology helps each child to develop new and positive attitudes toward school tasks that at one time were painful experiences. Increased learning occurs and self-esteem and self-confidence are bolstered.

An analysis of an individual communication disorders evaluation conducted by a speech/language pathologist provides data regarding the child's capacity to communicate effectively. Because the data also indicate the severity of the deficiency, the allied therapist can design an appropriate treatment schedule.

Similarly, the occupational therapist at CPH conducts evaluations of the children's sensorimotor functions. Specific areas of assessment include sensory system function, gross and fine motor development, neurophysiological maturity, ability to attend to tasks, perception, and daily living skills. Based on the identification of the sensorimotor problem areas, a treatment program is developed. The child participates in specific, purposeful activities directed toward improving sensory processing and facilitating sensory integration. This treatment is very important in a hospital population where 50% to 60% of the children have some central nervous system pathology.

At CPH, an Integration of Services Model has been developed to provide treatment approaches that will more effectively remediate the diversity of problems identified through the individual diagnostic assessments in communication disorders and occupational therapy (see Table 9.1).

STAFF DEVELOPMENT

In developing an effective educational program for severely disturbed children from diverse cultural backgrounds, the teachers, allied therapists, and other support staff must acquire considerable understanding of human growth and development, the values and beliefs of the varied cultural groups, and the art and methods of teaching.

Ongoing training is available through participation at rounds, case conferences, and professors' rounds. The Director of Educational Services also provides individual clinical supervision to the teachers and allied therapists on a six-week cycle. Additional individual supervision is provided as needed or as requested.

One aspect of the inservice training is focused on topics that will provide the staff with a greater understanding of clinical issues and treatment modalities; another is focused on topics such as cultural values and traditions in Hispanic and native American communities, to afford the staff a better understanding of a variety of behaviors, for example, why many native American children never look an adult in the face. The children's culturally determined behaviors require other teaching methods. Thus, inservice sessions deal with a variety of new educational techniques and methods. The inservice training program for the Mimbres School personnel has been developed through a collaborative effort among the teachers, allied therapists, child-care workers assigned to the school program, and Director of Educational Services. A needs assessment survey is conducted annually to identify the areas of common interest for inservice seminars and workshops. Such topics as how to use computer technology as an instructional tool, understanding the psychological impact of chronic illness on the very disturbed child, and strategies for stress management in teachers have been identified. The nature of the teachers' and child-care workers' attitudes that can help disturbed children is discussed from the viewpoint of the child's needs and disturbance, and the way the school can use the educational program as a treatment modality.

CONCLUSION

In the therapeutic educational environment of a children's psychiatric hospital school, the interrelationship of teaching and learning must remain fluid in order to effectively meet the cultural and emotional needs of the children. Skillful teachers, through acknowledging the children's different cultural experiences, are able to guide the children to safely share their culture with others as well as to acquire new knowledge and skills. Thus, an atmosphere is established in which children can achieve competence and develop positive self-esteem. Intrinsic to the therapeutic educational program are the beliefs that every child can learn and that through positive learning experiences each child's feelings of self-confidence and self-respect will increase.

Behavioral and psychodynamic concepts, when integrated into the structure and organization of the therapeutic school, support the overall clinical treatment goals for enhancing each child's self-regard and competence. Skilled and empathic teachers, allied therapists, and child-care workers help children to express their feelings, pain, and fears, and to try out new interpersonal relationships. Through a task-oriented instructional program, the teachers and allied therapists focus the children's attention on developing competencies in activities such as risk taking, decision making, and effective communication with adults and peers. Expressive arts activities, skillfully encouraged by the staff, engage most children in activities that lessen their cultural and emotional barriers to communication.

Children who have severe emotional problems often experience specific learning disabilities. Educational assessments can be exceptionally effective in identifying the extent of a child's learning disability. More effective approaches to the remediation of communication disorders and sensory integration dysfunction can be accomplished through a synthesis of treatments.

The teacher, understanding the child's pathology, adjusts each child's school program to incorporate instructional strategies and materials that will enable beneficial learning experiences to occur. Thus, a comprehensive therapeutic educational program enables each child to improve his or her skills in tasks such as reading, communication, and interpersonal relationships; in turn, the child's positive feelings about self are enhanced.

The school contributes in many ways to the total therapeutic program of the hospital.

REFERENCES

Aardema, V. (1975). *Why mosquitoes buzz in people's ears: A West African tale.* New York: Dial Books.

Berlin, I. N. (1980). Problem solving and creativity: A family–school collaboration. In *Children and our future* (pp. 53–58). Albuquerque: University of New Mexico Press.

Bettelheim, B. (1974). *A home for the heart.* New York: Knopf.

Fenichel, C. (1971). Psycho-educational approaches for seriously disturbed children in the classroom. In N. J. Long, W. C. Morse, & R. G. Newman (Eds.), *Conflict in the classroom: The education of children with problems* (pp. 337–345). Belmont, CA: Wadsworth.

Haring, N. G., & Phillips, E. L. (1962). *Educating emotionally disturbed children.* New York: McGraw-Hill.

Hewett, F. M., & Taylor, F. (1980). *The emotionally disturbed child in the classroom* (2nd ed.). Boston: Allyn & Bacon.

Hobbs, N. (1966). Helping disturbed children: Psychological and ecological strategies. *American Psychologist, 21,* 1105–1115.

Quattrone, D. F. (1989). A case study in curriculum innovation: Developing an interdisciplinary curriculum. *Educational Horizons, 10,* 28–35.

Redl, F., & Wineman, D. (1954). *The aggressive child.* New York: Free Press.

Taba, H. (1962). *Curriculum development: Theory and practice.* New York: Harcourt.

Tramontana, M. G., Hooper, S. R., Curley, A. D., & Nardolillo, E. M. (1990). Determinants of academic achievement in children with psychiatric disorders. *Journal of the American Academy of Child and Adolescent Psychiatry, 29,* 265–268.

CHAPTER TEN

Short-Term Psychiatric Hospitalization of Children and Adolescents

Lynn E. Ponton

Hospital-based psychiatric treatment of children and adolescents has changed dramatically during the past 10 years because of clinical developments such as the increasing use of psychotropic medications (Small & Perry, 1989), financial changes, exemplified by the decreasing length of stay (Sharfstein, Dunn, & Kent, 1989), and changes in the inpatient population of children and adolescents, made manifest by an increasing number of psychosocial problems (Jemerin & Phillips, 1988). Decreased lengths of stay, increased utilization review by third-party payers, and a rapidly developing body of clinical knowledge point to a need to redefine treatment goals for short-term hospitalization.

CATEGORIES OF SHORT-TERM TREATMENT

The determination of the kind of psychiatric treatment needed, based on the amount of time that a child or adolescent stays in a hospital, is arbitrary but necessary. Length of stay dramatically affects the type of care that can be given. For children and adolescents, the average length of stay in state psychiatric hospitals and psychiatric units in general hospitals steadily decreased from 1970 through 1986. In contrast, the average length of stay for children and adolescents in private psychiatric hospitals increased from 1980 to 1986. Most recently, data from all three categories of psychiatric units indicate that there is a decrease in the length of stay, even in private psychiatric facilities (Mandersheid & Millazzo-Sayre, 1990).

For the purpose of this chapter, I have divided short-term treatment into two categories: brief hospitalization and crisis hospitalization. *Brief hospitalization* is a treatment modality requiring longer than a week but less than a month to complete. In a version described by Blotcky and Gossett (1988), the focus of this type of hospitalization is often a diagnostic assessment including the completion of a written evaluation and the initiation of an individual treatment trial (i.e., psychopharmacologic, behavioral, or a combination of treatment modalities). *Crisis hospitalization* is a subcategory of short-term hospitalization, typically offering treatment for one week or less.

Although this chapter does not address intermediate and long-term treatment, it is important to know their definitions for comparison. Intermediate-term inpatient treatment is arbitrarily defined as a program that lasts one to three months and offers a comprehensive array of treatment modalities to meet both short- and long-term treatment goals. Long-term inpatient hospitalization is longer than 90 days and targets treatment of children and adolescents with severe, repetitive symptoms and illnesses unresponsive to other treatment modalities (Blotcky & Gossett, 1988).

REASONS FOR ADMITTANCE TO THE HOSPITAL

The subject of psychiatric hospitalization of children and adolescents arouses considerable controversy. The Joint Commission on Accreditation of Hospitals (1974/1988), the American Psychiatric Association (1976), and the American Academy of Child and Adolescent Psychiatry (1978, 1989), have each developed separate hospitalization criteria. The following recommendations integrate these different criteria.

1. Children or adolescents should be admitted to a psychiatric hospital when their behavior places them in situations of acute danger. The use of a short-term unit accomplishes several functions. It provides a "safer" environment for them while the staff rapidly assesses their behavior and family situation and then makes a recommendation regarding treatment. In this category are children and adolescents who are suicidal; who abuse drugs, alcohol, and other agents; who, as runaways, place themselves in situations of danger; or who have anorexia nervosa or bulimia and are in imminent danger. This category also includes psychotic children and adolescents, who may also be in imminent danger.

2. Children or adolescents should be admitted to a psychiatric hospital when their behavior presents a real danger to society. Juvenile facilities offer an alternative placement under certain circumstances. An assessment conducted to determine which type of placement is indicated should include both a mental status examination and a clearly defined treatment plan. Psychiatric hospitalization is indicated when children and adolescents have homicidal tendencies, set fires, sexually abuse others, or have a grave mental illness that has caused their behavior. Courts will not confine runaways even though their behavior often demonstrates a serious mental problem.

3. A child or adolescent who has failed in outpatient psychiatric treatment should be considered for psychiatric hospitalization. Such failure might include a period of severe disruptive behavior such as school failure, drug or alcohol abuse, physical violence, or running away. An acute hospitalization (Parmalee, 1980) might be used to develop strategies where outpatient treatment has consistently failed. An acute hospitalization may also serve to better engage the family in the child's treatment, although that is not always the case; a family may decide to withdraw at this point.

4. A court may order evaluation for psychiatric assessment via a request for assessment regarding criminal responsibility and assistance with placement.

Ponton and Hartley (1987) examined reasons for adolescent admission to an acute psychiatric hospital and found that 28% of all those admitted presented with drug and alcohol abuse, 26% with psychotic behavior, 24% with suicide attempts, and 19% with aggressive or violent behavior. The marked acuity of these presenting symptoms reflects an overall increase in acute behavior in the child and adolescent inpatient populations.

AIMS OF SHORT-TERM INPATIENT TREATMENT

The aims of short-term psychiatric hospitalization for a child or adolescent are very much affected by the expected length of stay. At the time of a child's admission to a psychiatric hospital, there should be a careful assessment of the presenting problem and of the financial resources available to the child for psychiatric treatment.

Crises units in psychiatric hospitals for children and adolescents have the following aims:

1. To provide a safe environment, ensuring that the children do not harm themselves or others or cause serious property damage.
2. To define a main problem to focus on during treatment. The choice of problem should consider stabilization of the child, to allow a transition to a less restrictive level of care or, if a longer period of treatment at the initial level is required, to determine and arrange for that treatment.
3. To maintain well-developed liaisons among longer-term and residential inpatient facilities and day treatment and outpatient facilities.

Units that primarily provide crisis treatment should focus their treatment philosophy and treatment planning meetings around stabilization and discharge. In a very preliminary assessment, a medication may be regarded as most useful. Medications, however, are frequently used only for stabilization in this kind of program. During a crisis hospitalization, paperwork should be concise and functional. A streamlined document that can accompany the child's entry and exit from the hospital is important. Parents and guardians should be involved in the child's treatment at the time of admission, and should be repeatedly alerted to the projected length of stay, in order to avoid surprise or disappointment at a later date.

The aims of a brief psychiatric hospitalization for children and adolescents may be more extensive. A program in this category must often accomplish the aims of a crisis psychiatric unit as well as perform a rapid, multidisciplinary assessment that includes a diagnostic formulation, beginning psychopharmacologic trials, which could not be conducted on an outpatient basis, and behavioral programs targeting specific symptoms.

The staff working in this kind of program must communicate well, and they must be flexible in their ability to work with sudden changes and varying lengths of hospitalization. Like the staff working in crisis units, they should be informed of the estimated lengths of stay for their patients, from the time of admission. The different members of the assessment team should be aware of the projected discharge date and there should be a well-developed mechanism to integrate and organize the different components of the evaluation so that the written report accompanies the patient at the time of discharge.

TREATMENT PHILOSOPHY

Developing a treatment philosophy for a unit providing short-term inpatient psychiatric treatment for children and adolescents is a task requiring courage, patience, and flexibility.

A unit that does primarily crisis psychiatric hospitalization of children and adolescents should integrate the principles of *acuity, advocacy,* and *active liaison* with the psychiatric and social service community into its treatment philosophy.

Acuity

The physical plant should provide a safe environment that can contain acutely suicidal or violent children and adolescents. Adequate rooms for seclusion and restraint should be available and there should be a keen knowledge regarding the use of psychopharmacologic agents for behavioral management. The staff must be trained in techniques for rapid restraint and close observation of suicidal patients. All staff, including temporary personnel, must be alerted to the fact that they are working in a facility where suicidal and violent behaviors are ongoing. They should be carefully educated about their role, especially regarding seclusion and restraint, safety measures, and their own physical protection. Inservice education, through discussion and practice in trial situations, can help build an *esprit de corps* among the staff—an important effect that should be carefully cultivated. Declining staff morale can become a serious problem when an inpatient unit faces pressures regarding clinical needs, financial limitations for treatment, lack of social services for assistance with follow-up, and rapidly changing legal regulations. In a multicultural setting, staff prejudice may contribute to declining morale, making the staff feel ineffective and helpless.

Advocacy

The principle of *advocacy* must be an active component of the treatment philosophy. Many of the children and adolescents hospitalized in inpatient psychiatric units are not funded for even minimal treatment. As care providers for them, the unit's staff members have a significant amount of contact with both public and private sources of payment for health care. Staff members who are in contact with agencies need to be trained both to assess the needs of the children and adolescents they are treating and to describe and justify these needs to the sources of payment. Being an advocate for hospitalized children and adolescents also necessitates working through organizations that establish health care policy. Certain staff, often the unit director or administrator, should participate in this activity and should appraise other staff about the results. Advocacy helps address problems with declining staff morale.

Active Liaison

The third principle to be integrated into the treatment philosophy is emphasis on an *active liaison with the community*. As the lengths of stay in psychiatric hospitals for children and adolescents have decreased, this principle has become increasingly important. The staff needs to have daily contact with referral sources and treatment facilities. The community needs to develop a network that connects acute facilities with residential treatment and group home programs. Educating staff about how to build and maintain these networks is important.

TREATMENT PLANNING FOR SHORT-TERM PSYCHIATRIC HOSPITALIZATION

Initiating concise, focused treatment planning at the time of admission to the hospital is particularly important when the child's expected length of stay in the hospital is less than a week. Priority must be given to the behaviors and symptoms that are most acute or most amenable to short-term treatment.

Nurcombe's method (1989) of "goal-oriented treatment planning" begins by abstracting (from the clinical material collected) the pivotal problems, or those problems that require the child to stay in the hospital. Harper (1989) critiqued Nurcombe's method, noting that it can result in more than a half-dozen "pivotal problems." He emphasized the focal problem, which he defined as the main reason for the child's hospitalization. Harper's recommendation for focusing on one problem per admission to streamline the treatment planning process is particularly practical during a short hospitalization (a week or less), although it is also relevant to long-term treatment planning.

Harper recommended rephrasing pivotal problems as goals that will contribute to the stabilization of the acute patient, then selecting therapies to assist in meeting the goals. He noted that specific objectives are needed for each goal and the objectives must be monitored. Other important steps include the design and implementation of a discharge plan and the negotiation of the entire discharge plan with family members or guardians. It is important to have an effective, simple method for conceptualizing, planning, and carrying out treatment when the time in hospital is limited. The treatment plan must be designed so that temporary staff can understand and implement it.

Harper also stressed the importance of using jargon-free language so that the plans can be easily communicated. The medical record should clearly indicate the length of hospitalization and, rather than prematurely or falsely close off certain areas, any ambiguities or unknown factors should be noted. A list of factors known to contribute to the illness helps avoid speculation. Diagnoses and formulations may be proposed tentatively, but their limitations should be stated.

Ponton and Green (1990) noted that medical records for short-term hospitalization of children and adolescents may include entire sections from previous reports, often without consideration of applicability to the present record. These grafted sessions are often misquoted and not attributed to the original author. This kind of charting is seriously misleading and is best replaced with brief, clearly documented statements in which the degree of speculation is defined.

IMPORTANT COMPONENTS OF SHORT-TERM PSYCHIATRIC HOSPITALIZATION FOR CHILDREN AND ADOLESCENTS

Admission, stabilization, evaluation, and discharge are the important components of a short-term psychiatric admission. They must be planned for in detail. In the discussion of these components, the cases of four inpatients from the Child and Adolescent Psychiatry units at Langley Porter Psychiatric Institute at the University of California, San Francisco (UCSF) are described, to illustrate principles of short-term treatment and how awareness of and respect for culture and ethnicity in a short-term setting can be integrated into treatment plans.

The Adolescent Psychiatric Unit at UCSF has a long history of working with adolescents from varied cultural and ethnic backgrounds, including many adolescent immigrants and refugees. The model used for psychiatric assessment and stabilization of adolescents at UCSF emphasizes several approaches that facilitate treatment from a multicultural perspective (Budman & Ponton, 1986).

Model Treatment Approaches

Staff Education. A multicultural perspective can be enhanced in all short-term units by case conferences and workshops that focus on cultural aspects of patient care. Important areas to discuss are clinical histories, the meaning of mental illness within different cultures, the impact of cultural background on discharge plans, and the attitudes toward medication in different ethnic groups.

The Use of Cultural Consultants. A cultural consultant is usually, but not always, a member of a mental health discipline who has a background and understanding of one culture or ethnic group. The cultural consultant provides expert advice about the background of the patient, advice that can aid in assessment and treatment. The cultural consultant must have a good relationship with staff and a history of being helpful to patients and families by increasing their understanding and acceptance of treatment modalities. Cultural consultants are different from translators, many of whom are not trained specifically in mental illness. The consultants have knowledge of a specific culture and of how its members might affect and react to a mental illness. Short-term units should compile a list of consultants as a reference that can be quickly activated.

Specialty Wards. Certain geographic areas with a high percentage of one ethnic group may develop a psychiatric unit for children and adolescents that focuses on one or several large cultural or ethnic groups (Lee, 1985).

Multicultural Program. Units located in geographic areas with a large variety of ethnic groups need to enhance staff awareness of each cultural group. When staff education employs cultural consultants and translators together with case material from different ethnic groups, a better understanding of the different kinds of transference and countertransference that can develop becomes an important staff experience.

Admission Phase

The admission phase is a very important part of a short-term hospital treatment for a child or adolescent. Several tasks have to be accomplished.

Assessment. The admission process must clarify the legal issues of the person's eligibility for admission and provide an opportunity for family members and leaders in the ethnic community to help determine and advocate for the needs of the child and the family.

Admission Paperwork.   One set of paperwork should follow the child from admission to discharge. Important items such as demographics, parents' or guardian's address and phone numbers, major admitting problems, treatment plan, and tentative date of discharge should be immediately obvious on the document. Review and consolidation of the medical record help to eliminate any unnecessary paperwork.

Obtaining Information.   Either the admitting psychiatrist or another staff member (a social worker or nurse) should meet with the child and the parents or guardian and determine any other information (for example, old admission records or school records) that may be needed. Releases of the information should be signed. Short-term admissions benefit greatly from obtaining this information quickly, and flexibility and ingenuity can be valuable tools. Former hospitals can be called, with the parents present in the room, to expedite acquisition of records, and FAX machines can be used to ensure a quick transmission of information.

Welcome.   There should be a standard method for welcoming children and their families to the unit. They should be introduced to the staff, shown the ward, and given a list of the rules, visiting hours, and daily routine. Families must be introduced to the different treatment modalities and helped to understand how important their involvement is.

The following case illustrates an admission that utilized both a multicultural approach and a focus on short-term principles. Peter, a 16-year-old white boy who had arrived in the United States from Russia only three months before, was being considered for admission to the inpatient adolescent psychiatric service at UCSF. Peter's school, which specialized in integrating immigrants to this country, had reported that he was "losing touch with reality, talking about people who were out to get him and spending much time isolated and withdrawn." The mother and stepfather, who had only recently been reunited with the boy after a six-year absence, had very little information about his recent history. They did have a copy of his medical history from Russia, which included notations about a prior psychiatric hospital admission. Important parts of his admission procedure included obtaining permission to talk to the school, a translator fluent in Russian (the only language the boy spoke), financial information, and permission from the parents to utilize a social worker from the Russian Community Center as a consultant to the family and the staff. Necessary parts of the record from Russia—history, diagnosis, and medication—were translated immediately. A case conference with teachers, parents, consultants, translator, and staff was scheduled even before Peter's admission occurred. This kind of consolidated admission process requires organized planning and a knowledge of the community resources available.

Stabilization Phase

"Stabilization" may constitute the major goal of an entire psychiatric admission for a child or adolescent, particularly in crisis hospitalizations where the entire stay is shorter than seven days. The aims of a crisis hospitalization are:

1. Providing a safe environment;
2. Defining a main problem, focusing treatment on alleviation of its symptoms, and achieving some stabilization; and
3. Providing continuity with the next treatment setting.

Integrating a multicultural perspective poses additional challenges, as illustrated in the following case.

Claire, a 17-year-old girl of Chinese background, was admitted to the inpatient adolescent psychiatric unit at UCSF after ingesting an overdose of aspirin. She was a good student and had been doing well in school and at her part-time job. During the year prior to admission, she had become depressed when the fighting between her divorced parents increased; she felt caught between them, wanting to be loyal to each. The overdose was a single gesture by a depressed adolescent girl living in two households with divorced parents who were fighting. Treatment of Claire's suicidality was chosen as the focus. The treatment goal was defined as decreasing Claire's suicidality and determining whether she could return to her present living situation. Claire was admitted to the unit initially on a close suicide watch, because she could not contract to not harm herself. As she became less suicidal, the level of monitoring was decreased until there was no determined risk. Four family therapy sessions involving both households were scheduled during Claire's one-week hospitalization. A family therapist who was experienced at working with Asian families worked with Claire and her two sets of parents during the hospitalization. The therapist served as a consultant, alerting the staff to general characteristics of Asian families and specific points relevant to Claire and her family, including a more reserved style outside the family and shame about divorce. Although the two families were angry, communication had been almost nonexistent. While Claire was in the hospital, the family therapist set up a treatment plan. She saw the families individually and together, working on the specific goals of decreasing the hostility and obtaining minimal communication. Claire left the hospital on the seventh day and outpatient family treatment continued with the same therapist.

Evaluation Phase

Inpatient psychiatric evaluation of children and adolescents requires a multidisciplinary team that has had experience working together and adequate time to allow the individual parts of the evaluation to be completed. The time required to complete an evaluation generally falls within the category of brief psychiatric hospitalization.

The following steps will assist in the evaluation process:

1. Define the problem that is the focus of the evaluation. An example of an evaluative question and plan might be: "Does this child exhibit psychiatric thought processes? If so, define the limitations and make treatment recommendations based on those findings."
2. Make certain that all members of the evaluating team—usually a psychiatrist, psychologist, nurse, teacher, rehabilitation therapist (i.e., art, drama, dance, or recreation), and social worker—understand the focal problem and the reason for the evaluation. Additional consultants might include medical specialists (e.g., a neurologist) and an education or language therapist.
3. Design an evaluation plan that is coordinated with objectives, whenever possible, and involves measurement rather than qualitative judgment.
4. Design an evaluation that allows for assessment and integration of cultural factors.
5. Observe time limitations. A date for a case conference and a tentative discharge date should be set up at the time of admission. All members of the evaluation team should be appraised of the discharge date.

Jean, a 7-year-old adopted boy of mixed black and white parentage, was admitted to a children's psychiatric unit for evaluation. For several months prior to admission, Jean had exhibited unusual behavior: he appeared to be not listening to his parents or teachers, often being withdrawn and unable to concentrate on his studies. In addition, his mother stated that she had trouble making him behave.

The evaluation was jointly requested by the school, the parents, and the boy's health maintenance organization, which wanted a carefully researched treatment plan in order not to waste his health care coverage. Evaluation questions included:

Is this behavior psychotic?

What appears to be interfering with his ability to do his studies?

What could help him attend to his studies and be less withdrawn?

How could the mother be assisted with caring for her son?

The members of the evaluation team (psychiatrist, psychologist, nurse, social worker, teacher, educational therapist, speech therapist, and movement therapist) met and discussed the admission history and the evaluation questions, and reviewed the possible answers. They agreed on a conference time on day 14 and a tentative discharge date of day 21.

At the evaluation conference, with Jean's outpatient psychiatrist and school teacher attending, several of the evaluation questions were answered. Psychological testing had shown psychotic thought processes. The observations of the nursing staff and the psychiatrist's mental status examination corroborated this finding. The educational therapist did not find any specific learning disabilities but noted that Jean's "disturbed thought processes seriously affected his ability to learn."

The members of the evaluating team discussed whether psychotropic medication would be helpful to Jean, carefully assessing the potential risks and comparing them with the benefits. A determination was made to initiate a trial during the remaining days of the hospitalization. In addition, several members of the evaluating team observed that the mother was quite inconsistent in her discipline of Jean. The mother, from Martinique, expressed difficulty understanding her son's problems and at times attributed them to "voodoo." Many staff found it difficult to work with this mother, believing that she was purposely sabotaging her son's treatment. The staff met as a group and discussed how they could work more effectively with the mother. The evaluating staff thought that it would be important to find an outpatient therapist who had an understanding of the mother's background and could work with her ideas about her son's illness and her inability to discipline him. Such a person was available to help. The staff's sensitivity to the mother's perception of her son's illness enabled them to address it with the family and to provide a resource for further treatment.

Discharge Phase

When short-term hospitalizations occur, a tentative discharge date should be determined at the time of admission. Many units specializing in short-term hospitalization sabotage entire treatment plans because they do not adequately prepare for the time of discharge.

It is critical to clarify the legal and immigration status of the child or adolescent before an admission takes place. The following case illustrates the problems that can take place when that does not occur.

Juan, a 13-year-old boy from El Salvador, was admitted for inpatient psychiatric evaluation to the adolescent psychiatric unit after making a suicide attempt. His immigration status was not clarified at the time of admission. Shortly thereafter, it was discovered that immigration authorities were in the process of deporting his mother and that Juan's own status was in jeopardy. Through staff efforts, his case was separated from the extradition proceedings concerning his mother, and Juan was able to continue treatment in this country. Juan's case alerted the staff to the importance of being aware of immigration status.

Necessary Alterations in Treatment Modalities in Crisis or Brief Hospitalization

Maintaining safety has become the main priority when inpatient units have a large percentage of suicidal and violent patients.

Inpatient psychotherapy during a crisis stay in a psychiatric hospital should be focused on the admitting problem. Patients who are acutely disorganized make best use of frequent brief meetings, perhaps several 10-minute sessions each day. These sessions are focused on monitoring the mental status and the medications. The child's amenability to future individual psychotherapy should be evaluated. Helping a child understand his feelings, particularly those associated with hospital admission and treatment, is an important part of psychotherapy in an inpatient setting.

Group therapies, including large (community meeting format) and small groups (selected patients), are still a traditional part of inpatient psychiatric programs, particularly for adolescent inpatients. In the short-term setting, the daily community meeting can provide a place to introduce new patients, give a community farewell to the patients being discharged, and foster discussion about how the unit is functioning. Small-group therapy allows an opportunity for a more focused exchange. A group focused on cultural understanding is valuable in a geographic area that is culturally mixed. Discussions of family expectations, peer group roles, and sexuality can occur in this context and provide important exchange. A culturally sensitive small group also serves to diminish racial hostility, prejudice, and "gang" division on the unit—an important benefit for psychiatric units located in areas where gang division and fighting are major problems.

A special-topics group designed to educate patients about the risk of HIV infection is an important addition to any adolescent inpatient program (Ponton, DiClemente, & McKenna, 1991). Adolescent psychiatric inpatients exhibit a much higher percentage of HIV-related risk behaviors than a geographically comparable school-based population (DiClemente, Ponton, Hartley, & McKenna, 1989). In a short-term setting, the group format must be designed to foster education and, probably, primary intervention in less than a week. The format can then be repeated as new admissions enter the hospital.

Both large- and small-group meetings on child inpatient units require adequate staffing. For example, a community meeting can be conducted in a child inpatient setting only if there is an adequate number of staff members (sometimes a one-to-one ratio is required) who provide structure and support. Physical holding is often required in this setting. Such a meeting can establish a sense of an organized community with rules and flexibility, but it requires planning and staffing.

Expressive therapies (art, drama, music, and recreation) are vital components of inpatient milieu programs. In a short-term setting, assessment and introduction are primary functions of expressive therapy groups. It is important to coordinate the entire group therapy program on a unit, so that all of the groups are designed to meet short-term aims, primarily stabilization and evaluation.

Family therapy is another treatment modality that can be modified to achieve short-term treatment goals. Several options are particularly useful. Claire's family was seen four times during her one-week hospitalization. Increasing the frequency of family sessions may help the team achieve "stabilization." With other patients, family therapy sessions may not be clinically indicated and should not be part of the treatment plan. In general, family sessions are useful in providing a place for considerable information exchange, a process that expedites the evaluation.

Psychopharmacotherapy has become a valuable and accepted part of child and adolescent psychiatric hospitalization. Physicians treating a patient during a crisis hospitalization most frequently utilize medication for stabilization. The most common target symptom is "aggressiveness" (Small & Perry, 1989). Brief hospitalizations may involve the initiation of a trial of medication for a variety of other target symptoms such as depression, hyperactivity, severely disorganized thought processes, enuresis, and tics.

Introducing a psychopharmacologic agent to a family is a complex and often difficult process. A child or adolescent who is acutely symptomatic may have been medicated directly prior to the admission. Obtaining an accurate acute and long-term medication history becomes an important part of the admission process. Educational handouts about neuroleptics, antidepressants, lithium, and other medications, written specifically for families, can be given to parents at the time of admission and serve to answer many practical questions. The handouts should be available in the primary languages used in the geographic area that the unit serves. Translators should also be readily accessible at this point. It is worthwhile to explain the use of medications to parents and guardians at the time of admission. The child or adolescent should be enlisted as an ally. Educational handouts and small groups focused on medication support serve to foster this alliance. Consents for medication should be signed at the time of initiation of treatment and should be periodically reviewed.

A unit philosophy must be developed about the use of medications. Standardized rating scales for detecting symptoms and abnormal involuntary movements (Simpson, Lee, Zowbok, & Gardos, 1979) should be readily available to the staff and they should be trained to administer the rating scales and appropriate medications.

COMMON MANAGEMENT ISSUES

An assaultive child or adolescent poses a significant challenge for the staff on an inpatient unit. Because admission criteria have become more defined by destructive behavior toward oneself and others, a large number of patients with recent histories of assaultive behavior may be in one unit at the same time. Careful planning is needed, to limit the number of violent episodes and the use of seclusion and restraint.

The physical plant should be thoroughly reviewed. Blind corners, bathrooms, closets, and laundry rooms should all be examined for their attention to safety measures. Ideally, there should be adequate visibility of the children and adolescents at all times and some degree of privacy. Small changes can be made without altering the entire physical facility: Mirrors can be added to blind corners, bathroom shower heads can be recessed into the wall, closets can be locked, and laundry facilities can be made clearly visible.

A critical area of planning concerns implementation of a program that manages aggressive behaviors. Kalojera, Bedi, Watson, and Meyer (1989) reported a 64% decrease in the number of episodes of seclusion and restraint on three inpatient adolescent psychiatric units when behavioral management programs were initiated. Under their protocol, staff classified disruptive behavior into four stages and used verbal and behavioral interventions to control the behavior at each stage. Patients were actively involved in negotiating discharge from seclusion and restraint, and this interaction appeared to effectively decrease the duration of time spent in those remedial activities.

In another area of planning, an individual risk management plan should be designed for each child or adolescent at the time of admission. Each plan should include a history of assaultive behavior, specific verbal interventions that limit each patient's escalation to violence, preferred medication, and a seclusion program. The age of the child will affect the method employed. Holding and seclusion blankets are commonly used to calm assaultive children. Camisoles and quiet rooms are more commonly used with adolescents.

A final area of planning involves an organized staff rehearsal of assaultive behavior management. Reviews of this procedure should be held at regular intervals and temporary staff should participate.

Management of group violence is another area that deserves attention. Riots have been reported on both child and adolescent psychiatric units. Units with a large proportion of patients from different cultural groups should be attentive to group division and associated violence. Utilizing experienced staff in adequate patient–staff ratios helps guard against group violence.

Suicidal behavior should be assessed and planned for in a manner similar to assaultive behavior measures. First, the physical plant should be reviewed, with attention to safety precautions. Next, a suicide levels system should be initiated. An individual risk plan should be developed for each patient admitted with suicidal symptoms. Staff planning should focus on how to manage one-to-one observations during a period of restricted staffing and what to do after a suicide attempt has occurred on the unit. Activities such as notification of key staff and parents, review of the risk plan, discussion of whether to tell other patients, and incident reports should be covered during planning.

The discovery of the use of drugs or alcohol on the unit poses a unique management challenge for the staff. Clearly defined rules proscribing the use of these agents should be distributed to all patients and their families. Staff should actively promote the concept of a drug-free environment. When drugs or alcohol are discovered, a frank discussion in a community meeting should follow. Under certain circumstances, usually when several patients are involved in prohibited activities, room searches are an option. However, the legal rights of the patients should be adhered to when this action is undertaken.

A number of units utilize a point system and/or a level system of behavioral management that encourages and rewards responsible behavior. Generally, a point system begins with the negotiation of a contract with the child or adolescent. Behaviors are described in positive terms and given a point value. Point systems during a short-term admission should be simple, focusing on one or two behaviors. A simplified level system, in which the patient's overall behavior determines his or her activity level, should also be used during short-term admissions.

CONCLUSION

During the past 10 years, the short-term psychiatric hospitalization of children and adolescents has been affected by a variety of clinical, financial, and social factors. Most prominent is the decreasing length of stay in hospital. A clear definition of the type of treatment that can be provided in a short-term psychiatric setting must be accepted by any program planning to engage in this activity. Determining the criteria for hospitalization for children and adolescents, the treatment philosophy, the aims of treatment, and the treatment plan is a challenging process for any facility. A program that values advocacy for hospitalized children and adolescents and provides a clearly defined service with good community outreach and aftercare is performing an important community mental health task.

A multicultural approach can be an integral part of short-term treatment. Here again, limiting and defining the kind of services that will be provided are important; stabilization and rapid assessment are the major functions. Multicultural sensitivity through the use of cultural consultants and translators, inservice education, multicultural group therapy, and the development of community liaison that emphasizes cultural issues can modify the character of a program, to permit the development of a sharply defined acute inpatient service that accurately perceives and assesses the multicultural factors.

REFERENCES

American Academy of Child and Adolescent Psychiatry. (1978). *Guidelines for treatment resources, quality assurance, peer review and reimbursement.* K., Stevenson & M. Maholick (Eds.). Washington, DC: Author.

American Academy of Child and Adolescent Psychiatry, Committee on Adolescent Psychiatry and Adolescent Psychiatric Hospitalization. (1989). *Inpatient hospital treatment of children and adolescents: Policy statement.* Washington, DC: Committee on Adolescent Psychiatry and Hospitalization.

American Psychiatric Association. (1976). *Manual of psychiatric peer review.* Washington, DC. Committee on Peer Review.

Blotcky, M. J., & Gossett, J. T. (1988). Psychiatric inpatient treatment for adolescents. *The Psychiatric Hospital, 20;*85–93.

Budman, C., & Ponton, L. E. (1986). A model for psychiatric evaluation of the adolescent refugee. *Society Proceedings, Annual Meeting of the Academy of Child and Adolescent Psychiatry* (pp. 2–8).

DiClemente, R. J., Ponton, L. E., Hartley, D. E., & McKenna, S. (1989). Prevalence of sexual and drug-related risk behaviors among psychiatrically hospitalized adolescents. In J., Garrison, I. L., Lourie, P. Magrab, & D. Coherty (Eds.), *Issues in the prevention and treatment of AIDS among adolescents with serious emotional disturbance.* Washington, DC: Georgetown University Press.

Harper, G. (1989). Focal inpatient treatment planning. *Journal of the American Academy of Child and Adolescent Psychiatry, 28,* 31–37.

Jemerin, J., & Phillips, I. (1988). Changes in inpatient child psychiatry: Consequences and recommendations. *Journal of the American Academy of Child and Adolescent Psychiatry, 4,* 397–403.

Joint Commission on Accreditation of Hospitals. (1974, update, 1988). Accreditation manuals for psychiatric facilities serving children and adolescents. Chicago, IL: Author.

Kalojera, I. J., Bedi, I., Watson, W. N., & Meyer, A. D. (1989). Impact of the therapeutic management on use of seclusion and restraint with disruptive adolescent inpatients. *Hospital and Community Psychiatry, 40,* 280–285.

Lee, E. (1985). Inpatient psychiatric services for Southeast Asian refugees. In T. Owant (Ed.), *Southeast Asian mental health: Treatment, prevention, services, training and research* (pp. 307–329). Washington, DC: U.S. Department of Health and Human Services.

Mandersheid, R., & Millazzo-Sayre, L. (1990). Provisional unpublished data. Washington, DC: NIMH, Survey and Reports Branch, Division of Biometry and Applied Sciences.

Nurcombe, B. (1989). Goal directed treatment planning and the principles of brief hospitalization. *Journal of the American Academy of Child and Adolescent Psychiatry,* 28, 26–30.

Parmalee, D. X. (1980). The adolescent and the young adult. In *Specific aspects of inpatient psychiatry.* New York: Knopf.

Ponton, L. E., & Green, J. (1990). *Ethical issues in inpatient adolescent psychiatry.* Unpublished manuscript.

Ponton, L. E., & Hartley, D. E. (1987). Premature termination from adolescent inpatient psychiatric treatment. *Society Proceedings, Annual Meeting of the Academy of Child and Adolescent Psychiatry* (p. 8).

Ponton, L. E., DiClemente, R. J., & McKenna, S. (1991). An AIDS intervention for psychiatrically hospitalized adolescents. *Journal of the Academy of Child and Adolescent Psychiatry.*

Sharfstein, S. S., Dunn, L., & Kent, J. J. (1989). The clinical consequences of payment limitations. The experience of a private psychiatric hospital. *Psychiatric Hospital,* 19, 63–66.

Simpson, G. M., Lee., J. H., Zowbok, B., & Gardos, G. (1979). A rating scale of tardive dyskinesia. *Psychopharmacology, 64,* 171–179.

Small, A. M., & Perry, R. (1989). Pharmacotherapy. In R. D. Lyman & S. Prentice-Dunn (Eds.), *Residential and inpatient treatment of children and adolescents* (pp. 163–185). New York: Plenum.

CHAPTER ELEVEN

The Therapeutic Matrix in the Inpatient Treatment of the Adolescent

E. James Anthony

In my previous professional career (which I now refer to as B.C. or before Chestnut Lodge!), I worked with adolescents who were tangentially malad-justed, prone to anxieties, neurotically conflicted, vaguely confused about their developing selves, or underachieving at school, and I was often able, with the help of developmental change, to bring about spontaneous cures, although I would not argue with parents who attributed the great improve-ments to treatment. One of the cognitive pleasures in seeing such cases was that they fell neatly into place theoretically, as the details of history under-went elaboration. The stages and transitions appeared clearly demarcated according to psychoanalytic theory, and it became one's professional task to circumvent the next hurdle.

After I came to Chestnut Lodge and began to deal with seriously dis-turbed adolescents suffering from depressions, borderline states, schizoid or schizotypal personality disorders, disorders of conduct, substance abuse, and types of psychosis, I discovered a blurring of classical stages. The sexual aggressive responses of the first five years of life continued unabated into latency. The preadolescent and adolescent became simply hungrier, greedier, crueler, dirtier, more inquisitive, more boastful, more egocentric, or more inconsiderate than before, with an escalation of infan-tile elements. The changeover from pregenital to genital functioning, the latter element being so much more pleasing to work with therapeutically, was conspicuous by its absence.

From a psychodynamic point of view, these adolescents seemed like oversized babies. Incestuous thoughts were no longer latent but manifestly related to actual sexual abuse during childhood in significant numbers of cases. In place of individuation and clear-cut identity formation, there was an ambivalent merging with primary objects; parents and adolescents were inextricably locked in endless love–hate struggles. I wondered, with doubt and trepidation, what could be done for such cases, and I found myself, as in the opening lines of Dante's great allegory, "in a dark wood." Actually, my "wood" was the lovely campus of Chestnut Lodge, in an area, at the far end, given over to the containment and treatment of these seriously dis-turbed young people whose outward semblances lived in close and work-ing conjunction with their unrestrained primitive selves. The question that arose in my inexperienced mind was: How does one hold, in Winni-cott's sense, these monstrous babies in whom sexuality and aggression, coupled with enormous neediness, floundered unpredictably and awk-wardly all over the place?

When I took a closer look at the holding environment, I became even more surprised. Not even pretending to be a rose garden, it was a well-structured facility that seemed to be an anachronism in today's psychiatric world, where treatment is short and mindless, in the sense that the brain is the target of therapeutic endeavor and chemical treatment. Here, I had found myself in a place that offered an Eriksonian moratorium, lasting years, perhaps offering a chance to recover an orderly sequence of developmental stages in lieu of chaos and confusion. Chestnut Lodge had a long-term staff with long-term therapeutic perspectives. For them, the mind, especially the unconscious mind, was a living and operating reality and they were talking to and understanding and making meaningful connections between different parts of a patient's life.

Central to the program was psychoanalytically oriented therapy conducted four times a week by analysts, or those in analytic training, or, in rare circumstances, those who had been analyzed. It was primarily a psychoanalytic world, in which there was an abiding belief in the major tenets of psychoanalysis but where psychoanalysis was carried out with a great deal of flexibility, finesse, and skillfulness. Psychoanalysis was carried out in a special milieu and the milieu itself was saturated with the dynamic understandings with which the program was pursued.

Some would regard this approach as a dodo in a highly technological world; others, as a Utopia from psychiatry's frenetic chase of quick cures; others, as a last-ditch stand in a fast disappearing world. But the staff is not defiant; they do what they do best and what they have long learned how to do, and they do it well, humanely, and quite successfully. In spite of insurance difficulties, the patients are still referred to the Adolescent Unit at Chestnut Lodge from all over. They still remain for years, not months, and still continue to keep the hospital, including the adolescent division, relatively full. Chestnut Lodge may be an anachronism that reappears constantly in the history of the world as a revival of man's humane spirit.

THE LOGIC OF PLACE

When I speak of logic, I am thinking, often at one and the same time, of an operational sequencing tied to secondary process and reality testing on the one side and what Freud referred to as the "logic of the unconscious," in which apparently meaningless productions could be demonstrated to have their own connectedness, meaningfulness, and convincingness. At different times in the progressive–regressive cycle of human living, one or the other mode is predominant, although, at all times, puzzling admixtures may coexist, depending on the situation to which the individual is exposed. Different places range from the psychoanalyst's office to a task oriented session in the schoolroom. The therapeutic milieu at Chestnut Lodge comprises the family cottage unit, the school, the room used for group therapy, the office of the family therapist, the art therapy studio in the rehabilitation section, and the private office in which individual therapy takes place. The place seems to determine, in an almost uncanny way, the level of logic, rationality, and realism characterizing the transactions, and even the most disturbed patients appear to gauge the levels of regression appropriate to the particular situation.

The most extreme examples occur in group therapy, when regressive acting-out spreads contagiously from member to member with individuals vying with one another and exhibiting themselves for the benefit of the group therapists. In family therapy, the presence of the parents is highly provocative for extreme oppositional reactions; rebelliousness is worked out stormily at times during the sessions. At such times, the temper tantrums of the adolescent are not unlike those observed in the toddler. At the unit meetings in the cottage, the power struggles with the unit psychiatric administrator are very much in evidence as the administrator sets about dispensing privileges—weighing reported behaviors, good and bad, delicately in the balance. Feelings of injustice are rampant, and angry arguments, challenges, and confrontations dominate the proceedings. On these occasions, conscious logic is pursued, but faultily.

It is quite surprising how much self-control reigns within the psychoeducational atmosphere of the schoolroom, where conscious logic is at work in relative tranquillity and depressions, rages, and regressions are put temporarily "between brackets" so that learning can proceed. In the rehabilitation and recreation settings, one notes how the rules of the game are adhered to and how much the joys of creative expression and other activities are relished. Finally, in the daily individual session, there seems, at first, so little to say, no one to interact with, no one to challenge for privileges; there are no lessons to be learned, no parents to be abused and demeaned, and no fellow group members to regress with, fight with, or panic with. It is essentially boring but, at the same time, somewhat frightening. This one-on-one relationship is highly taxing; it appears so purposeless, lacks an agenda, and is especially mysterious because the whole of the community regards it as the central experience to be obtained at the Lodge. The patients will often deny this and talk about the usefulness of family therapy where they are brought closer to understanding or being understood by their parents, of group therapy where so many of their peer problems are worked out so dramatically, of the unit meetings where the system of privileges allows them to measure their progress through help and responsibility in a concrete way, of the special education where academic successes are fostered by the teachers and help to raise their self-esteem, and of their wonderful houseparents whom they begin to call "mom" and "dad" and treat with filial love and hate.

The place creates its own spirit, and certain cases are suited to certain places so that some sense of matching has evolved, but still far from precisely. Some adolescents, especially the younger, immature, and impulsive ones, may find themselves more at home in a children's unit, where the emphasis is on learning and mastery of techniques based on the principles of play, especially in terms of activities, and where insight is not at the heart of the treatment. This kind of ego-building, in a highly structured environment wherein *consistency* is the key word, has been successful with adolescent patients who are still striving to undergo latency and seemingly respond to latency techniques.

The generic milieu where adolescent and adult patients commingle, except in group therapy, and where the focus is on the adult–adolescent relationship, has been deemed suitable for adolescent patients who are psychotic, organically affected, or impulse ridden. It is claimed that this generic type of place is beneficial not only to the patients but also to the staff; the adults have a calming effect on the adolescents so the degree of turmoil is lessened. However, the energetic, provocative, and loud behavior of the adolescents may be hard for adult patients to take, and disturbed adult patients do not present good role models for the younger group. Those who favor this setting regard it as a richer and more realistic milieu but, on reading protocols from such environments, the arguments offered are post hoc because of the absence of adolescent and special school facilities. My own experience has been that apart from a few isolates who will cross the campus to seek out adult patients, the adults are glad, for good developmental reasons, to be exclusively together.

In the third type of facility, an adolescent world is created, with its own campus, its own school, its own residential units, and its own recreational opportunities. In this setting, borderline cases, affective disorders, and personality disorders are inclined to flourish and the general trend today seems to be toward the development of specialized adolescent units of this nature where group cohesion and group support play a vital part in the treatment.

THE LOGIC OF RESPONSE IN ADOLESCENT AND STAFF

Most of the adolescents who are admitted to hospitals manifest a serious ego weakness resulting in the continuing use of primitive defenses such as splitting, projective identification, denial, and acting-out. Certain consequences follow these tendencies:

1. There is a low tolerance of anxiety and frustration, with poor impulse control. This, in combination with a heightened drive pressure, is rapidly transformed into action that may be relieving for the patient but extremely troublesome for his environment.
2. The patients experience difficulty in taking responsibility for their feelings, their activities, and their lives.
3. Because of understandable counterreactions from the environment, the patients feel continually judged, exploited, victimized, and abandoned.

4. The splitting defense causes the patients to polarize people with whom they are in contact into "good" and "bad" individuals; because of superego projections, they themselves feel bad and worthless and they may try to compensate for this low self-esteem by developing grandiose and omnipotent fantasies in place of a realistic sense of competence and achievement; and because of their failure to neutralize sexual and aggressive drives, they are led into excesses of erotic and bellicose behaviors that still further lower their self-esteem, increase their sense of shame, depress them, and compel them to distract themselves through drugs, antisocial activities, and confrontations with authoritative figures. Since they are not able to learn from experience, this cycle often leads to repetitive, fruitless encounters.

There is also a logic of response, both conscious and unconscious, for the staff. It is surprising and uncanny how the staff may replicate parental and familial responses in their interactions with the adolescent patients. These responses are so compelling that they cannot be traced to factors of age, sex, or past experience. The more idiosyncratic types of staff reaction are traceable to resonances and reflections from their own adolescent experiences and to adolescent struggles with siblings and parents. The staff members may also react to the intensity of the adolescent, to what Anna Freud referred to as the iridescence, to the awful impulses at work at this stage, to the sense of urgency, and to the imperatives that drive the adolescent. Experience may lead them also to regard the adolescents as dangerous or as dangerous-seductive. They may, out of such fears, attempt to placate the patients in an effort to keep a good relationship going. The most disturbing experience for the community is when the splitting tendencies of the patient polarize the staff into good and bad figures, or into liked and hated ones, so that they become conflicted among themselves. Still another problem for certain staff is their inability to deal verbally with the patients. Words, in fact, seem to them awkward, unwieldy, and ineffectual, while action is commanding and gets things done. On an action–reflection spectrum, the patients stand heavily at one end and the staff may weaken and move helplessly toward the same side. At this point they may experience feelings of failure, exhaustion, and "burnout," or may resort to high-handed and somewhat punitive tactics. Staff members who become adept at dealing with the "here and now" and can confidently conduct "life space" interventions with patients "on the wing" are particularly useful in the therapeutic community.

THE FAMILY AS A MIRROR

Families of disturbed adolescents reveal complementary defensive structures and are equally engaged in continuous struggles over issues of autonomy and dependence. These struggles have their roots in shared unconscious fantasies that derive from parental internalized childhood experiences. "Splitting" occurs in all parts of the family so that there are good and bad parents, good and bad siblings, good and bad children. These distorted and polarized perceptions may not be characteristic of all family relationships at all times, but they appear to represent a pattern of family regression in the face of acute adolescent anxieties. The parents may equally engage in struggles with the unit administration that recapitulate the important family struggles, allowing the adolescent to observe and to learn during the family meetings. The staff may also be caught up with the parents in similar struggles, again allowing the child to observe and learn. The issues that are so acute in the current life of the adolescent may awaken smoldering and unresolved pathogenic conflicts from the parents' own adolescence struggle. Thus, the parents may often look at their adolescents and see remnants of themselves that they had quite forgotten about.

THE INTERACTIONAL NETWORK OF THERAPIES

The Chestnut Lodge experience provides, as previously noted, an Eriksonian moratorium for the adolescent patient in which experiments in thinking, feeling, and acting can be tried out in a safe and accepting environment before being put to the more demanding test of life. The experience requires conditions that are steady, stable, and secure and, especially, a sensitivity to the complex needs of confused and conflicted individuals. The therapeutic aims are to replace action with words, to help with the cultivation of relationships, and to meet some of the adolescents' dependent yearnings together with the rageful responses to them. If limits are set, they are imposed with understanding and not arbitrarily.

To carry out long-term treatment, a facility requires long-term staff, especially long-term therapists accustomed to long-term psychotherapy. This is true for individual, family, and group psychotherapists. Consistency also necessitates that long-term and short-term patients are not mixed in the same unit. In the cottages, the "family" cooks its own meals, does its own chores, and provides its own recreations.

The Chestnut Lodge tradition has certain characterizing emphases. It recognizes the primacy of the individual psychotherapy that the patient receives, insisting that this is where the deeper conflicts of the patient are worked through within a psychoanalytic frame of reference, and that through the psychotherapy, structural changes are made in the personality. It separates the role of therapist from that of administrator, to allow the therapist to work therapeutically unhampered and at the same time to keep a wary eye on the dangers of splitting that can act as a strong defense against the resolution of transference resistances.

In practice, the ancillary therapies are often given primary place by the patient, who may manifest a heavy resistance to the psychoanalytic process and experience it as unpleasantly intrusive, boring, unhelpful, and unconcerned with real-life issues. Some patients will talk of their therapeutic group with high approval, maintaining that the peer discussions are highly significant to their lives and deal with a stigma and shame of being psychiatrically hospitalized; of missing out on all the joys and excitements of adolescence in the outside world; of finding out who is relating intimately to whom at the present time. They will wonder why they were ever admitted, why they are still being kept in, and how they can ever get out (unless their insurance lapses). The groups at the Lodge are conducted along the lines of group analysis; focus is on the group process in both its manifest and latent forms. There is little doubt that the interpersonal behavior of the patient generally improves with the group experience.

Family therapy is valued as the primary experience. Family problems and current family relationships become the sources of acute tensions that occasionally disrupt the family meetings. The dynamic viewpoint deals with the here-and-now and makes little effort to uncover latent conflicts. Sometimes the parents are seen in couples treatment therapy but more frequently their therapy includes the adolescent patient. Administrative therapy occasionally dominates the psychological horizon of the adolescent patients who become engaged in a power struggle with the administrative psychiatrist, to whom they very easily transfer a lot of negative parental feeling because privileges are handled exclusive by the administrator.

Does this therapeutic interactional network succeed in practice? When functioning smoothly, that is, with minimal rivalry among the various therapists, the intrapsychic, the interpersonal, the familial, the psychoeducational, and the rehabilitative may work synergistically and the patients may appreciate the various therapy times. However, there is no question that when patients speak of a therapist, they are referring to their own individual therapist; when they speak of therapy, they are referring to individual therapy; and when they speak of not wanting to go to therapy, they are speaking of a resistance to the individual psychoanalytic approach. They regard the approach negatively because of its probing, its threat to their independence and autonomy, its demand for reflectiveness and introspection (which to many of them is anathema), and its exploration of intimacies (which is surprising because in the units and in the groups they will often talk profanely and in pornographic terms about sexual impulses). In the one-to-one situation, individual therapy becomes strangely scary.

When the inpatient sojourn is ended by general agreement among the therapists, the patient continues first as an outpatient with his individual therapist, and then as a private patient with the same individual therapist. In fact, the outpatient rarely seems to continue into private practice.

Termination most often comes by mutual agreement rather than as a natural ending of the long-term therapeutic process.

A CASE EXAMPLE

Lisa, age 16, transferred from another hospital that did not have the resources to treat her, and said so. She was the offspring of a mixed-religion marriage (Roman Catholic and Jewish) and was born, after considerable perinatal trauma, by cesarean section because her mother became toxic. She was 6 pounds 11 ounces at birth and jaundiced. As a small child she began having "spells." After investigation, a diagnosis of temporal lobe epilepsy was made and she was put on Carbamayepine. The parents, now ages 41 and 40, had divorced when she was eight and the father had taken up with a young and rather attractive girl. When I interviewed Lisa on admission, I thought that she fell into a borderline category on the more benign side of the continuum, and that her condition was complicated by the epileptic factor and its psychological repercussions, since it made her feel different and deviant. She told me that life had never been the same since her brother was born when she was four, and that her mother seemed to make him into a tin god. She had turned to her father for solace but, at the time, he was raging an ongoing battle with his wife and Lisa was often caught in the hostilities between them. She told me that if she was kept in the hospital, she would either run away or commit suicide. When she arrived for admission, the front of her clothing was drenched with tears. I received the impression of a very immature and frightened girl who had a great deal of underlying separation anxiety.

In family therapy, the parents continued their marital conflict and seemed more involved in this than in their unhappy daughter. Her openness in the unit was somewhat surprising. She had immediately told her roommate that she had a vaginal discharge and suffered from herpes—an announcement that caused alarm and repulsion among the other children. She then complained bitterly of being shamed, even though the revelation had come from her. She drank some cleaning fluid in a suicidal gesture.

In family therapy, it emerged that she felt damaged by her mother who had done everything good for her brother but had given her nothing except a defective brain. In her earlier years, she had been functioning at a superior intellectual level, but now she was more or less average. She felt that something had gone wrong with her, that her brain was addled. At times, it seemed that she could self-induce an epileptic seizure by hyperventilation and that she did this as an attention-seeking device. At other times, she would fake mental retardation, acting stupid and dragging one foot behind her.

In group therapy, she seemed confused about her sexual identity and would vaguely suggest that she was androgynous. She felt that people did not like her and that she did not know how to get them to like her. Her affects were labile but she could control herself and present a good facade of smiling equanimity that covered over her helpless and impotent rage.

The whole question of accepting help was at the core of her treatment. "I just want to be somewhere else than were I am," she said, in attempting to describe her restlessness. When asked about loving relationships in her life, all she could say was that she had never been number one for anybody. Her father had his "floozie" and her mother had her "wimp" of a son. All she experienced from her mother was a smothering, a suffocating mold that always attempted to make her what she was not and make her feel what she did not feel. She thought that her mother wanted to be a "dick" like her father and do better than him. Her father also wanted to run the show. "He thinks that just because he can put people to sleep [as an anesthesiologist] that he can knock me out too. He tells me that I am not going to run the show with him around, but he's the one that attacks me."

In group therapy, she said that her big problem was not being in with the right people. People did not like her because they were put off by her depression. "They don't like me when I am depressed and they don't trust me." She was outrageously flirtatious with the boys in the group (as well as outside the group) and took great pains about dressing up and presenting herself elegantly, often having to borrow clothes from others to do so.

In family therapy, her intense need to merge with either parent who would have her was very much to the forefront. As she approached her parents emotionally or physically, they would retreat behind some prohibition, criticism, or demand, but there was no consistency on their part, only conflict and remembered bitterness. The absence of warmth and affection was striking and she would sometimes turn to the family therapist and ask pathetically: *"You're* for me, aren't you?"

The administrator was struck by her immaturity, her abysmal self-esteem, her self-defeating proclivity, and her overall vulnerability. "She reaches out constantly but cannot accept the hand that you offer her," he said. She would run rapidly through her narrow repertoire of "little girl" flirtatiousness, suicidal threats, copious weeping, imperious demanding, and hopeless self-commiseration. "I'm so completely fucked up and none of my cuts have been healed." Yet, there was an appealing "black humor," a self-denigration that was much more Jewish than Italian. She had told her boyfriend, she said, that she was going to throw herself off the building, and he had said to her in return: "If you do that, I'll come to the funeral, open the casket and pee on your face." She laughed and remarked that this had put her off suicide.

Her individual therapist was a male psychoanalyst who had not previously treated an adolescent but had an adolescent daughter. Because, at the start of Lisa's treatment, she was thought to be at risk, the psychoanalyst saw her in her cottage and attempted to form a working relationship with her. She tried to make him into an ally who would help her to leave the hospital, but when he said that he was there to help her live more happily with herself, she became enraged and refused to see him until she was induced to do so by the administrator, who told her that her therapist was an "okay guy." She wondered whether she could see the administrator instead of the therapist but was told that one aspect of her treatment was dealing with her angry feelings for her therapist. "I'm angry with everyone," she said. "And that's it?" the administrator replied. "You need someone whom you can get angry with and who can help you with your anger." She decided to see her therapist.

After a brief phase in which she gave him a good deal of back history, the therapist questioned her about the details of her life, clearly at a loss to know how to begin with this moody girl. "I though that I would work within the limits of her comfort," he later explained. At first, he offered to drive her to his office at the other end of the campus, and she accepted, turning on his radio and telling him not to talk shop while they were driving. She was interested in his office and took down his pictures and examined them. He told her that they were reproductions by Picasso, and she asked who that was. She later wanted to walk back and so they took to walking across the campus. When they passed two other patients, she thought she hear them saying, "Look at that top-heavy bitch." She objected to the therapist's carrying an umbrella when it was drizzling, because people would think that he was queer. On one occasion following the session, he watched her clutch at the air with one hand and then hold it as if she had caught something. At first he thought this was an epileptic attack, but she told him that it was "Arthur," an imaginary insect that she always had with her to play with. He jokingly repeated the action and told her that he had caught "Alfred," and they both laughed. He felt that he was making headway, but soon discovered this was a very premature conclusion. She began to complain that she was bored coming to see him, that he was old, and that he had nothing interesting to show and tell. She became increasingly abusive and called him obscene names. "You're not sensitive. You don't know how to respond to me. You're just stupid." Her rage at him escalated and she once again complained to the administrator that she wanted a change of therapist. He encouraged her to continue, using a mild threat of privileges.

The analyst felt quite inadequate at this point and wanted to throw in the towel. He said that he did not know how to give her what she needed, and that he had no experience with adolescents.

After a lapse, she returned to give him "another chance." She asked him questions as if in a test and if he failed, as he generally did, she rejected him and told him that he was no good. She said that her administrator had told her that she had come back to therapy and that was the only reason that she was coming. She seemed very withdrawn from the therapist. He in turn went to his supervisor, who encouraged him to trust his therapeutic instincts and to be more spontaneous and less tight and controlled. "She is a human child—treat her humanly."

She was now clearly regressing in the treatment situation. She would sit or lie sucking her thumb and rubbing her eyebrow or twirling a piece of her hair. She would bring a small bear with her that had been with her since childhood and would snuggle up to it. She would chew little pieces of paper. She would play at times with "Arthur" and ignore the therapist. When he asked her for her fantasies, she said, "Bitch! If I told you, my dreams would go away, and then I would have nothing to look forward to."

At this time, she made a suicidal pact with two other girls and took some detergent fluid which made her sick. The therapist, once again, began to feel incompetent. The supervisor recommended a lighter touch, something playful and even humorous. When Lisa came in for her next session, she was carrying a book and at one moment she complained of feeling very depressed. "Even 'Arthur' has left me." The therapist inquired where he had gone, and she said to her father's home. She then assured him that "Arthur" was not real but only something that she imagined. He said that he understood that. Things began to get more heated and once again she attacked him, physically throwing a book at him but missing; the book landed on the floor. She said to him: "You pick it up." He stared at her smilingly and said: "Lisa, you must be kidding!" She seemed surprised, then turned to the "itsy-bitsy bear" that she had brought with her. After a while, she began to sob and presented a picture of almost total despair. He came and put an arm on her shoulder and asked: "Did your mother ever hold you?" She replied: "I hate my mother." She began to pick at her toenail and to wind the removed nail onto her finger. She said that her father would often do this for her. She held out her toe and the therapist said: "We must rush you to surgery!" She laughed and began to deal with him much more benignly. She said that her father had done many funny things with her and also told her a lot of very gross jokes. She then said to him appealingly: "You know, I want someone to beat the hell out of me, just like my father did. I just want to be beaten." This seemed to stem from a nuclear fantasy that had strong elements of the unresolved oedipal relationship with the father buried in it. Also stemming from it were her masochism and minor self-destructive tendencies.

Following this exchange, there was a breakthrough in her individual therapy. As a direct consequence, some of the immaturities in her behavior began to subside, her social contacts with her peers improved, she began to do better at school and to take more interest in her work, and she began to emerge in group, like a cicada coming out of a 17-year quiescence. She began to look less borderline and more neurotic, even though there seemed to be a strong mixture of preoedipal and oedipal dynamics. She was gradually becoming more popular in her unit and more accepted by the whole adolescent community.

Winnicott's playfully creative approach appears to have been the turning point in Lisa's therapy and, in bringing about the shift, to have affected all therapies in a synergistically positive manner. She said, insightfully, to her therapist: "I know we have fun together sometimes, but I also know that you take me seriously and I like that." As a strong therapeutic alliance and transference relationship developed, the therapist's countertransference was reduced and he began to feel more self-confident.

It is difficult to say of Lisa that there was a Mastersonian "natural therapeutic design," comprising a testing phase during which the therapeutic alliance was established by confronting her with the defenses against her feelings of depressed abandonment and dealing with these in memories, fantasies, dreams, and transference during the second phase. Lisa certainly did come face to face with hopelessness and helplessness and wishes for unconditional love, and she did verbalize the fantasy that if she dealt realistically with and separated from primary and transitional objects, she might well die or they might die. It's too early yet to say whether she will enter a final separation phase in which she is much better adapted, much less depressed, and on the way to becoming individuated. Again, in her insightful way, she talked about being a boy–girl and thought that this was why she had so much trouble with her menstrual periods.

CONCLUSION

Lisa is what we call a "good" Chestnut Lodge patient because her disturbance was of such an order and such a nature that she was gradually able to take full advantage of the therapeutic forces at work in the milieu, to use one therapy in the service of another, and yet, at the same time, to extract a maximal amount of therapeutic benefit from each therapeutic mode. This meant that as her neurotic and borderline processes were resolved in the daily psychoanalytic mode of treatment through full use of the transference, her peer relationships improved with the help of group therapy and her family relationships improved with the help of family therapy. She developed a warm relationship to the houseparent and when she was given privileges to go out, spoke of coming home. Adolescents in this type of setting have a second chance to rework their earlier conflicts within a holding environment peopled with understanding professionals whose purpose it is to make sense of the patient's life, offer him or her the sensibility that comes with ingoing therapy and raise the hope (that often looked previously as if it had been extinguished) for a brighter future.

CHAPTER TWELVE

Multicultural Aspects of Countertransference with Children and Adolescents in Milieu Settings

Deane L. Critchley*

* The author is grateful to Irving N. Berlin, M.D., for providing the clinical examples in this chapter.

Transference and countertransference feelings and thoughts are probably ubiquitous among human beings. They usually represent, in the present, unconscious and preconscious feelings, thoughts, and behaviors experienced with important people in one's childhood. The stimuli evoked in interpersonal relations are often similar to those experienced in childhood. For example, feelings, attitudes, and behaviors toward authority, especially toward one's supervisor, frequently occur because the supervisor reminds an individual of his or her parent. In a common countertransference experience, a child's behavior reactivates in an adult feelings the adult experienced as a child toward one parent or the other. Thus, an experience of reciprocal love between a child and a parent may flood the parent with loving feelings toward the child that are far in excess of a reaction to the child's actual behavior. Similarly, an angry, hostile child may cause an adult to withdraw or to feel retaliatory anger, depending on the adult's own recollected experience with angry parents.

In the milieu, countertransference reactions by staff members are common and may either be detrimental to the therapeutic work with the children or, if understood, may in fact enhance such work. In this chapter, countertransference is discussed theoretically as it relates to milieu treatment. Common countertransference issues that occur in the milieu setting are described, with special focus on multicultural issues. Finally, possible ways of dealing with countertransference within the milieu are suggested.

PAST EXPERIENCES AND PRECONCEIVED IDEAS AND FEELINGS

Most humans behave with others as they learned to behave in their early relationships with their parents, siblings, and other significant people in their lives. Their reactions to individuals and situations are largely the result of past learning and of the insights gained through life experience, education, and/or psychotherapy.

Children, adolescents, and milieu staff often have experienced similar life situations and may share similar preconceptions. Some of these include the following:

1. Children and adolescents often remind staff of aspects of themselves. They then react, or overreact, with anger or withdrawal or excessive comforting because of memories of how their parents and other significant adults responded to them and to their needs.
2. Prior experiences within a hostile, aggressive, and punitive family lead to distrust of others and easy arousal to anger and resentment.
3. In the absence of early attachment and nurturance as an infant and child, intimate relationships are frightening to contemplate and

difficult to achieve. A hunger for closeness and a fear of striving for it remain.

4. Experiences with overly lenient, unrealistically praising adults who were unable to be clear, firm, and truthful in their appraisal of efforts as a child may lead to an unrealistic view of one's efforts as an adult. One then tends to express warmth and praise toward a child or adolescent patient's behavior or productions, no matter what their merit, in a manner that is usually felt by others to be insincere. Such an adult typically uses the same exaggerated tone of voice he or she experienced as a child.

5. Children and adolescents, because of their egocentrism, often lack the capacity to "hear" adults. This "inattention" makes the children difficult for many staff to deal with in the home or to work with in treatment.

GENERAL THEORETICAL IDEAS

The concepts of transference and countertransference originated in psychoanalytic theory and were quickly incorporated as explanatory concepts in a variety of psychotherapeutic approaches. In its original context, transference described the patient in the analytic hour when he or she assigned to the analyst thoughts and feelings that previously were and presently are identified with significant people in the patient's life.

Transference was originally assumed not to apply in work with young children because their parents were alive and were part of the children's daily life. Therefore, children were not thought to transfer upon the therapist the attitudes, fears, desires, and wishes experienced with important figures from their past, as is characteristic in the treatment of adults.

It is now commonly accepted, as clarified by both Anna Freud (1946) and Melanie Klein (1932), that the transference experience with children is similar although not identical to that of adults. The child, like the adult, has no alternative but to project upon the therapist, in a disguised or not so disguised form, the attitudes, expectations, and feelings engendered in the child by both verbal and behavioral interactions with the parents. Especially transferred are those attitudes and feelings which are destructive, conflict-inducing, and threatening to the child and his or her development and which usually bring the child to therapy.

Kernberg (1976) described two concepts of countertransference, the "classical" and the "totalistic." In the classical concept, countertransference thoughts and feelings are aroused in the therapist by behaviors, thoughts, and feelings of the patient which bring into focus figures or events and experiences from the therapist's own past. The therapist needs to be aware of countertransference feelings so that they will not be acted upon and hinder the treatment. Alertness to and awareness of countertransference thoughts and feelings are useful in clarifying the meaning and context of the patient's behavior, which elicits the countertransference.

Through the use of countertransference data, one can better understand unexpressed feelings, thoughts, and attitudes of the patient that remind the therapist of attitudes or experiences with persons in his or her past.

In milieu settings, the totalistic concept of countertransference is very applicable; it is the total emotional response of the therapist or milieu worker to the patient. This concept includes both the conscious and unconscious reactions of the clinical worker to the real life behaviors of the patient as well as to his or her transferences. The concept of totalistic countertransference also permits discussion of how repressed and unresolved staff conflicts may be elicited by contact with certain patient behaviors and subsequently acted on in staff relationships.

An 11-year-old boy was admitted to the unit. He had regressed severely after losing his mother in an auto accident, which he witnessed. The milieu staff reacted in two quite different and exaggerated ways. On admission, the boy needed to be dressed, fed, taken outside, and led around to get exercise. The boy's frightened startle reactions and screaming when he heard very loud noises, or car tires screeching, or a child screaming, made staff feel helpless in their desire to comfort him. Part of the staff group felt certain that only by being loving, patient, and comforting would they help the boy. The other staff members felt equally strongly that only by requiring and demanding more age-appropriate behavior and insisting that the boy not scream in reaction to loud noises would he be helped.

The oversolicitous staff members had probably experienced exaggerated concern from their parents regarding their pains and hurts. As adults, they tended to overemphasize the debilitating effects of even minor illnesses. The "need to be tough" staff members feared regression. Some described their parents as having denied the reality of the child's pain and having made their signs of caring contingent on the child's denying the amount of pain or "being very brave." Each staff contingent felt anger toward the other group, certain that its own way was best. A middle-of-the-road approach was slowly worked out. Expectations of the boy were gradually increased and recurrent attempts were made to help him verbalize his panic and fear of loud noises and obtain comfort rather than scream. Much discussion time was spent in allowing staff to express their own feelings and to listen to each other.

Countertransference to Parents

The recognition in reality that work with children and adolescents necessarily includes the parents is the clinical reflection of the psychological reality of the parent–child unit within the transference and countertransference. This phenomenon is illustrated frequently when we observe how milieu staff working with children and adolescents commonly express fantasies of magically rescuing the child from the "pathology" or "neglect" of the parents. Such fantasies reflect the professionals' defense against the feelings of guilt and anxiety generated in reaction to the fantasied replacement of the child's parents and of "parents" more generally. Such fantasies usually reflect the professionals' need for an all-loving and all-giving parent as well as their need to show that they are better parents than were their own parents. These feelings may be reinforced if the child or adolescent responds to their nurturance and improves.

Such categorizations as good and bad, loving and rejecting, eager to help and uncooperative, which are used to subtly dichotomize treatment staff and parents, are current in some measure in all settings where children and adolescents are treated. Displaced feelings such as those described have been given support over the years by those who view the sick child as the helpless victim of psychological trauma inflicted by the parent. At its extreme, this view was expressed in the concept of the "schizophrenogenic mother." Although this concept and similar ones have been discounted, their emotional roots remain and continue to find expression within the countertransference.

Some of the many insurmountable difficulties that often beset the relationship between the real parents and the milieu staff can be linked to feelings similar to those just described. Generally, children who have endured a particularly unhappy life, for example, with a psychotic parent, or whose condition is due to physical or sexual abuse, call forth immediate pity. These children are more likely to evoke fantasies among the staff and concomitant rage against the parents. Sometimes the impact of a particularly traumatized and withdrawn youngster can evoke these feelings and fantasies in an entire staff with extraordinary swiftness and intensity.

Identification with the good and loving parent and the living-out of the magical helping fantasy often represent a useful attitude in milieu treatment. Therapeutic optimism and a willingness to begin treatment with youngsters with very severe pathology are typical results. However, when the expected change in the youngster does not appear, bewilderment and anxiety may arise, along with the helplessness that underlies every magical rescue fantasy. When the magic of the staff's "concern and caring behavior" does not work, the anger and disappointment elicited by the child cannot readily be displaced on parents who are not in sustained, daily contact with the youngster. New displacement objects may be sought. Certain staff who are perceived as having special relationships with the child, such as the child's primary milieu worker or the child's therapist, often become the focus of countertransference feelings. In such splitting, some of the staff generally hold unspoken thoughts such as, "If only he wanted to, he could really cure that child," or, "Why doesn't she work harder and do a better job of treating the child?" (Berlin, Boatman, Sheimo, & Szurek, 1951).

COUNTERTRANSFERENCE ISSUES IN THE MILIEU

Disagreement is expressed in the literature regarding whether counter-transference is a major factor in short-term milieu treatment of children and adolescents. Halperin et al. (1981) believed that brief inpatient treatment periods permit staff to adopt more objective and disengaged attitudes and do not allow staff to develop relationships that lead to unconscious reactions or intense affect.

Greenberg, Haiman, and Esman (1987) argued that equally intense countertransference occurs within staff who work with adolescents during acute hospitalization and that the unique constraints and demands of a brief hospitalization may actually exacerbate countertransference reactions.

A number of points are supportive of the position taken by Greenberg and her colleagues. Children and adolescents are more likely to express their sexual and aggressive feelings through their behavior than are adults. Exposure of the staff to such direct behavioral expressions of these feelings in children is much more likely to evoke painful memories from their past than are the same impulses expressed verbally as wishes or fantasies, as is more likely to occur with adults (Bettelheim, 1950; Redl & Wineman, 1957).

Second, in short-term milieu treatment, there is potential for staff frustration and burnout related to limited patient contact and stay, which often does not permit the staff to see major changes in the child prior to discharge (Nurcombe, 1989). When youngsters come and go quickly, staff members tend to use detachment and disengagement to defend themselves from getting too close to patients (Bonier, 1982). When anger, guilt, helplessness, and frustration color staff reactions to clients, countertransference is intensified. Without measures to help milieu staff deal with these feelings, the likelihood of reverberating and reoccurring countertransference reactions is enormous. If the issues are not dealt with around one client and family, they will arise around subsequent youngsters and families who activate similar feelings.

To understand the complexities of countertransference in milieu treatment, one needs to study the problems encountered in treatment, including treatment failure (Ekstein, Wallerstein, & Mandelbaum, 1959). The task is an unwelcome one, for a variety of reasons. First, no one likes to acknowledge either difficulties or failure. To reexamine a clinical process that in itself was painful and traumatic to all concerned is also painful. Largely, however, the reluctance stems from the discomfort of the experience, which reawakens painful failure experiences in the past and thus persists long after the patient has been discharged. In effect, countertransference creates a barrier to its own examination.

The essence of the milieu treatment process is that as each child or adolescent projects his or her needs, hurts, and distortions upon the milieu, by and large the staff members will need to find within themselves the under-standing and strength to resist slipping into the roles the youngster projects on them. To the extent that patients succeed in evoking from the staff the responses they evoked within their family, treatment will fail. The greater the child's disturbance, the more difficult it becomes to resist the push of countertransference and to resist emotional entanglement with the youth and family.

Younger disturbed adolescents and children evoke feelings of anger, re-taliatory hostility, indifference, and withdrawal from many adults. These same reactions commonly occur within milieu settings. In addition, violent, assaultive children and adolescents may evoke retaliatory anger and a sense of helplessness in many adults within the milieu. These feelings may then be acted-out toward the youth and family or in staff relationships (Berlin, Critchley, & Rossman, 1984).

Harry at 14 was a severe behavior disorder and was admitted following an attempted suicide. On the unit, Harry's skillful splitting of staff into good and bad guys and his unpredictable, violent outbursts of invective and assaultiveness made the diagnosis of borderline personality likely. Harry's repetitive behaviors in several residential settings as well as on the unit made him an unwelcome patient. Harry alienated most of the staff but he also successfully charmed a few staff who supported him. His behavior controlled the environment. In order to remove his control, a unit proce-dure was begun. Any effort by Harry to split staff, rage at or hurt peers or staff, or con others to escape responsibility for his acts was instantly met with team restraint and an escort to the quiet room.

Despite the effectiveness of this method with other borderline and narcissistic personality disordered adolescents, the staff were so enraged with Harry's unpredictable, vicious, and violent behavior that they wanted him out of the unit even before the method was tried. Nevertheless, a trial of the procedure was initiated. No matter what Harry said or did after his behavior initiated it, the restraint procedure was completed. Harry be-came wary of his actions and began to stutter in his effort to control his verbal abuse.

Harry's parents had given their consent to this procedure because noth-ing else had worked, and the hate he engendered in all adults raised their fear that he would end up being killed. By the end of a month, Harry's behavior was beginning to change. He looked more neurotic and sought out his therapist and milieu worker to talk for the first time.

One of the signs we look for as indicative of progress toward conflict resolution is a borderline child's or adolescent's ability to empathize with or express sympathy toward a peer. Harry's reaction to a suicide attempt by a new, very depressed girl was to look at the bandages on her wrists and to say, "Boy, that must hurt and you must have been in lots of pain to do that." Although Harry was repeating comments that he had heard from staff members, his voice sounded concerned. Days later, he was heard saying to this depressed young woman, "I think you can really get help here."

Feelings of anger and helplessness are commonly evoked by violent, assaultive youngsters, such as those who have been severely neglected or physically or sexually abused. A sense of helplessness often arises from the staff's inability to deal effectively with the impulsive and violent behavior. Suicidal and passive aggressive youngsters also evoke feelings of anger and helplessness. In his classic paper, "Hate in the Countertransference," Winnicott (1949) vividly described reactions to unpredictable, hostile, and "conning" behavior of youngsters. The violent youth has usually been severely abused, physically, sexually, and psychologically. Violence toward peers and adults is often a way of being in control of an environment in order to avoid being controlled by violent, abusive adults.

A major purpose of milieu treatment is to remove control of the environment from the youngster. Therapeutic, that is, nonretaliatory and sometimes noncontingent use of restraint and seclusion is also needed to help the patients realize they are no longer in control. The milieu becomes a "holding environment" (Winnicott, 1965); its structure and consistency provide the child or adolescent with opportunities to deal more positively with developmental crises and conflict resolution. The ultimate goal of milieu treatment, regardless of its length, is to positively enhance the "goodness of fit" (Chess & Thomas, 1984; Woolston, 1989) or the nature of the interactions between the child and his or her environment.

MULTICULTURAL ASPECTS OF TRANSFERENCE AND COUNTERTRANSFERENCE

When working with children or adolescents and families who come from cultures other than those represented by the majority of mental health professionals, it is critical to understand not only the traditional beliefs and customs of that culture but also its theories in relation to health and illness and intervention.

If one is a member of a prevailing or majority culture, it is far too easy to accept and express one's own cultural beliefs as universals and as "the truth," with the implication that beliefs and customs that are different are "strange" and "invalid." Prejudice, an almost universal phenomenon, is absorbed via one's family and community.

Multicultural Aspects of the Milieu

During short-term treatment, milieu staff need to have the ability to quickly establish therapeutic relationships with the patients and their families. They need a basic understanding of what symptomatic behaviors in the child or adolescent and what parental attitudes are culturally determined.

Common problems related to treatment staff prejudice involve hostility toward the family because of their refusal to acknowledge they are part of the youngster's problems and defensiveness about the patient's and family's initial lack of trust in the milieu staff.

Other countertransference issues that often arise include blaming parents for their youngster's difficulties, especially when the staff finds the child's behaviors particularly difficult to manage. When English is the second language for a family, parents' difficulty is communicating sometimes arouses feelings of anger and contempt in staff members. These feelings often result from the staff's inability to communicate milieu plans and to respond to the parents' questions about their child, and from their difficulty in engaging the parents in a collaborative effort to resolve certain issues involving the child or adolescent or to deal with situations such as passes. Many parents are reluctant to question aspects of the child's treatment even though they may not understand them. Difficulties such as these increase the staff's sense of helplessness with the family, further alienate the staff and parents, and increase the staff's prejudice against the family.

Some staff members perceive the family's wishes to include the use of native healers and the application of native herbs and treatments as a refusal to understand the "real" etiology of the problems. These staff members conclude that the family wants to avoid any real understanding of their child's problems.

Some parents may be substance abusers; others are not very well organized, or keep few appointments, or are difficult to engage. Staff members often write these families off as unworkable and give up, even though these may be the only families to whom the patients can return. Unfortunately, a vicious cycle occurs because the staff's covert contempt, anger, and prejudice encourage increased noncompliance by the family. Any of these countertransference feelings, if unrecognized and if not repetitively explored, will disrupt treatment. If unresolved, they lead to treatment failure.

Massive unemployment and poverty; disruption of the extended family; increasing divorce rates with more single-parent, female-headed families; alcoholism and drug use; chaotic family life-style—all of these contribute to the destruction of cultural traditions in Hispanic and Navajo families and affect the capacity for nurturance in these and Anglo families (Leighton & Hughes, 1961; Van Winkle & May, 1986). Unfortunately, treatment effectiveness is greatly reduced with such families. However, if one can find older, stable, tradition-oriented people such as tribal elders or godparents, who demonstrate sustained interest and have regular contact with the child or adolescent, treatment effectiveness is dramatically improved.

Dealing with Countertransference Issues in the Milieu

Unrecognized and unresolved countertransference feelings among milieu staff lead to increased anxiety and inappropriate and uncontrolled anger, which create an ever increasing psychological burden and burnout for staff.

The special stresses that occur in milieu settings demand supportive staff structures for containing and correcting destructive countertransference situations. In addition, these structures encourage staff members to monitor their own reactions to the youth and family, to ensure that they are accurately perceiving and interpreting the feelings and behaviors of both.

Of critical importance are the acceptance and acknowledgment by all milieu staff of the inevitable occurrence of countertransference. Only when such a philosophical orientation is acted upon rather than given lip service will staff members be able to explore the possibility of such feelings and behaviors without fearing that their existence denotes incompetence or "unprofessionalism."

Second, a milieu treatment staff needs to develop an overall philosophy and integrating theory that can encompass differing individual and family treatment, educational intervention, and psychopharmacologic and milieu approaches. An orientation that focuses on the interplay among specific developmental failures, their effects on the child's feelings, thinking, and behavior, and their impact on the milieu treatment staff will enhance staff awareness of critical issues for the clients and families as well as for the staff. This increased clinical sensitivity may then be used diagnostically to address both psychodynamic issues and their behavioral manifestations.

Once a treatment philosophy is developed, it can be used to address milieu issues from the perspective of both the child's or adolescent's treatment environment and the staff's working environment.

To create a milieu that is conducive to acknowledging and resolving countertransference issues, nursing administration and the unit leadership need to take steps to provide milieu staff with the time and space to deal with their own feelings and reactions to clients and their families and to other staff members (Critchley & Berlin, 1979). In this era of emphasis on cost containment and cost effectiveness, this may seem an impossible feat. However, there are a number of ways to work toward this goal:

1. Maintenance of a specific, specialized milieu staff to work with children and with adolescents;
2. Ongoing staff education, at all levels, dealing with developmental, psychodynamic, transference, and countertransference issues, and multicultural variables and their interactions;
3. Regularly scheduled conferences on evaluation, treatment planning, and clinical management for individual clients and families;
4. Regularly scheduled staff meetings to deal with specific milieu issues such as interstaff conflicts;

5. Ongoing, regular individual and small-group meetings with senior staff, in which milieu staff members are free to discuss their intense ambivalence and feelings of frustration and hostility toward difficult clients and families.

Staff meetings and clinical supervision are among the most effective tools available to help staff members deal with their own feelings and behavior. Staff members need to develop sufficient trust among themselves so that they feel more open to revealing and accepting supportive objective comments about their feelings and behaviors with each other and with the youngsters. Such a use of staff discussions is facilitated when staff members are provided with ongoing, regularly scheduled clinical supervision which helps them look at their own childhood relationships with significant others as they impact on the staff persons' current attitudes, feelings, and behaviors in the treatment setting (Critchley, 1987). When crises occur within the milieu or when "problem" patients are encountered, these discussions are also helpful to explore which components of staff reactions in these situations are derivatives of their countertransference attitudes.

Certain feelings and behaviors that arise frequently and always need discussion and resolution are those related to staff members who have themselves experienced physical, sexual, or psychological abuse or have been substance abusers. These staff are most at risk when working with children and families with similar problems. If staff members are not helped to deal with their own issues, especially the pain they experienced and their resulting hate and mistrust of others, they will be unable to work effectively with those who have experienced similar problems.

Anita, an 11 1/2-year-old Hispanic girl, was hospitalized after taking all of her mother's Valium in a suicide attempt. Anita had been sexually abused by an uncle since she was 2 1/2 years of age. Her sexually provocative behavior with males, seductive looks, and touches resulted in further sexual abuse. Her suicide attempt occurred when her girlfriends at school ostracized her after she made a "pass" at one of her friends' boyfriend.

On the unit, Anita could not help but be seductive with male staff and peers. To several male and female staff members, this blatantly sexualized behavior in one so young was so disturbing that they wanted to have her sent to the state psychiatric hospital despite the fact that the treating hospital ran a program for sexually abused girls and boys of all ages.

In both staff discussions and supervisory sessions, it became clear to some staff members that Anita's seductiveness aroused feelings of envy in several female staff. Many of these women, raised in households where sexuality was repressed, felt constricted about sexual matters. Some of the male staff members perceived Anita's seductive behavior as a threat and were fearful they might lose control of their impulses. These men could also recall seductive behavior exhibited by their mothers or sisters, in their dress or lack of it, as well as these women's forbidding anger if, as boys, the men became aroused and demonstrative.

The attitude of most of the staff toward Anita's mother was one of great anger for permitting her brother to abuse Anita, despite the mother's ignorance of these events and her prompt action when told about it. Some staff saw in the mother's sedate manner some sexual overtones. The emergence in the present of old sexual conflicts interfered with the staff's perceptions of both Anita and her mother and thus their ability to work with them effectively.

Ongoing discussions dealing with both the theoretical issues of countertransference and the issues aroused by specific youngsters are required to help staff members understand the difference between their perspectives and the youngsters'. For example, a youngster may at one moment be laudatory and loving toward a staff member but may quickly and inexplicably move to verbal and physical assault of the same person. Because they see their own behavior as relatively constant, staff members are often at a loss to understand the youngster's shifting perceptions. Staff need to be helped in their struggle with their reactive feelings of anxiety, hurt, and anger. It is helpful at such times to clarify how the child's or adolescent's past experiences with adults have fostered a perception that they are inconsistent, unpredictable, and untrustworthy. Such perceptions lead the youth to believe that only being tough and aggressive will prevent others from inflicting hurt or taking advantage. In turn, this line of reasoning leads the youth to believe that changing his or her behavior is for someone else's benefit, and that it is better to con the staff to make them perceive a behavior change because somehow this perception will keep the youth in control.

Staff members must understand how the client's and family's projections, while unreal, are vital aspects of the therapeutic process. Positive transference is part of the motivation to trust the staff, to view them as benign and helpful, and to begin the work of treatment. When positive transference is lacking, as with clients who have never developed trust, the clients' view of staff members from the outset may be hostile. Staff members need assistance to become aware of how a patient's behavior is demonstrating positive or negative transference and of ways to deal with the transference in order to facilitate treatment. One can, for example, ask mistrustful children to critically examine staff behavior to determine whom they can trust.

CONCLUSION

Countertransference reactions within the milieu are to be expected. Milieu staff need to understand both the dynamics of the phenomenon and how to use it effectively in their work with patients and families.

This chapter has dealt with a range of treatment variables and their implications for countertransference in the milieu treatment of children and adolescents. Clinical examples provided illustrations of typical countertransference reactions. Mechanisms such as splitting, projective identification, and intense displacement are reactions commonly experienced by milieu staff. Feelings that would be minimal or could be avoided in outpatient treatment are intensified in milieu treatment. Expectations and disappointments are intensified as well.

An understanding of the multicultural variables that add complexity to the psychodynamics of the interactive process is critical. Countertransference reactions are also triggered by cultural variables and need to be recognized and resolved in order to promote effective treatment.

Staff burnout is much greater if countertransference problems are not recognized and resolved. The inevitability of countertransference reactions must be acknowledged and specific steps taken to increase the likelihood that countertransference can be used to enhance rather than hinder the treatment process. Supportive structures that will help staff recognize and resolve their countertransference reactions are necessary in milieu settings, to enhance therapeutic effectiveness.

REFERENCES

Berlin, I. N., Boatman, M. J., Sheimo, S. L., & Szurek, S. (1951). Adolescent alternation of anorexia and obesity. *American Journal of Orthopsychiatry, 21,* 387–419.

Berlin, I. N., Critchley, D. L., & Rossman, P. G. (1984). Current concepts in milieu treatment of seriously disturbed children and adolescents. In M. Shore & F. Mannino (Eds.), *Psychotherapy of children: Vol. 1. Psychotherapy: Theory, research and practice* (pp. 118–131). Washington, DC: American Psychiatric Association.

Bettelheim, B. (1950). *Love is not enough.* Glencoe, IL: Free Press.

Bonier, R. J. (1982). Staff countertransference in an adolescent milieu treatment setting. *Adolescent Psychiatry, 10,* 382–390.

Chess, S., & Thomas, A. (1984). *Origins and evolution of behavior disorders from infancy to early adult life.* New York: Brunner/Mazel.

Critchley, D. L. (1987). Clinical supervision as a learning tool for the therapist in milieu settings. *Journal of Psychosocial Nursing and Mental Health Services, 25,* 18–22.

Critchley, D. L., & Berlin, I. N. (1979). Day treatment of young psychotic children and their parents: Interdisciplinary issues and problems. *Child Psychiatry and Human Development, 9,* 227–237.

Ekstein, R., Wallerstein, J., & Mandelbaum, A. (1959). Countertransference in residential treatment of children. *Psychoanalytic Study of the Child, 14,* 186–218.

Freud, A. (1946). *The psycho-analytical treatment of children.* London: Imago Publications.

Greenberg, L., Haiman, S., & Esman, A. (1987). Countertransference during the acute psychiatric hospitalization of the adolescent. *Adolescent Psychiatry, 14,* 316–331.

Halperin, D., Lauro, G., Muscone, F., Rebhan, J., Schnabolk, J., & Schachter, B. (1981). Countertransference issues in a transitional residential treatment program for troubled adolescents. *Adolescent Psychiatry, 9,* 559–577.

Kernberg, O. (1976). *Borderline conditions and pathological narcissism.* New York: Jason Aronson.

Klein, M. (1932). *The psychoanalysis of children.* London: Hogarth Press.

Leighton, A., & Hughes, J. M. (1961). Cultures as causative of mental disorders. In A. Leighton & J. M. Hughes (Eds.), *Causes of mental disorders: A review of epidemiological knowledge* (pp. 131–148). New York: Milbank Memorial Funds.

Nurcombe, B. (1989). Goal-directed treatment planning and the principles of brief hospitalization. *Journal of the Academy of Child and Adolescent Psychiatry, 28,* 26–30.

Redl, F., & Wineman, K. D. (1957). *The aggressive child.* Glencoe, IL: Free Press.

Van Winkle, W. W., & May, P. (1986). Native American suicide in New Mexico, 1957–1979: A comparative study. *Human Organization, 45,* 293–301.

Winnicott, D. W. (1949). Hate in the countertransference. *International Journal of Psychoanalysis, 30,* 60–75.

Winnicott, D. W. (1965). *The maturational process and the facilitating environment: Studies in the theory of emotional development.* New York: International Universities Press.

Woolston, J. L. (1989). Transactional risk model for short and intermediate term psychiatric inpatient treatment of children. *Journal of the Academy of Child and Adolescent Psychiatry, 28,* 38–41.

CHAPTER THIRTEEN

Multicultural Issues in the Milieu Treatment of Violent Children and Adolescents

Irving N. Berlin

No child or adolescent elicits from the inpatient staff as much hate and anger or as many feelings of violent retaliation and helplessness as the hostile aggressive child or adolescent. Many of these youngsters, even though only 8 or 9 years old, have an uncanny skill to split staff, to cause staff to fight with each other, and to avoid responsibility for their actions. These behaviors frustrate staff efforts to be helpful.

Unless both the child's transference feelings and the staff's counter-transference feelings are constantly dealt with, the patient, by his or her behavior, remains in control. According to Winnicott (1945), the ability to "hate objectively" and, thus, to "act decisively" in most instances is not realized.

From the work of Kernberg (1979), Kohut (1972), Masterson (1972), Rinsley (1980), Mahron (1982), and Offer, Ostrov, and Howard (1984) in self psychology, and that of Friedman, Arnoff, Clarkin, Corn, and Hurt (1983), Mahler and Kaplan (1977), and Stern (1982) in infant and child development, comes an understanding of the etiology of some of these severe and trying disorders. Nielson (1983), Keith (1984), and others who have been associated with secure treatment of these violent children and youths, have clinically validated the development of borderline and narcissistic children. Their work is a beginning for both understanding these children and thinking through some possible treatment approaches (Bleiberg, 1984).

The developmental problems appear to center on the separation–individuation stage of development. The practicing substage, the rapprochement phase, and, especially, the rapprochement crises seem to have been particularly poorly worked through. According to these authors' description of the practicing phase, the child experiences a mother whose symbiotic ties are so great that the child's experimenting with new discoveries and exploring a new world to find out how everything works are sharply restricted. In contrast to the "normal" child, whose parents dote on him or her and praise every new discovery, such as finding out how to turn the lights on and off, the symbiotic mother can neither allow such freedom nor praise the exploration and new discoveries.

During the rapprochement crisis, the mother is unable to succor the child when it experiences periods of high anxiety. The symbiotic mother feels threatened by any separation or observation of the child's taking pleasure in new discoveries and becoming master of its universe. Thus, the mother not only thwarts separation–individuation efforts, but is withdrawn, nonsupportive, and punitive about any pleasures the child shows toward mastery; the child's anxieties are met with anger and hostility. Since healthy separation is thwarted, the child appears fixated at the point of trying to establish autonomy and separation. The child has no real sense of a separate self. In the face of the mother's controlling behavior, the child may feel angry, depressed, and helpless. The child certainly feels very hostile toward the rejecting mother and the rage, combined with her image, is internalized and forms a hostile introject. These feelings toward the symbiotic mother, which risk further loss of all support from her, are unconsciously kept from awareness. The child then has to live with the unconscious images of a good and bad mother, the origin of the need to split people in the environment and individuals in closer interaction into good and bad persons. However, feelings of depression and worthlessness are increased. To defend against the severe and painful depression, the child may project the bad introject of the mother on individuals in the environment and attack them. Both Keith (1984) and Nielson (1983) described this defensive maneuver as the fundamental dynamic that fuels the violent acting-out. The critical separation-individuation issues brought to the fore by the onset of adolescence serve to greatly amplify the previous problems and the need to split others, to never be satisfied with what is offered, or to be unpredictably violent. The seductive adulation of one moment reflects the need to be liked and cared about; the hateful behavior of the next is unconsciously designed both to deny the need for the caring and to test the caring. A repetition of previous experiences with the mother not only reinforces the poorly experienced separation-individuation process but also thwarts the achievement of object constancy, a contributor to the testing process just described.

Early abuse may interfere with the attachment process, especially where one or both parents have been alcoholic, depressed, or schizophrenic. Thus, many children have experienced both very early neglect and later abuse (Lewis, Pincus, Shanok, & Glaser, 1983; Lewis, Feldman, & Barrengos, 1985).

The early experiences of many borderline children include being totally controlled by adults through fear of physical hurt or sexual abuse. Later, these children are controlled through a symbiotic process whereby the disturbed parent cannot permit the child's independent functioning for fear of losing control over the child's behavior. Parents may especially need to keep the child physically close and, thus, to validate the parents' importance to the child (Imber, 1984; Noshpitz, 1984).

It is extremely difficult to plan a treatment program in the milieu to deal with the violent child's overwhelming distrust of adults, rapidly vacillating love–hate relationships, and unprovoked and often unanticipated violence. The degree of control that the patient exercises over the environment and in the therapeutic relationship with the psychotherapist by such behavior is one of the critical issues (Benalcazar-Schmid & Berlin, 1986; Rosenthal & Doherty, 1985).

The child's transference projections and the staff's countertransferences are major milieu problems; overcoming them can become a major objective. Some experienced staff members may confront both the adulation and overwhelming anger as unrealistic behaviors, without reacting personally to the patient's attitudes. Over time, such confrontations may be effective. Staff who are not too overwhelmed by a violent young person's behavior can sometimes ask the young person what beliefs and feelings, in their opinion, underlie certain behaviors, especially their hostility and violence. For the first time, the child or adolescent may begin to feel that someone understands the turbulent feelings beneath his or her behavior and the yearning for unambivalent and continuous nurturance. Such clearly enunciated insights into the patient's actions may also, in time, become effective in reducing both the angry and the seductive behaviors. The need to control others in order to feel safe and unlike the small child of the past who was hurt and controlled by adults is not easily dealt with (Bettelheim, 1967).

As a first step in trying to contain the violent borderline, conduct-disordered, or antisocial young adolescent, the staff should try to eliminate the patient's use of violence as a way of controlling any environment, wherever he or she might be. A new patient should receive a careful explanation that any behavior that is a threat or a con, any avoiding of responsibility for behavior, or any conduct that sets other patients off to behave in a violent or antisocial way will lead to instant isolation in the quiet room. As many staff as are required should be used to bring an assaultive patient to the quiet room. The aim of this treatment is to help the patient to become aware of the antecedent tension, feelings, and thoughts that resulted in violent behavior so that they can control themselves and not require others to bring them under control. Only the inevitability of clear consequences for aggressive, violent behavior leads to the development of anxiety and a capacity to look within, as the young person perceives that previous controlling mechanisms do not work.

SOME MULTICULTURAL ISSUES

Several issues around violent behavior in young male adolescents relate to their particular cultural backgrounds. Many Hispanic male adolescents who come from Hispanic communities that have gangs learn that fighting and being violent and assaultive toward authority figures or toward other adolescents are considered macho by the gang and sometimes by the male parent. Hispanic mental health workers and professionals can be effective in helping the adolescent and his family to examine some origins of such behavior and its possible end result. The milieu's methods of dealing with violent assaultive behavior can reduce that behavior and help the Hispanic youth to find, through athletics, music, school, or leadership in group activities, other ways to feel effective and competent. These methods are especially effective as the boys begin to relate to particular unit staff members and seek to please them and to model their attitudes and behavior after them.

Among some American Indian tribes, there are few operative cultural traditions. The various clans and extended family groups are not available to initiate ceremonies of puberty and adolescence, and to define the new responsibilities which young adults should be given. There are also few models of effective traditional adults. Adolescents may thus grow up without many behavioral constraints and with alcoholic adults as their models.

Thus, in many tribes and pueblos, alcoholism among parents who tend to physically and sexually abuse their children and adolescents may lead to their children's becoming depressed or violent in reaction to such treatment. When the treatment of a depressed adolescent becomes effective, the underlying hatred and anger may emerge as violence. Such violence can usually be contained in the therapeutic work, using both individual and milieu therapy. Indian youths who are hospitalized because of their violent behavior and substance abuse require some help from an elder of their tribe to learn what is really expected of them by the tribe and to feel that, with help in the hospital, they can become a valued member of the tribe. When such help from a tribe is not forthcoming and the parents will not participate in family therapy, little that is of therapeutic value occurs in the hospital.

THE IMPACT OF MILIEU PRACTICES

The prejudicial feelings of staff and other patients may also precipitate violent behavior. The following vignettes describe two different kinds of violent behavior stemming from similar abuse in childhood.

The Case of Allen

Allen, a 13-year-old boy from a southwest pueblo, had been physically abused by an alcoholic father since age 1 ½. Allen's mother drank, though not quite as much as his father; she also was abused by the father and could not defend her son. Allen was 5'8" and weighed 180 pounds. He had been hitting children and teachers since he was in the third grade. A few months prior to Allen's hospitalization, he beat up an abusing uncle who had cared for him after his parent's death. (His parents had died in a drinking-related auto accident a year before.) His attack on a tribal police officer, who was returning him to a group home from which he had run away, led to his hospitalization.

Allen was hospitalized with the proviso that there would be weekly visits by a social worker and an elder who would assume the role of Allen's *tribal advocate,* a program recently begun by the court and social services in that pueblo (Manson, 1982). The social worker promised a decision with regard to a discharge plan, targeted for six months after Allen's hospitalization; a couple in the pueblo would be sought to become the foster parents to this large, strong, impulsive boy.

In the cottage for 13- and 14-year-olds, Allen was the biggest and strongest and one of the most impulsive adolescents. There was a question of how he would be contained; only one of the male child-care staff was his physical match. The cottage clinician, a child psychiatrist, and the cottage staff coordinator, an M.A. in counseling, wisely chose a very petite, pretty, young woman as Allen's individual staff person and a young, male, child psychiatry trainee as his individual therapist. It was hoped that Allen would not attack his female staff person when she had to confront him with an uncompleted task or an aggressive behavior toward his peers.

Allen quickly dominated the cottage after knocking down the cottage leader. When his female staff person told him to stop his aggressive behavior and to study rather than to just sit in school, Allen laughed and said, "What are *you* going to do about it?" On a particular day, Allen would not accompany the female staff person to his room or stay on room restriction. During a meeting, the staff decided that Allen had to experience real, but not retaliatory or punitive, consequences for his behavior. The cottage coordinator, a tall, thin man, called in the milieu director, who was a specialist and trainer in nonpunitive physical restraint. When the milieu director understood the problem. he quickly gathered together two more staff and the coordinator; all were trained in physical restraint. They worked out a signal system that would bring them to the cottage, and additional early evening and night restraint teams were activated.

The day restraint team did not have to wait long for action. That afternoon, Allen struck a peer who would not yield to him in the lunch line. The team quickly came and together they approached Allen. In an instant, he was lying spread-eagled on the floor. The team members were in complete control. Restraining one of Allen's arms, the cottage coordinator pointed out that, first, they would not hurt him but intended to keep him on the floor until he could control himself, and, second, that this would occur every time he hit someone, broke the rules, refused to work in school, or otherwise became violent.

In the next four days, Allen experienced 13 restraints in various settings—cottage, school, cafeteria, and campus. He was aware that he was never hurt, but learned that he would not be permitted to use his strength to control others.

Allen grew to like his young therapist, who sympathized with his terrible early life and taught him to play games. For the first time in his life, he played dominos, checkers, and board games, which he was capable of enjoying like a small child. Because the restraint team reacted so rapidly and in unison to Allen's threats, he was thwarted in any attempt to beat up anyone. Allen began to complain that he was losing face by the restraints, which left him helpless. His therapist offered a suggestion: When Allen felt he was losing control, he could ask to go to the quiet room for

15 minutes or until he regained control; thus, he would both exercise self-control and save face.

Because Allen did not recognize his own welling-up of anger or his readiness to strike out, the staff cued him in to the feelings he seemed to be showing them. At first, he looked anxious and suspicious when a staff member told him he was showing signs of becoming angry. However, he controlled himself most of the time so that he would not be restrained, and gradually avoided violent behavior. He began to learn to trust the staff members' observations, especially those of several staff toward whom he was developing friendly feelings. Eventually, Allen identified his own early cues of tension and quickly asked for the quiet room. Over a period of six weeks, Allen slowly gained control of himself. His self-control made it possible for him to learn to play effective basketball and volleyball. He began to achieve in school and received a great deal of praise. He formed friendships with several residents of the cottage; one became his "girl-friend." He spent a great deal of time with his primary staff person, who warmly congratulated him each time he avoided trouble. He also regarded his therapist as a wise and helpful friend to whom he could bring his troubles, for problem solving together.

During this period, the social worker and the tribe elder visited Allen every week. They had a family-like conference at which Allen could talk about his hatred toward his father, mother, and uncle without fear of being rebuked for parental disrespect or disrespectful language. As the social worker and elder noted Allen's improvement, especially his efforts to avoid serious problems of assault on his peers and staff, they began to express their approval of his new wisdom. They recognized that violence had been the method Allen had used to control a hostile and noncaring environment and that control in the hospital setting had to be dealt with as the first phase of treatment. When Allen was discharged at the end of 6 months, he went to live with the elder who was his advocate and his wife. He has continued to do well in school. The pueblo has promised to finance his college education since he has continued to get good grades in the pueblo high school. There has been no further violence.

In Allen's case, as in others, once an adolescent's control over the environment is no longer possible, changes in attitude, new learning, and increased trust in others slowly emerge. The assertion of benign (not hurtful) parental control allows some restructuring of the personality to occur.

The Case of Pablo

Pablo, a 14-year-old Hispanic boy, was hospitalized after a frenzy of hostile, violent behavior toward his abusing father and deriding older brother. Pablo broke his brother's arm and knocked his father unconscious with a serious depressed skull fracture. He used the baseball bat that his father had often used, to beat him on his body and legs.

Pablo was known alternately as a quiet, cooperative teenager who could do well in school for teachers who evidenced their interest and were pleased with his efforts. When teased by his peers, by his brother, or, on one occasion, by a *cholo* gang, his extraordinary frenzy of violence frightened everyone and they began to leave him alone.

At 14, Pablo was 5′9″ and weighted 190 pounds. He was an all-state tackle in his first year in high school.

The attack on his father and brother occurred when the father slapped the mother for demanding money and the brother laughed; he and the father had been out on a drinking spree the night before. Pablo could only state that, in an angry fog, he grabbed the bat and lashed out.

Pablo, his brother, and his younger sister had all suffered severe physical abuse when his father was drunk. His mother passively protested but did nothing about it.

Because of the episodic nature of Pablo's violence, a psychiatric and neurological work-up was indicated. There was some apprehension on the young adolescent unit about admitting someone who had been so violent, but the general feeling was that Pablo could be helped.

Pablo willingly signed himself into the hospital, somewhat shaken at the terrible results of his violence. After two weeks, the father was discharged from the general hospital. The mother, older brother, sister, and Pablo then met in family therapy. The father had to work out a time when he could be away from his work as a machinist; it was four weeks before he joined family therapy. The father was very angry about the discussions that had occurred previously, mainly concerning his drinking and physical abuse of his children and wife. He maintained that Hispanic men ruled their families and could treat them any way they wanted. When asked if this permission meant that he could get his family to hate him so much that one member crushed his skull and others had, from time to time, threatened to leave home or to kill him, the father grunted, "Well, that wasn't good," under the angry eyes of his family.

On the unit, Pablo flourished. He did well in school, liked his teacher and aide, and felt close to the male mental health worker, a fine athlete whom he admired. The first incident of violence occurred when the unit acquired Sandy, a borderline 13-year-old boy who taunted everyone and hit some staff and, more frequently, peers. At the same time, Hal, a new mental health worker, was hired—an Anglo man in his forties who, after 10 years as an army medic, returned to civilian life and worked effectively in several residential treatment centers.

With consummate skill, the borderline youngster made cutting and anti-Hispanic remarks to Pablo where few others could hear him. He flattered Hal, who also made anti-Hispanic remarks toward Pablo.

After a week of these insults, Pablo walked up to Sandy and hit him several times, knocking him down. Hal came to Sandy's aid and also got slugged and hurt. There was general chaos but Pablo followed his mental health worker to the quiet room.

In the effort to process these events, staff commented on Sandy's teasing Pablo and on Hal's anti-Hispanic comments. A number of questions were raised about how to work with all three individuals.

Violence resulting from the baiting of others by borderline adolescents was not new. At issue was how to work with all persons concerned. It was agreed that if Sandy covertly bad-mouthed Pablo, Pablo was to tell Sandy's mental health worker, who would without any discussion isolate Sandy. Any public bad mouthing, conning, or disruption caused by Sandy would result in his prompt isolation.

Hal was seen by the unit chief and the unit milieu coordinator together. They tried to help him see that he had been manipulated by a borderline adolescent who was skilled in such manipulation and asked whether he had any awareness of anti-Hispanic, anti-Indian, or anti-black feelings and attitudes. He admitted that his family and community in West Texas were very prejudiced, but said he had tried hard in the army to get along with all the minorities. He promised to try to become aware of his feelings and was informed that he would be closely monitored and supervised during his probationary period.

Pablo met with his staff person and the unit coordinator, who made clear that he was to be censured for hitting Sandy and Hal. Although perhaps justified in his anger, he would be penalized by being demoted from level 3 to level 2 in the behavioral management program. (Level 3, the highest level, indicated exemplary behavior in all activities and leadership in group programs and resulted in many privileges and freedom of the hospital grounds.) This enabled Pablo to feel understood but he also felt hurt that, despite exemplary previous behavior and being set up by Hal, his violence had led to a consequence. He was able to begin to talk with his therapist about the hate he felt toward his father and toward everyone who teased him and hurt his feelings. His rages at such times scared him. Through the therapy and the ability to turn to his milieu staff person when he began to feel upset and angered, he was able to contain his violence.

In family therapy, the anger Pablo and his sister felt toward their mother for her helpless retreat when they were abused by their father began gradually to emerge. The mother's background as an abused child was revealed. She feared that nothing less than killing her husband would help, because calling the police had not changed things when her husband hit her early in their marriage and later hit their first son. As the father became aware of how much hatred and murderous feeling his drunken assaults on his family members had caused, he became acutely afraid that he might lose his family and he began to attend AA meetings.

Pablo's hospitalization continued for 6 months. His only other violent episode was in defense of a younger boy who had been attacked by a newly admitted, violent, psychotic adolescent. On discharge, Pablo had learned to control his anger and to think through the alternatives that were open to him when he was teased. He had done exceptionally well in every activity including school and was idealized as a model by other male adolescents.

DISCUSSION

Children and adolescents who have suffered serious physical abuse tend toward violent acts themselves. It is not an accident that 65% to 75% of inmates in state and federal prisons for violent crimes against persons suffered severe physical abuse in childhood (U.S. Department of Justice, 1986). Because the number of violent youths is increasing, adolescent units are finding it necessary to develop methods of handling violent, conscience-less patients.

Violence, as seen in the children's psychiatric hospital setting, is noted mostly in Anglo youth because the number of Anglo patients is above 50% of the hospital population. By contrast, 70% of the prison population is Hispanic, black, and Indian. Borderline and narcissistic personality disorders are frequently admitted for hospital treatment; they too are mostly Anglo and have not yet come into contact with the courts. Additionally, more minority adolescents and adults arrested, prosecuted, and jailed than are Anglos, especially middle-class Anglos (U.S. Department of Justice, 1986).

Hispanic youths who are violent experience both severe physical abuse and sanction for their violent acts, in their gangs and, perhaps, at home. Violent acts usually occur after heavy drinking. These youths seem to have an open hunger for relationships and caring by others, which makes treatment more likely to be effective.

American Indian patients come to our hospital from various tribes and pueblos in the state. Two of the tribes were formerly very warlike. The forced living on the reservation, the destruction of their culture and traditions, and the lack of employment, which might have replaced hunting as a means of providing for the tribes, make the adults bitter, angry, and alcoholic. Violence against friends while drinking is common among the families of the adolescent population of these tribes. There is less overall violence among the Pueblos and other tribes, but the increased general unemployment and alcoholism among adults and the chaotic family units spawn abused, neglected, and sexually abused children, some of whom tend to be violent as a way of protecting themselves from further abuse by adults.

As mentioned earlier, the tribes need to be more concerned with finding adequate adult models for adolescents, if their traditions are to be carried on. A number of tribes have initiated efforts to deal with poverty, unemployment, family disintegration, alcoholism, and violence against self and others. Some of these efforts have been effective in restoring family cohesion. They have begun to emphasize tribal traditions on one hand, and are dealing with employment by using Anglo techniques of creating businesses, small industries, and farming cooperatives on the other. Young people from these tribes have the most hope for the future.

CONCLUSION

The individual dynamics leading to violent behavior are essentially similar in children and adolescents of all races, but some multicultural factors must be acknowledged and given special vigilance by the hospital milieu staff. The prejudices of milieu staff against American Indians, Hispanics, blacks, and other minorities will aggravate violent behavior and delay the therapeutic effectiveness of a milieu intervention program and of family and individual therapy. Prospective milieu staff must be screened vigilantly so that those hired are minimally prejudiced and, even more important, are open to discussion of their feelings and beliefs both in the milieu meetings and in individual or group supervision. Only then can continued learning occur.

The development of a behavioral program that includes isolation and restraint where necessary is important. Violent youths must not be allowed to control the environment. When an adolescent can no longer use violence, cunning, and flattery, and is unsuccessful at splitting staff and individuals into good or bad persons to respond to the pathology of the moment, he or she becomes more responsive to a therapeutic milieu. An increase in anxiety usually indicates that the process of controlling others is ineffective. The anxiety then motivates the adolescent to participate in individual or family therapy. The next likely steps are to engage in the treatment programs, to participate in the milieu program, to begin learning in school, and to becoming socialized and responsive to peers. This is a difficult and very demanding program for the milieu staff. The extra efforts required initially to restrain and isolate violent adolescents, when carried out with consistency, seem like one of the few ways to help these youths to make some character changes.

REFERENCES

Benalcazar-Schmid, R., & Berlin, I. N. (1986). Violence in the hospitalized adolescents: Some considerations in the management of aggression in the long-term hospital unit. *Bulletin of the Menninger Clinic, 50,* 480–490.

Bettelheim, B. (1967). *The empty fortress.* New York: Free Press.

Bleiberg, E. (1984). Narcissistic disorders in children. *Bulletin of the Menninger Clinic, 48,* 501–517.

Friedman, R. C., Arnoff, M. S., Clarkin, J. F., Corn, R., & Hurt, S. W. (1983). History of suicidal behavior in depressed, borderline patients. *American Journal of Psychiatry, 140,* 1023–1026.

Imber R. R. (1984). Reflections on Kohut and Sullivan. *Contemporary Psychoanalysis, 20,* 363–380.

Keith, C. (1984). *The aggressive adolescent.* New York: Free Press.

Kernberg, P. F. (1979). Psychoanalytic profile of the borderline adolescent. *Adolescent Psychiatry, 7,* 234–256.

Kohut, H. (1972). Thought on narcissism and narcissistic rage. In A. Solnit et al. (Eds.), *Psychoanalytic study of the child* (pp. 360–400). New Haven: Yale University Press.

Lewis, D. O., Feldman, M., & Barrengos, A. (1985). Race, health and delinquency. *Journal of the American Academy of Child and Adolescent Psychiatry, 24,* 161–167.

Lewis, D. O., Pincus, J. H., Shanok, S. S., & Glaser, G. H. (1983). Homicidally aggressive young children: Neuropsychiatric and experiential correlates. *American Journal of Psychiatry, 139,* 882–887.

Mahler, M. S., & Kaplan, L. (1977). Developmental aspects in assessment of narcissistic or so called borderline personalities. In Hortocollis (Ed.), *Borderline personality disorders: The concept, the syndrome, and the patient* (pp. 71–85). New York: International Universities Press.

Mahron, R. C. (1982). Adolescent violence: Causes and treatment. *Journal of the American Academy of Child and Adolescent Psychiatry, 21,* 354–360.

Manson, S. M. (1982). *New directions in prevention among American Indian and Alaska Native communities.* Portland, OR: National Center for American Indian and Alaska Native Research.

Masterson, J. (1972). *Treatment of the borderline adolescent: A developmental approach.* New York: Wiley.

Nielson, G. (1983). *Borderline and acting-out adolescents: A developmental approach.* New York: Human Sciences Press.

Noshpitz, J. (1984). Narcissism and aggression. *American Journal of Psychotherapy, 38,* 17–34.

Offer, D., Ostrov, E., & Howard, K. (1984). *Patterns of adolescent self image: New directions for mental health services.* San Francisco: Jossey Bass.

Rinsley, D. B. (1980). Diagnosis and treatment of borderline and narcissistic children and adolescents. *Bulletin of the Menninger Clinic, 446,* 147–170.

Rosenthal, P. A., & Doherty, M. D. (1985). Psychodynamics of delinquent girls' rage and violence directed toward mother. *Adolescent Psychiatry, 12,* 281–289.

Stern, D. N. (1982). The early development of schema of self, of other, and of various experiences of self with other. In J. D. Lichtenberg & S. Kaplan (Eds.), *Reflections on self psychology.* New York: International Universities Press.

U.S. Department of Justice. (1986). *Profile of state prison inmates.* Washington, DC: Bureau of Justice Statistics.

Winnicott, D. W. (1945). Hate in the countertransference. *International Journal of Psychoanalysis, 30,* 69–75.

Part IV

Professional Issues

Rindner, in Chapter 14, raises the important issues involved in interviewing and selecting the best candidates for milieu staff and hiring those who will work effectively in a multicultural setting. She emphasizes the need for prevention of burnout, especially through inservice education. Because rewarding staff is difficult in most hospital structures, she describes some ways in which administrators can help staff to feel valued and important.

In Chapter 15, Critchley describes the development of child psychiatric nursing as a specialty and the unique contributions nurses can make to the milieu. Nurses' clinical training in patient observation, important in all clinical work, becomes especially helpful when pharmacotherapy is used. The tradition of supervision and the direct provision of a treatment model in work with patients are given as methods of increasing the competence of nursing and other milieu staff.

Hendren and Berlin, in Chapter 16, focus on the hospital administration's role in facilitating treatment of severely disturbed, often poor, minority patients. Acute awareness and knowledge of mental health economics and government policies facilitate planning treatment and efforts to obtain funding. Health insurance and managed health care are discussed. Hospital regulation by accrediting agencies, credentialing of staff, and quality assurance are among the other issues reviewed. Ethical considerations and the role of clinical leadership are important elements of effective clinical administration of a hospital that serves children and adolescents from different cultures. The human problems faced by clinical administrators are briefly explored.

In Chapter 17, Berlin shares some principles of clinical administration that have been personally distilled over some 35 years of experience in both clinical administration and psychotherapeutic work with children, adolescents, and families. The evolution of some clinical administrative principles from certain repeated experiences is discussed. While these principles are derived from the author's own experience, they have interesting general applications.

Vargas's chapter on outcome evaluation is a thoughtful exposition of how the evaluation of children from different cultures might be more carefully considered. The issues of how the dominant culture's clinical diagnoses influence evaluation of individuals from other cultures are examined. The problems of determining norms—adapting various standard tests and questionnaires to the requirements for each culture versus using each individual from a minority culture as his or her own control with respect to original pathology and improvement—are described. Finally, a more pragmatic evaluation method is briefly outlined and discussed.

CHAPTER FOURTEEN

Recruiting, Developing, and Training Staff for Work in a Multicultural Setting of a Children's Psychiatric Hospital

Ellen C. Rindner

This chapter addresses several factors that impact the availability, recruiting, training, and retention of children and adolescent psychiatric or mental health nurses and child-care workers for work with child and adolescent inpatients. Persons who are responsible for hiring, orienting, and providing ongoing supervision to these two groups of staff members face a formidable challenge because of a lack of trained and qualified personnel, ethnic minority applicants, and formalized training programs, and the nationwide nursing shortage.

To function safely, a novice psychiatric nurse or child-care worker typically requires six months of training within the milieu setting. Furthermore, a new staff member requires approximately two years to become an expert. The hiring institution, therefore, must carefully develop hiring criteria and a training curriculum, to reduce staff turnover and enhance employee retention.

RECRUITMENT ISSUES

Several availability problems face an employer attempting to recruit mental health professionals for work with emotionally disturbed youth from ethnically diverse populations. The need for professionals in this area has multiplied because of expanded youth services, a more widespread use of child and adolescent psychiatric hospitals and milieu therapy, and the nationwide nursing shortage (Harris, 1990). The nursing shortage, which began in the 1980s, had direct impact on the number of people going into nursing and on those who specialize in psychiatric and mental health nursing. A primary source of the shortage, besides the reduced numbers of students entering baccalaureate programs since the mid 1980s, has been the ever increasing need for nurses for general hospital settings, especially in intensive care, emergency room, dialysis, psychiatry, and other specialty areas. Child and adolescent psychiatric and mental health nursing is considered a subspecialty of psychiatric nursing and requires advanced training. As a result, even those nurses drawn to the field require substantive training before they can be considered competent.

Fewer students, however, are interested in working with disturbed youth (Pothier, 1988) and few of those who do enter the field represent ethnic minorities. This constitutes a major problem because the mental health needs of ethnic minority populations far exceed the current availability of trained professionals to care for them (Yager, Chang, & Karno, 1989). In addition, compared to nursing opportunities, there are presently fewer educational opportunities for child and adolescent child-care workers, primarily for two reasons:

1. Services for troubled youth have been fragmented and government funding for child and adolescent mental health services has been cut.

In addition, the government has sharply limited educational funding for mental health professionals, and the lack of scholarships and financial support has had an adverse impact on recruitment efforts.

2. Although nurses' salaries have been substantially increased to meet the shortage, child-care workers' salaries continue to be low by comparison. Low salaries contribute significantly to the high turnover rate of child-care workers.

Another major problem facing the recruiter is that the majority of mental health professionals are from dominant-culture backgrounds. For work with an ethnically diverse patient population, ethnically diverse mental health professionals are desirable. Patient care can be severely compromised if the mental health professionals have little or no knowledge of how cultural factors impact upon the youths' and families' health beliefs and health-seeking behaviors. Cultural factors directly influence both transference and countertransference issues among the therapist, the client, and the family. Cultural bias can adversely affect the ability to assess pathology and to treat it.

Culturally insensitive or poorly trained mental health professionals can adversely affect the quality of patient care (Moffic, Kendrick, Reid, & Lomax, 1988). Conversely, mental health professionals with backgrounds culturally similar to the clients' often have greater success in establishing a therapeutic relationship with the client and family and in working with them to modify their dysfunctional patterns of behavior. Such professionals also have an increased tolerance for cultural idiosyncrasies that impact treatment and may understand the behavior within the cultural context. Speaking in the client's native tongue also serves to improve communication with the family, especially the extended family. Therefore, every effort to recruit mental health professionals with cultural backgrounds similar to the patient population's should be made by the hiring institution.

The hiring of a culturally diverse staff needs to be implemented by a supplemented multicultural training program, in order to educate and sensitize the workers to the cultural differences that exist. Training in this area must involve content (how cultures differ) as well as process (how workers can develop their ability to be empathic with ethnically diverse clients).

USE OF CAREER LADDERS

Various career ladders or career tracks are proposed for psychiatric nurses and child-care workers. Career ladders can be a valuable recruitment and retention tool, to enable staff to grow professionally and to increase the overall quality of patient care (Evans & Lewis, 1985). The use of a clinical career ladder for nurses and child-care workers recognizes the staff members' clinical expertise in providing direct patient care and rewards them through increased leadership responsibilities, advancement in grade, monetary benefit, and other forms of recognition. The ladder should reflect the institution's and treatment program's overall purpose and objectives. As the staff member is able to advance up the ladder, the promotions must be associated with recognition of increased ability, accountability, and responsibility. To be successful, the clinical career ladder must distinguish among beginning, intermediate, and advanced levels of practice and must provide advancement opportunities at each level.

One of the potential drawbacks of a clinical career ladder program within inpatient hospital settings is a tendency to focus exclusively on an "administrative track" and to ignore or negatively reinforce staff members who are interested in developing their clinical and/or teaching skills. Motivation to enhance clinical expertise needs to be rewarded through the provision of a "clinical track" that promotes increased acquisition of knowledge and skill level in milieu therapy and other forms of treatment. A "teaching track" is recommended for those interested in patient and/or staff education as a means of advancement and increased job satisfaction.

Some inpatient settings have designed introductory curricula for neophyte child-care workers and psychiatric nurses and advanced curricula for experienced milieu workers. Strategies to make the clinical track relevant include developing a curriculum that combines didactic material with illustration via case presentation and seminar discussion. Those interested in the teaching track can develop teaching modules under the guidance of the staff development instructor and can then be supervised when teaching the module to the staff and/or patients.

STAFF BURNOUT

Burnout is characterized by gradual disillusionment with a job, combined with increased feelings of powerlessness and frustration that lead to decreased job performance. In the field of inpatient child and adolescent milieu therapy, the staff member deals on a daily basis with the aftermath of traumatic events in the children's lives, for example, physical, sexual, and emotional abuse. Staff burnout must be anticipated as inevitable because of the tremendous emotional needs of this population. Working with deprived, abused children and adolescents puts the staff members in constant touch with their own unresolved issues from their family of origin. The young people also will try to engage the staff member in reenacting the role of their parents, especially in their acting-out behavior, which creates increased staff stress.

Multiple methodologies can be utilized to prevent staff burnout. The best cure for burnout lies in the area of prevention.

Staffing patterns that provide an adequate staff-to-patient ratio are essential, to promote patient safety and to relieve staff stress. Work schedules should also provide the staff with sufficient time off so that they can relax and regenerate. If possible, staff should have a minimum of two days off at each break, and should not work a long period of successive days without adequate breaks.

Weekly support groups conducted by qualified persons who are not part of the management team (Evans & Lewis, 1985) have often proven successful. The group leader needs to be nonjudgmental and supportive, to enable the staff members to ventilate their feelings during the initial phases of the support group. During the working phase of the group, the leader should facilitate the group's adoption of stress-relieving strategies and problem-solving skills.

Staff education about verbal and physical acting-out of clients can alleviate employee stress, because the threat of patient aggressiveness is always an ongoing stressor in the psychiatric milieu. Education and workshops about patient pathology can also help to reduce staff countertransference and increase staff insight. Allowing staff to participate in seminars away from the institution may provide temporary relief from the intensity of the workload and an expanded knowledge base. The staff can also share their new knowledge with their peers.

Team-building strategies such as peer supervision, retreats, and staff parties may contribute to team spirit and be an important antidote to burnout. Open communication between management and team members about the stress level in the milieu can be maintained during rounds and supervision, and is crucial to identifying stressors and taking steps to resolve them.

CRITERIA FOR HIRING MILIEU WORKERS

The recruitment and selection of child and adolescent psychiatric or mental health nurses and child-care workers is becoming an increasingly complex and critical decision for administrators. Recruiting and training staff members is a time-consuming and expensive proposition. It is therefore imperative that the hiring institution carefully decide, prior to recruitment, on criteria for interviewing and hiring and strategies for screening to find the most appropriate candidates for the position.

A psychiatric nurse is a licensed, professional nurse who has both clinical experience and expertise in the specialty of child and adolescent psychiatric or mental health nursing. The nurse's expertise is measurable through a formal review process, usually an examination conducted by the American Nurses Association. The minimum recommended educational preparation for the child and adolescent psychiatric or mental health nurse is a baccalaureate degree in nursing (Bulbrook, 1980). The nurse may further specialize at the master's level and become a clinical nurse specialist in child and adolescent psychiatric or mental health nursing in a program geared to the subspecialty.

A psychiatric nurse's performance yields learning that exceeds the knowledge acquired or required in basic nursing education or the credentials of a beginner in the field. The value of advanced preparation has hiring implications. If one hires a new baccalaureate graduate who has no previous psychiatric nursing experience, he or she will fall below the skill level required to fulfill the position. It is incumbent on the hiring institution, therefore, to supplement the nurse's deficits by providing education and supervision, to ensure the safety of the psychiatric milieu.

The nursing shortage is a reality (Roberts, Minnick, Ginzberg, & Curran, 1989) and few available nurses, especially those prepared at the baccalaureate level, are interested in child and adolescent psychiatric or mental health nursing. Associate degree graduates are sometimes the only available nurses to fill positions. Hiring them can complicate the inservice training process because academically these graduates are weaker in their knowledge of growth and development and their psychiatric theory base than baccalaureate nurses. However, associate degree graduates who are given proper training and supervision can make excellent child and adolescent psychiatric or mental health nurses if they possess a love for children, an openness about revealing their feelings in the clinical work, and a tremendous amount of motivation to supplement their educational deficits.

In addition to education, the traits one should look for when attempting to hire a child and adolescent psychiatric nurse are: direct psychiatric patient care experience, direct psychiatric inpatient experience, experience with emotionally disturbed youth, interpersonal skills, experience in an interdisciplinary setting, psychological mindedness, appearance, writing skills, self-knowledge, pediatric nursing experience, experience working with parents, problem-solving skills, and ability to resolve conflict.

A child-care worker, often referred to in other settings as a mental health worker or psychiatric aide, is considered to be a paraprofessional who may perform activities within the scope of nursing practice in the milieu. Few educational programs exist that adequately prepare individuals to fulfill this role.

The educational preparation for the child-care worker varies dramatically from institution to institution; typically, the minimum education requirement is a high school diploma. Many new baccalaureate graduates prepared in psychology, social work, or other behavioral science areas select the child-care worker position as a point of entry into the mental health system. The baccalaureate worker is likely to utilize this work experience to help him or her decide whether to pursue further study at the graduate level. This is usually the first job experience for these workers. They tend to be impressionable, have limited life experience, and are prone to having rescue fantasies. They therefore need substantial inservice and supervision to compensate for their lack of training.

The high school graduates who seek a child-care worker position typically are older and possess more life experience. They are more likely to be representative of the ethnic minorities. These workers tend to be extremely invested in their work and to stay in the field for long periods of time. They are the "heart and soul" of the milieu.

One of the major problems facing the hiring institution is retention of both types of child-care workers. The turnover rate in this position is exceedingly high because of a lack of job status, limited opportunity for job advancement, low salaries, and high burnout rate. Every effort should be made by management to help the child-care workers feel valued, via requesting competitive salaries for them, recognizing outstanding contributions at yearly award ceremonies, and instituting career ladders.

Management also needs to be cognizant of the ever present discrepancy between salaries and child-care salaries. Nurses who may have far less education and/or experience than child-care workers may be making almost twice as much in salary. Needless to say, this can create feelings of resentment.

When hiring a child-care worker, many of the criteria used for hiring a nurse apply. The recruiter needs to evaluate the worker's appearance, alertness, friendliness, writing skills, conversational ability, decision-making skills, and self-knowledge (Harris, 1990). In addition, the recruiter must establish that the potential staff member has a love of children, an ability to be patient, and a willingness to perform bathing and hygiene, recreational, and educational tasks. Every effort should be made to recruit workers from culturally representative minorities.

The recruiter should try to assess the worker's sense of personal boundaries, limit-setting abilities, and understanding of personal expressions of anger and fear. The worker's reaction to such feelings in others is also important.

Perhaps recruitment of psychiatric nurses and child-care workers has to begin at the high school level, with vocational programs specifically designed to recruit ethnic minority students into the field. The hiring institution should reinforce this recruitment and retention effort by participating in community health fairs, lecturing at local high schools and colleges, offering student scholarships, and forming a standing recruitment and retention committee.

INTERVIEW PROCESS

There are several steps in the interview process. Prior to the interview, the recruiter has to have a clear idea of what type of employee will make the best milieu–employee fit. Factors such as the preexisting employee constellation or employee mix need to be considered. For example, the milieu should contain a mix of novice and experienced mental health professionals as well as staff from divergent age groups and ethnic backgrounds. The personalities of the milieu staff should be complementary, to avoid a rigid and punitive or an overprotective and lenient milieu.

In the initial interview with the person responsible for recruitment, it can be valuable if the applicant is given several case scenarios that are likely to occur within the particular milieu (e.g., staff splitting, confidentiality issues, patient rights, handling aggressive patients), to determine how the candidate reacts. The recruiter can then assess the applicant's judgment, philosophy of treatment, honesty, and decision-making skills.

Applicants should be asked about their preference for age groups of children; they may have positive or negative countertransference to a particular age group. Wherever possible, the applicants' preferences should be honored because their ability to assess those with whom they fit best demonstrates insight into themselves. For example, one would not want to hire an applicant to work with teenagers if the applicant makes derogatory statements regarding this group or says that they "drive me crazy just like my teenagers do and I am liable to retaliate against them." Applicants should be asked whether they have children of their own, and their ages, because they may have a positive or negative countertransference to this same age group of patients. Applicants should be asked directly if they believe this similarity would bias their performance.

It is very helpful to have a potential employee interviewed by several milieu staff representatives from different disciplines. The interviewer should observe the applicant's reaction to a group interview and should determine the consistency of replies to the individual interviewer and to the group. Another helpful screening technique is to invite an applicant to spend some time observing the unit, to get an overview of the patient population and of the job responsibilities. Pairing an applicant with an experienced nurse or child-care worker can give the interviewer direct feedback regarding the applicant's interpersonal skills and comfort in the milieu. This additional clinical experience should be scheduled only when there is a good possibility of hiring the applicant and the interviewer wishes to assess the milieu–staff member fit, or when the applicant has some doubts about the patient population. Prior to scheduling any observational or work experience, the issues of confidentiality need to be thoroughly discussed with the applicant. In some cases, it is helpful to "try out" employees in a per diem or "on-call" pool prior to permanent hiring. This trial relationship allows both the temporary employee and the employer to assess the employee's competency and to determine the milieu–worker fit. Hiring and training can prove expensive and emotionally exhaustive work. It is therefore well worth the interviewer's time to carefully screen employees and to check their references (Wolf, 1989).

Terminating an employee who turns out to be a poor performer, or is a poor fit, ultimately is costly, takes additional supervisory time, and adversely impacts the milieu.

MILIEU MODELS

There are essentially two models for milieu management. In the first model, nurses are responsible for milieu management and child-care workers are under their direct supervision. In the second model, child-care workers manage the milieu and report to a Milieu or Program Director and nurses work within the milieu but report to the Director of Nursing. There are advantages and disadvantages to each model.

In the first model, nurses manage the milieu and delegate milieu responsibilities to child-care workers, who are part of the nursing department. Nurses and child-care workers are under the domain of nursing and therefore have one philosophy and set of hospital policies to follow. In addition, a professional, licensed, registered nurse is in charge of the milieu and its maintenance and is accountable for crisis management.

The disadvantages of this system are twofold. First, because the nurse manages the milieu, the amount of time she or he has for direct patient care is restricted. Generally, nurses go into the profession to spend quality time with patients. Being tied up with administrative tasks is seen as a deterrent by most nurses.

Second, the "charge" nurse is likely to have less education and/or experience than the child-care workers assigned to the unit, because of the dearth of trained child and adolescent psychiatric nurses. This situation (which occurs often in this model) can jeopardize the safety of the milieu and lead to resentment among the child-care workers.

In the second model, where nurses and child-care workers work side-by-side, the major advantage is that nurses get to spend much more time in direct patient care, which in turn increases their job satisfaction. Child-care workers who have leadership and management skills are able to advance administratively and "run" the milieu whereas in the first model only nurses can advance administratively.

There are disadvantages to this model as well. The major disadvantage is that child-care workers and nurses report to and are supervised by different department heads. This can lead to splitting as well as confusion as to who is ultimately accountable, should there be a problem within the milieu. Another disadvantage is role blurring, since there is a tendency to duplicate roles of child-care workers and nurses within the milieu.

For the second model to work, role differentiation needs to be made clear and there must be open lines of communication between the nursing and milieu program directors regarding the focus and responsibilities of each discipline. Both nurses and child-care workers are responsible jointly for the day-to-day management of the milieu on a 24-hour basis. Although each discipline's focus may differ, ultimately they should complement each other as long as the goal of both disciplines is to provide quality milieu treatment for inpatient emotionally disturbed youth.

ASSIGNMENT OF MILIEU WORKERS TO CHILDREN AND FAMILIES

Several variables should be taken into account when assigning staff to work with children and their families. One variable is the nature of the child's and family's pathology, which must be matched to the skill level of the worker, in order to successfully engage the child/family system. Another variable is the type of staff temperament best suited to the child. For example, under certain conditions it might be helpful to pair a hyperactive child with a calm, low-keyed staff member. Children who have a number of complicating medical issues are typically paired with a nurse, to best meet their medical and psychological needs. Finally, if the skill level or temperamental match is not an essential issue, staff who request to work with a particular child and family should be given preference, to satisfy a significant motivational variable in the assignment process.

STAFF DEVELOPMENT

This section discusses orientation, needs assessments, continuing education, teaching strategies, curriculum development, supervision, and the evaluation process.

The hiring organization, according to the Joint Commission on Accreditation of Healthcare Organizations' criteria, must conduct a formal orientation for psychiatric nurses and child-care workers hired by the institution. The primary purpose(s) of any inpatient psychiatric hospital orientation is to familiarize the new employees to their new job responsibilities, environment, and coworkers.

Orientation is also an important process for staff who are promoted and/or change from one position to another within the milieu setting. Transferring employees generally can be oriented in an informal, individualized manner. New employees are usually oriented in larger groups or by utilizing a formal didactic core of orientation classes supplemented with a clinical preceptor experience (Finkelman, 1980). A preceptor is an experienced nurse or child-care worker (to orient each discipline respectively) who has had training in clinical supervision techniques, knows the hospital's policies and procedures, and desires to precept. Most career ladders (Evans & Lewis, 1985) enable employees to advance by becoming preceptors. For a senior staff member, teaching new employees through the process of role modeling can be a wonderful experience.

The minimum didactic courses that need to be covered during the initial orientation period in a child and adolescent psychiatric inpatient hospital are listed in Table 14.1.

Many of the orientation classes can be taught simultaneously to nurses and child-care workers; however, classes that address specialty areas need to be taught separately.

The hiring institution must ensure that the milieu staff members' training continues throughout the entire period of employment. Continuing education programs help improve the overall quality of care, prevent employee burnout, and improve overall hospital morale. There are many different approaches to continuing education for the employee. According to Lewis (1978), a minimum of three sources of learning are available to the new employee (trainee): individual supervision, personal psychotherapy, and instruction in psychotherapeutic theories and treatment modalities. Unit-based inservices, case conferences, daily rounds, and outside conferences and/or college courses are additional sources of continuing education.

To make an accurate assessment of the employee's learning needs, the staff educator should make a learning needs assessment at least every six months, to provide for staff development attuned to the needs of the employee. It is extremely useful to get specific requests for classes about

Table 14.1. Orientation Curriculum

All Incoming Milieu Workers
Hospital Philosophy
Organizational Structure
Fire and Safety
Universal Precautions
Control of Aggressive Patients
Therapeutic Communication and Relationships
Developmental Assessment

Nurses: Job Duties / Responsibilities	*Child Care Workers:* *Job Duties / Responsibilities*
Documentation	Documentation
Cardiopulmonary Resuscitation	Vital Signs
Psychopharmacology	Hygiene/Care of Patients
Legal Aspects of Patient Care	Legal Aspects of Patient Care

Table 14.2.   Advanced Training Curriculum

DSM-III-R Criteria/Diagnoses
Developmental Theory
Psychodynamic Theory/Therapy
Humanistic Theory/Therapy
Behavioral Theory/Therapy
Family Systems Theory/Therapy
Group Theory/Therapy
Psychopharmacology
Impact of Culture on Mental Health/Mental Illness
Multicultural Seminar
Transference/Countertransference

children and adolescents from the milieu staff; they are more likely to benefit from a class that they have selected rather than a class that is mandated.

A seminar approach to staff training can be more useful than a lecture format because experienced child-care workers or nurses may have as much knowledge about the topic as the instructor. Unless the educator makes use of their expertise, staff members may be "turned off" to the material. When actual case histories are used to illustrate theory and/or interventions, worker involvement and interest in the class content are enhanced. The use of multimedia modalities provides heightened learner interest and retention. The author finds videotaped sessions and made-for-television movies about a specific topic, such as child abuse, useful methods of initiating group discussion and facilitating comprehension of theory.

Basic content needed for the safe treatment of emotionally disturbed youth was addressed in Table 14.1. A more in-depth educational program should be planned by the staff development department for the continued growth of its employees. Advanced training topics are listed in Table 14.2.

It is extremely helpful to seek consultants or experts in the field who can develop and teach the advanced curriculum and bring their expertise into the training area to increase the staff's theory base. In addition, structured exercises should be developed to improve interpersonal skills, empathy, warmth, genuineness, and self-disclosure (Lewis, 1978).

STAFF SUPERVISION

Each department within the children's inpatient hospital should have a clearly delineated model outlining who performs supervision, with whom, and how often. Supervision may be performed on an individual basis, in a group setting, or by utilizing both modes of supervision.

Supervision of the milieu worker should address the following variables on a continuing basis:

1. Attitude;
2. Level of initiative;
3. Interpersonal skills;
4. Quality of work;
5. Quantity of work;
6. Adherence to hospital policy;
7. Understanding of the dynamics of the assigned patient population;
8. Interface with multidisciplinary team members.

Intervention strategies and their implications also should be part of the supervision, so that the employee can accurately evaluate the effectiveness of the treatment strategies with the young person in day-to-day contacts.

Finally, the issues of transference and countertransference and the "normalization" of these phenomena must be addressed with the employee. Workers need to be assured that they are not "crazy" or "shameful" for experiencing intensely negative and/or positive feelings toward the patient (Grayer & Sax, 1986). In addition, the worker needs to be taught to recognize and resolve countertransference issues on an ongoing basis in the milieu. A major cause of burnout and high turnover is the failure of the institution to address and help the worker to deal with the emotional sequelae created by emotionally disturbed youth. Every effort should be made to support the employee emotionally through an increased knowledge base about the care of troubled youth.

Evaluating the effectiveness of inservice education and training in relation to employee needs must be a continuing process that is coordinated between the staff development person and the program director. The program director can alert the staff development person to the learning needs of the employee and to areas for improvement and growth. The staff development person will also find it useful to conduct a formal evaluation of each employee's performance on a semiannual basis. The evaluation should specifically assess the success or failure of the courses offered, the instructors' teaching abilities, and the teaching strategies that have proven effective. This information can then be shared with staff and used to modify staff development. The instructor can also informally assess the success of each class by asking for direct feedback about the relevance of the topic and the teaching style at the close of each class and by assessing the interest of the group on an ongoing basis.

RETENTION AND MORALE ISSUES

Retention of employees is an extremely important indicator that the institution's investment in training has proven successful (Wolf, 1989). Education is one antidote to sagging staff morale; it can rekindle the flame in a burnt out employee. Education alone, however, is not sufficient to motivate employees to stay with the organization. To improve the staff members' overall morale, milieu staff must be empowered through role differentiation, formal recognition of the importance of their work, provision of ongoing clinical supervision, and programs designed to reduce burnout.

Administrative attitudes play a tremendous role in sanctioning the role and importance of milieu staff members. If the administrative staff values milieu work, so will the rest of the hospital. The administration needs to acknowledge workers' importance through a commitment to providing safe staff-to-patient ratios, competitive salaries, ongoing training opportunities, and ongoing clinical supervision.

The milieu staff workers' morale is the life force of the unit and thus must be nurtured and tended on an ongoing basis through all of the strategies discussed here.

CONCLUSION

Successful recruitment, development, and training of staff to work in a multicultural inpatient children's and adolescents' psychiatric hospital take planning and coordination; they relate directly to the milieu workers' overall delivery of patient care. Careful screening and selection of nurses and child-care workers will decrease the amount of training and supervision time required and will assure a better milieu–staff fit.

REFERENCES

Bulbrook, M. J. T. (1980). *Development of therapeutic skills.* Boston: Little, Brown.

Evans, C. S., & Lewis, S. K. (1985). *Nursing administration of psychiatric mental health care.* Rockville, MD: Aspen Systems Corp.

Finkelman, A. W. (1980). *Staff development for the psychiatric nurse.* Thorofare, NJ: Charles B. Slack.

Grayer, E. D., & Sax, P. R. (1986). A model for the diagnostic and therapeutic use of countertransference. *Clinical Social Work Journal, 14,* 295–309.

Harris, T. (1990). Wanted: Psychiatric technician: Assessing decision-making skills. *Journal of Psychosocial Nursing and Mental Health Services, 25,* 23–26.

Lewis, J. M. (1978). *To be a therapist: The teaching and learning.* New York: Brunner/ Mazel.

Moffic, H. S., Kendrick, E. A., Reid, K., & Lomax, J. W. (1988). Cultural psychiatry education during psychiatric residency. *Journal of Psychiatric Education, 12,* 91–101.

Pothier, P. C. (1988). Graduate preparation in child and adolescent psychiatric mental health nursing. *Archives of Psychiatric Nursing, 2,* 170–172.

Roberts, M. J., Minnick, A., Ginzberg, E., & Curran, C. R. (1989). Strategies: The hospital nursing shortage—an examination of supply and demand factors influencing registered nurses' labor participation. *Nurse Executive Management Strategies, 13,* 1–7.

Wolf, J. R. (1989). Human resource management. *Psychiatric Annals, 19,* 432–434.

Yager, J., Chang, C., & Karno, M. (1989). Teaching transcultural psychiatry. *Academic Psychiatry, 13,* 164–171.

CHAPTER FIFTEEN

Nursing's Contributions to a Psychiatric Inpatient Treatment Milieu for Children and Adolescents

Deane L. Critchley

This chapter provides a brief overview of the development of the psychiatric nursing role in inpatient treatment, from the earlier traditional nursing roles to the implications for the psychiatric nursing role of the 1990s. The role of clinical supervision is described in terms of its contribution to milieu treatment and staff development.

The belief that the immediate environment in which the psychiatric patient functions is a significant variable in treatment is not new. The concept of milieu treatment and the psychiatric nurse's contribution to that treatment process depend on the site; thus, fluctuations in the degree of understanding and level of acceptance they receive are inevitable. For example, during the emphasis on community mental health programs and the proliferating family therapy movement, the importance of inpatient treatment was questioned. However, inpatient treatment shows no indication of disappearing. Any hospital experience must still be assumed to have an important meaning for patients and an impact on staff.

TRADITIONAL PSYCHIATRIC NURSING ROLES IN INPATIENT SETTINGS

Psychiatric nursing has evolved from participation as a "handmaiden" toward interdependent and independent collaboration as a clinically competent colleague. Initially, in inpatient settings, nurses were primarily used to carry out physicians' orders, to dispense medications, and to serve as the physicians' eyes and ears in observing and reporting patient behavior. These are significant nursing functions, but nurses and other mental health professionals realized that there were other roles that psychiatric nurses were competently prepared to carry out.

Following the period of custodial care for psychiatric patients, which ended in the 1950s, psychiatric nursing moved toward the concept of the one-to-one nurse–patient relationship recommended in the work of Peplau (1952). Her writings and teaching have significantly influenced the evolving practice of psychiatric nursing.

Peplau believed that the interpersonal process within the nurse–patient therapeutic relationship promotes a healthier adjustment for clients and helps to reduce their symptoms of anxiety, depression, and insecurity. Although Peplau developed her approach in an inpatient setting (a large state mental hospital), her focus was on the individual nurse–patient relationship rather than on the therapeutic potential of the interactions occurring within the total treatment setting.

Concurrently with the psychiatric nurse's increased involvement with the individual patient, enhanced use of the patient's environment for treatment purposes began. The environmental treatment components that were identified included restructuring the physical environment to make adjunct therapies more readily available; developing or encouraging specific attitudes and behaviors of staff, patients, and families; and coordinating planned activities that are ego-strengthening and that include a variety of work, recreational, and educational efforts.

Skinner (1979) noted that, although creation and management of a therapeutic milieu are the responsibility of nurses, there is a dearth of nursing literature devoted to the topic. Milieu treatment is a general term, and there are disagreements among those who espouse a milieu treatment philosophy. Some programs emphasize group interaction and process to such an extent that individual staff–patient time or treatment is seen as undermining the patient's experiences with the group and is thus contraindicated.

The role of nurses is both broad and diverse in a milieu setting. Nurses need to be supportive to the patients even as they encourage them to be self-reliant. Activities that will help relationships to develop and will enhance the patients' sense of self-worth must be planned. The ability to initiate and maintain normal social relationships needs to be fostered through a reduction of self-defeating, hostile, and rejecting peer relationships and an increase of adaptive ways of responding to stressful events. Nurses in milieu treatment teach self-help and interpersonal skills and foster prescribed attitudes, especially in attitude therapy and reality orientation.

Nurses function with particular effectiveness because of their professional experience as case managers and coordinators of services that children and adolescents may need. Nurses also work effectively with the patients' immediate and extended family members, counseling, teaching, and providing support to caregivers who are responsible for children and adolescents who have acute or chronic mental illnesses. Clinical supervision is also a task that nurses can carry out successfully in milieu settings.

Child and adolescent psychiatric nursing education has never been widely available. Because child psychiatric nursing is considered a subspecialty, it is not available in undergraduate programs. Currently, there are only eleven graduate child psychiatric nursing programs in the country; the annual number of graduates ranges from one to five (Pothier, 1988). A general decrease in university financial support has placed programs with low enrollments and intensive faculty–student involvement, such as one-to-one supervision, at risk.

The perception in the field has always been that there are too few nurses prepared to work with emotionally disturbed children and adolescents and that those who have appropriate preparation are not well-utilized. A study by Pothier, Norbeck, and La Liberte (1985) indicated that there is in the field a cadre of adequately prepared child and adolescent psychiatric nurses, but only about half of them are in positions that permit them to function in direct or indirect practice with children and adolescents. For a significant number of these nurses, no positions are available or access to children and adolescents who need their services is inadequate.

Current Inpatient Nursing Roles

The specific implications for psychiatric nursing's contribution to milieu treatment will depend on the organizational role assumed by the nurses. Currently, advanced educational preparation, knowledge, and skills enable nurses to contribute to the milieu in many ways. Their typical functions include the following:

1. Provide clinical supervision to other staff to assist them in identifying their own conflicts and difficulties in work with patients and families;
2. Participate in treatment planning for individual clients and families;
3. Participate in program planning for the unit as a whole;
4. Serve as a role model for being a milieu team member and for using therapeutically the everyday life events in the milieu;
5. Identify and carry out clinical nursing research and practice problems.

Many clinical questions that could be of value in improving patient care require further study. For example, what are the early warning signs for violent episodes? How is nursing service best organized for an acute adolescent unit? How can effective communication be encouraged with an autistic child who has few verbal language skills?

Within nursing and within hospital administration, there is currently a debate as to how best to prepare nurses for administrative positions. Should clinical knowledge or administrative and management skills be emphasized? As health care organizations have become more complex, their direction requires greater managerial skill; yet, the most effective nurse–administrator is one who has strong, *current,* clinical knowledge along with basic administrative skills. Effective administrative decisions can only be made when they are based on an understanding of the clinical goals and the issues they include *and* an appreciation of the interaction among staff and how their attitudes and behaviors affect patients, family behaviors, and clinical progress. Similarly, the contribution of the patients' and families' attitudes and behaviors to staff reactions and to the entire milieu must be understood. Administrative decisions significantly affect staff and patient attitudes and behavior.

Psychiatric nursing in a therapeutic milieu appears deceptively simple. Staff and clients talk a great deal, in pairs and in groups. Staff members involve themselves in educational and recreational activities as well as in activities of patients' daily living. The significance of a behavior needs to be examined in terms of its psychological meaning for a given context. For example, at times a behavior needs to be understood literally but at other times it is symbolic of a symptom and must be responded to in that context.

The sensitivity and thoughtful intervention that are required over long periods of time are both physically and emotionally fatiguing and demand a high level of self-awareness and a strong knowledge base (Schwartz & Shockley, 1956).

Tudor's article on mutual withdrawal (1952), a nursing classic, describes the detrimental effect on a patient of a nurse's behavior pattern. Stanton and Schwartz (1954) found a relationship between low staff morale, and the resulting behavior, and an increase in disturbed patient behavior. More recently, Cherniss (1980a, 1980b) argued that organizational structure can either enhance or diminish job stress and burnout. Stanton and Schwartz were discussing a group phenomenon, and burnout is usually an individual phenomenon, but the two concepts appear closely related.

The psychiatric nurse–administrator not only contributes significantly to creating and maintaining a particular organizational structure but, through an effective relationship with the staff, also influences the level of job stress and of staff coping skills.

CLINICAL SUPERVISION

Supervision, in human services fields, generally serves two distinct functions. First, it provides a means of administrative overview; the supervisor monitors and evaluates the work of subordinates and ensures conformity to organizational policies. Second, supervision fulfills a development function; it supports professional learning and growth. Clinical supervisors are expected to help staff to understand and constructively integrate emotional responses to clinical and other work-related situations. To be most effective, the administrative and professional development functions should be separated. In many settings, however, especially in administrative positions such as head nurse, these roles are combined.

For the major mental health professions, clinical supervision is a critical means of clarifying treatment problems. Supervision increases the staff members' understanding of therapeutic interactions as well as of the interpersonal dynamics among staff, patients, and families. Milieu staff who come from disciplines other than the major mental health professions usually have little or no experience with clinical supervision. If they join the staff as supervisory personnel, they are often unable to help staff members deal with their internal conflicts and their obstacles to working effectively and collaboratively with patients, families, and other staff. This problem is compounded when supervision is intermittent or crisis oriented and when the supervisor has not personally experienced clinical supervision that was directed toward professional and personal growth and enhanced self-assessment.

Clinical supervision in psychiatric nursing is derived from the traditional nursing practice of influencing the work of others via modeling. Discussions and general overseeing are combined with the knowledge of process that came initially from psychoanalysis. Clinical supervision provides an understanding of the environmental and intrapsychic factors that need to be integrated to achieve clinical competence.

Assistance in ongoing professional development is an absolute necessity for milieu staff, for several reasons. Staff members belong to a variety of disciplines; they have varying levels of education and professional experience; some may be new to the demands of work with emotionally ill children and adolescents or to the milieu treatment environment. Professional staff development is essential, to assist the staff in identifying their own as well as clients' conflicts and difficulties; to increase the staff's knowledge of growth and development and of psychopathology; and to create meaningful staff participation in treatment planning and implementation. The process also helps in the evaluation of the functioning of individual patients and families as well as of the total unit. Staff development serves to enhance clinical skills in utilizing everyday milieu events therapeutically.

Multiple Definitions of Supervision

Supervision can be technical or administrative, or it can be an intensive clinical therapeutic process. Haller (1976) defined supervision as a process in which a therapist—often, but not necessarily, a beginner—is helped to become an effective clinician. Loganbill, Hardy, and Delworth (1982) defined supervision as an intensive, interpersonally focused, one-to-one relationship in which one person is designated to facilitate the development of therapeutic competence in the other person. The following discussion of clinical supervision is based on this definition: Clinical supervision is an intensive, interpersonally focused professional function in which one person who is, hopefully, skilled, knowledgeable, and empathic is designated to facilitate the development of clinical therapeutic competence in another person (Critchley, 1985).

Clinical Supervision as an Organizing Framework

Clinical supervision can provide a means to describe and organize data that are critical to understanding the concepts and behaviors that form a part of the therapeutic process. This organization may be done within a particular theoretical framework such as a developmental perspective. Through supervision, this conceptual process can be integrated with an empathic understanding of the client and family and the dynamics of treatment. Using an integrated approach makes it possible to examine how the behavior of the supervisee has influenced the observations, interpretations, and overall quality of the interactions. Using supervision as an organizing framework permits examination of complex, multiple behavioral elements in a way that permits identification of antecedents, connections, and meanings.

Clinical Supervision Versus Therapy

A common misconception is that clinical supervision is personal therapy. Clinical supervision and therapy have some commonalities, but their goals and purposes are quite different. Supervision's goals do not include therapy for the supervisee. Rather, its goals are to help the supervisee develop greater clinical competence through the discussion of issues encountered in therapeutic work and to stimulate the supervisee's creative and therapeutic use of self. Therapy's goals are to help clients understand themselves better through recognition and resolution of conflicts and to ultimately move clients toward growth and increased autonomy. Therapy is based, in almost all cases, on the client's or family's recognition of a problem and their seeking of assistance to deal with that problem; they must acknowledge its existence, explicitly agree as to its nature, and have an interest in alleviating its pain, dysfunction, and conflict.

The purposes of clinical supervision are to teach psychotherapeutic skills and to deal with the problems the supervisee may experience in the supervisory and therapeutic relationships, but only to the extent that these problems affect the ability to learn and to work effectively.

Clinical Supervision Versus Consultation

Consultation and supervision have some similarities, but they also have important differences. The clinical supervisor carries administrative responsibility for the supervisee and thus can hold the supervisee accountable for her or his clinical work. The supervisor facilitates the professional development of the supervisee by providing theoretical knowledge and therapeutic techniques and by supporting the working-through of transference and countertransference reactions affecting clinical work. When this administrative responsibility is absent, the process is consultation, not supervision. Typically, consultation denotes a peer or collegial relationship. The consultee is free to use or to dismiss the outcomes of the consultation.

Clinical Supervision as Learning

The supervisory process can be an effective learning tool. Rather than answer all questions or provide all necessary information, the supervisor can use the problem-solving method, raising pertinent questions for the supervisee to think about and reformulate for further discussion. An equally important task is to help the supervisee enhance the ability to observe more closely and to describe more exactly both the clients' and his or her own behaviors. During this process, the supervisor can be helpful in pointing out any blind spots the supervisee may have about the interactions.

An important focus of supervision is to help the supervisee differentiate between a social and a professional role. Pointing out how a client or family is making inappropriate requests of the staff member may help to change a social response into a professional one.

Supervisory Methods. All clinical supervision requires recording interactions with patients and staff. Verbal recall, written process notes, and audio or video tapes are all possibilities. The most accurate and complete information is provided by video tapes. At the other extreme, verbal recall is the least reliable method. Observation and understanding of nonverbal behaviors are perhaps the most difficult tasks. Video tapes permit repeated, joint observation of interactions. Writing proper records of both the verbal and nonverbal aspects of interactions is extremely difficult to learn. Constant encouragement is required to move the supervisee from recording only the patient's verbal communication to recording patient–staff verbal communication and then to recording patient–staff verbal and nonverbal communication. No matter what method is used, it is necessary to analyze the data, extract themes, and identify problems relevant to the patient–staff relationship. It then becomes possible to evaluate the interventions used and formulate plans for the next session.

A form of participant supervision is particularly helpful in milieu settings. The supervisor may find it useful to observe an interaction between a staff member and a patient, in order to understand the impact of other patients and staff on the staff–patient relationship. The supervisor may also demonstrate a particular intervention with a patient. This kind of participant supervision may be especially effective because the supervisor is less involved with the patient and can look at his or her behavior more objectively.

Issues in Supervisory Development

Certain issues recur frequently in milieu treatment and are extremely problematic because of their ability to create conflict and massively disrupt the treatment process.

The symptomatic behaviors of children and adolescents need to be understood within the context of their illness and their efforts to cope with their own anxieties and conflicts. The intense, primitive behaviors of psychotic children, the impulsive, aggressive, and violent behaviors of behaviorally disturbed youngsters, and self-destructive or suicidal behavior in both younger children and adolescents are some of the most difficult behaviors for milieu staff to deal with because of the feelings and conflicts these behaviors arouse in them.

To effectively help these patients, milieu staff need to be helped to deal with their own patient-initiated feelings. These include anger, rage, retaliation, vulnerability, sexuality, helplessness, and a sense of failure. It is helpful to clarify how the child's feelings and attitudes, derived from past relationships, have influenced his or her current perceptions of the behavior of the treatment staff.

Persistent clarification of the purposes and limitations of the current treatment setting, along with recognition of the child's previous experiences of disappointment and rejection, helps staff feel less guarded and less vulnerable to the child's behavior. Staff members often find it difficult to appreciate the degree to which disturbed children and adolescents continuously project feelings and attitudes derived from earlier, emotionally hurtful experiences with adults and to be able to respond based upon the child's needs rather than on the basis of the adult's own reactions of anxiety, hurt, and anger.

Because these are ubiquitous feelings aroused in milieu treatment, they also are grist for the work of supervision. Other issues that tend to recur involve professional competence, emotional awareness, empathy, professional identity and autonomy, self-worth, self-determination, respect for individual differences, and professional ethics. Two particularly important issues are transference and countertransference. Clinical supervision must deal with the patient's and family's projections to the staff member of both good and conflicted aspects of old relationships and with the anxieties evoked in the staff member by the patient and family or as a result of the staff member's own unresolved conflicts.

A 10-year-old boy with a conduct disorder was thought to be ready for discharge after several months of treatment. The boy's discharge had been discussed with his parents many times. The parents, especially the mother, were extremely reluctant to consider discharge. They began reporting incidents that supposedly occurred when the boy was home on pass but were not consistent with the boy's behavior either on the unit or in school. The therapist discussed with the parents the issues that could be contributing to their reluctance: fears about separation, lack of protection, and loss. These discussions were not only unsuccessful but resulted in the referral of a younger brother by the parents. The mother reported that the 8-year-old child had problems identical to those of his older hospitalized brother. She presented a psychological evaluation of the 8-year-old to support her request for hospitalization of the second child.

The treatment team reviewed the evaluation of the younger boy and saw him for a brief outpatient evaluation. The results did not support a need for hospitalization. At this point, a staff conference was called to review the family's and children's needs.

The therapist reported that the mother had been in treatment for a number of years prior to her 10-year-old's hospitalization. The therapist felt that the woman had become very dependent on therapy, that she was using therapy to avoid facing the realities of her life situation, and that she was reacting to current situations in terms of her childhood experiences. She reacted to her husband as she had to her father. She constantly made psychological interpretations of his and the children's behavior. When confronted with her behavior, she reacted with violent temper outbursts, accusations of being misunderstood, and statements of a need to work harder in therapy.

The mother seemed clearly to have identified with the role of patient and was carrying her whole family along with her. The parents' (particularly the mother's) reluctance to have the older son discharged and interest in hospitalizing the 8-year-old seemed more understandable in the light of this new information. After discussing these issues, the staff felt more secure in their not agreeing to the mother's wishes. They planned to discharge the child and to continue seeing the parents, to help them deal with their relationship and to assist the mother in looking at her need to be a patient.

The supervisee needs to understand that the patients' projections to the staff, although unrealistic, are vital to the therapeutic process. Positive transference contributes to the youngsters' trust of staff and to their viewing staff as benign and helps parents in beginning therapeutic work. When positive transference is missing, establishing a therapeutic alliance becomes more difficult.

The patients' negative transferences lead to projections to the staff of feelings of hostility, lack of caring, criticism, and perceived dissatisfaction with progress. Supervision can help to identify the negative transferences expressed in the patients' behavior. Recognition of these behaviors reinforces the staff members' understanding that the behaviors are projections from the clients' past experiences rather than the results of staff responses. A major task in supervision is to understand that the reduction of negative transference in patients leads to their more integrated behavior. Supervision helps the supervisee become aware of the evidence of transference in a patient's behavior and how the transference may be used to further treatment.

Countertransference attitudes and feelings are elicited by patient, family, and staff behaviors that bring into awareness experiences from the past. Positive countertransference helps to consolidate the therapeutic relationship. Negative countertransference arouses a level of anxiety that most staff find difficult to recognize and resolve. Although initially difficult, discussion of such feelings in supervision permits an understanding of behaviors that have elicited the feelings. The supervisor does not interpret the supervisee's feelings but raises questions for consideration. "What is it in the behavior that makes you uneasy or angry or anxious?" Feelings such as helplessness, anger, obsequiousness, and passive-aggressive behavior make most people uneasy. The origins of such behavior in most people can be explored, which can help the supervisee to identify both the origins of his or her feelings and possible interventions. The exploration often has dramatic results in terms of staff growth and client progress.

A milieu staff person had begun working with a 5-year-old Hispanic girl whose previous worker had left the unit. The worker was challenged by this hostile, impetuous, and imperious child with whom no one seemed to get along. She began her work with the child around the issues of anger, limit setting, and anxiety. She seemed to be making no progress in establishing a positive relationship with the child. The worker was feeling increasingly frustrated and irritable, especially as she noted that both parents, but especially the father, treated the child as the family princess. Though the child's behavior was impossible to live with and her depression was frightening, both parents gave in to her every wish. The child had been sexually molested by a male cousin. The family was unable to act for fear of causing disruption and ill will in the extended family. The girl's severe depression and great hostility, and the family's paralysis in charging her cousin with sexual abuse, were being worked on in family therapy.

In supervision, as the worker was expressing her impatience and disappointment and describing how all her desires to help the child were repulsed, certain themes became more clear. The supervisor suggested that the worker's feelings about being repulsed might give a clue about the child's feelings. The worker said, "You mean she won't let me like her." This insight led to a discussion of the girl's negative self-image (she saw herself as being a bad person) and of her serious depression. The worker could then see the interaction that she and the child were caught up in: the child saw herself as worthless and bad and the worker was acting negatively, as if the child were worthless. The worker also recognized that some of her negative feelings were aimed at this strange Hispanic family, in which the need not to disturb the extended family seemed more important than obtaining justice for their daughter.

The worker was able to say to the child, "You won't let me like you and you're trying not to like me, too." The dynamics of both the child's and the worker's behavior were clarified through the discussion of their interactions, which then permitted the worker to move beyond the impasse in her work with the child. The worker also found that, as she understood the cultural aspects of the family's behavior, she could work more effectively with the child.

Crisis Supervision

Ideally, clinical supervision occurs on a regular basis and few situations that require extra supervision arise. However, actual emergencies do occur.

Supervision around a crisis is an opportunity for learning. It is part of the supervisor's responsibility to be available at such times.

If supervision is intermittent, or occurs only around crises, supervisees will find it difficult to define for themselves the learning goal of supervision or their own strengths and areas for growth. Without these definitions, development of a nonhostile yet questioning atmosphere is especially difficult. Crisis supervision is usually technical rather than process oriented and tends to exaggerate the negatives of behavior rather than concentrate on the excitement of continued learning in understanding of self and others.

CLINICAL ISSUES REQUIRING STAFF DEVELOPMENT

Given the severity of dysfunction in the inpatient population and their families, the diversity of personality, background, and experience of the milieu staff, and the sustained intensity of the emotions experienced, it is understandable that interstaff conflicts are common and recurrent. Regardless of the treatment philosophy or function, the milieu staff members often feel a sense of perplexity or a lack of understanding of the exact nature of the child's problems and the ways to respond most effectively.

Certain conflicts are common among milieu staff. To be resolved, they need to be made overt and discussed openly and nonjudgmentally. A typical, often covert, issue involves whose contribution to the treatment process is of most value. Often there is competition among psychotherapy, education, and milieu staff about the importance of their particular contribution to the child's or family's treatment. Frequently, this competition is expressed in disagreements regarding the patient's primary treatment needs. Only over time and through constant clarification of the issues involved with specific children and families do staff come to realize that all interventions are of value when they are therapeutic and that they are therapeutic when they result in conflict reduction, growth in self-esteem, and adaptive behavioral change over time, regardless of the context in which they occur.

Staff members may disagree about the degree of strictness or the unconsciously punitive behaviors the child's or adolescent's behavior elicits. Some staff members, as a result of their own personal experiences, may see the child as needing strict and restrictive behaviors. Other staff members may believe the child needs a nurturing, permissive relationship. Such conflicts are compounded when it is discovered that the child presents problem behaviors only in certain types of activities or with certain staff members.

Clarifying staff roles with different patients is a sensitive and time-consuming process. Staff members with strict or authoritarian backgrounds may find it difficult to learn to be more permissive and nurturant with a child because of their need to be "in control." Other staff members from backgrounds with little discipline or structure often find it difficult to be clear, firm, and consistent in their expectations of the patient, without feeling that they are being harsh and noncaring.

Ongoing staff discussions are helpful in clarifying the needs of the child, the origins of symptomatic behavior, and possible interventions. To be truly helpful, such discussions also need to identify staff members' feelings, the possible reasons for these feelings, and the methods of dealing with the feelings that will be in the best interests of the child or adolescent and the family.

CONCLUSION

This chapter has highlighted the development of psychiatric nursing's role in milieu treatment. The contributions of clinical supervision and staff development to milieu treatment were explored. Both clinical supervision and staff development function as support systems for those providing care; they are essential elements in maintaining therapeutic relationships. One must learn to care about oneself and experience being cared for before one is able to give care to others. All those who engage in clinical work experience some degree of emotional stress. The stress is evoked in listening to the troubles of other human beings, and it is inherent in the intimacy and responsiveness required in a therapeutic relationship. Clinical supervision and staff development can provide support and enhance the quality of the care provided.

REFERENCES

Cherniss, C. (1980a). *Staff burnout. Job stress in the human services.* Beverly Hills, CA: Sage.

Cherniss, C. (1980b). Human service programs as work organizations: Using organizational design to improve staff motivation and effectiveness. In R. H. Price & P. Olitser (Eds.), *Evaluation and action in the social environment.* New York: Academic Press.

Critchley, D. L. (1985). Clinical supervision. In D. L. Critchley & J. T. Maurin (Eds.), *The clinical specialist in psychiatric mental health nursing: Theory, research and practice,* (pp. 495–510). New York: Wiley.

Haller, L. (1976). Clinical psychiatric supervision: Process and problems. In C. R. Kneisl & H. S. Wilson (Eds.), *Current perspectives in psychiatric nursing. Issues and trends* (pp. 36–43). St. Louis: Mosby.

Loganbill, C., Hardy, E., & Delworth, U. (1982). Supervision: A conceptual model. *Counseling Psychology, 10,* 3–42.

Peplau, H. (1952). *Interpersonal relations in nursing.* New York: Putnam.

Pothier, P. C. (1988). Graduate preparation in child and adolescent psychiatric and mental health nursing. *Archives of Psychiatric Nursing, 3,* 170–172.

Pothier, P. C., Norbeck, J. S., & La Liberte, M. (1985). Child psychiatric nursing: The gap between need and utilization. *Journal of Psychosocial Nursing and Mental Health Services, 23,* 7.

Schwartz, M. S., & Shockley, E. L. (1956). *The nurse and the mental patient.* New York: Russell Sage.

Skinner, K. (1979). The therapeutic milieu: Making it work. *Journal of Psychiatric Nursing, 17,* 38–44.

Stanton, A. H., & Schwartz, M. S. (1954). *The mental hospital.* New York: Basic Books.

Tudor, G. (1952). A sociopsychiatric nursing approach to intervention in a problem of mutual withdrawal on a mental hospital ward. *Psychiatry, 15,* 193–217.

CHAPTER SIXTEEN

Administrative Issues in Present-Day Inpatient Care

Robert L. Hendren
Irving N. Berlin

The administrative issues described in this chapter are especially important in child and adolescent psychiatric hospitals that serve a large number of children and adolescents who are poor and/or come from various minority cultures. Families of these young people often have had a number of destructive experiences with bureaucrats from the dominant culture. Negative experiences with schools, welfare agencies, and health services, originally considered as sources of help, are especially traumatic and demeaning. The clinical administrator must, therefore, be alert to how every element of the hospital interacts with the minority families and their children. Other chapters in this book offer detailed discussions of sensitivity in working with minorities.

The clinical administrator needs to be knowledgeable about how the health system works and what efforts and methods are required to obtain the maximum funding and the greatest number of hospital days for those who require them. Awareness of the most successful current treatment processes for short-, medium-, and long-term stays helps the hospital to provide effective service for all its patients. This chapter focuses on those aspects of clinical administration which place in historical perspective the reimbursement patterns of private and government health insurance and the trends in quality assurance. This perspective may help in anticipating changes and in working out methods of dealing with them so that provision of the best possible services for patients and their families is uninterrupted.

Attention to administrative issues is increasingly important for the success of inpatient child and adolescent psychiatry programs. The rapid growth in the hospital treatment of psychiatric disorders during the past 20 years has led to increasing requirements for efficiency and accountability. Also, a much more competitive marketplace has developed. Today, because a successful hospital psychiatric unit depends not only on a good clinical program but also on a sound administration that is integrated into the entire program, clinical staff must have greater awareness of and involvement in the administrative issues facing the hospital. This chapter covers several of these important issues.

MENTAL HEALTH CARE ECONOMICS

Health care costs have grown from a consumption rate of 6.1% of the gross national product (GNP) in 1966 to 11% of the GNP in 1990 (Abramowitz, 1986; United States Department of Commerce, 1990). Although the percentage of the total health care cost represented by mental health care is relatively low (approximately 15%), this amount is more than double the percentage it represented in 1955 (approximately 6.1%) (Sharfstein & Beigel, 1984). The federal and state governments pay over 50% of mental health costs; for other health care costs, they pay approximately 43%. Private insurers pay 12% of mental health costs and 30% of total health care costs (Staton, 1989). Approximately $50 billion was spent in 1989 on hospital-based psychiatric care, compared with $19 billion in 1985. Of the 1989 total, 67% was paid by private insurance, and 17% of the total was reimbursed by Medicaid and Medicare (Kim, 1990).

In an effort to control costs, both the public and the private sectors are imposing limitations on the nature and extent of the mental health services they will fund. These limitations often result in restricted access to mental health care for minorities, the disadvantaged, and the seriously emotionally disturbed.

Governmental Policy

Governmental policy for the inpatient psychiatric treatment of children has reflected three different and variably important goals: "1) to provide treatment of last resort for the most impaired, 2) to foster the development of comprehensive services according to need and 3) to contain the costs of health care" (Harper & Geraty, 1987). In 1986, Congress passed Public Law 99-660, authorizing grants to states to develop and implement state comprehensive mental health plans for community-based mental health services for adults with severe and persistent mental illness and children and adolescents with serious emotional disturbances. To receive federal funds, states must develop a plan and demonstrate its implementation. Providing a community-based comprehensive plan is complicated in many states because multiple agencies are involved in various aspects of identification, planning, reimbursement, and treatment. Separate agencies may be responsible for social services, Medicaid, hospitals, residential treatment facilities, health services, community mental health facilities, and education, to name only a few.

Medicaid benefits are limited in most states. Limitations may be placed on prospective reimbursement per discharge, the number of days allowed for an inpatient stay, the number of outpatient visits, and the type of facility that can receive reimbursement. Prior approval of treatment and independent certification for necessity may be required. Many states are looking to increase Medicaid eligibility because the federal government provides a certain percentage of the reimbursement and states then pay what is often a smaller remaining percentage of the total bill. Restrictions and limitations are likely to increase; the amount of money being spent through Medicaid programs is increasing yearly. Several likely mechanisms for restrictions include peer review organizations (PROs), the resource-based relative value scale (RVS), diagnosis-related groups (DRGs), and managed care.

Health Insurance

In 1987, 37 million Americans were without health insurance. Children represented 32% of this uninsured population (Current Population Survey, 1989). Approximately 15% of adolescents aged 10 to 18 were without public or private health coverage in 1987 (Office of Technology Assessment, 1989). The proportion of adolescents without private or public health insurance coverage increased by 25% between 1979 and 1986, an increase due largely to increased poverty and decreased Medicaid coverage. Younger children are slightly more likely to be insured. The poor are the most likely to be uninsured. Hispanic adolescents are much more likely than others to be uninsured, regardless of family income, and black adolescents are much more likely than white adolescents to be uninsured, a relationship that is almost entirely dependent on family income ("Preliminary analysis . . . ," 1989).

Higher deductibles, increased copayments, and other restrictions are commonly associated with mental health insurance benefits. Compared to other illnesses, only 39% of employer health insurance plans provided inpatient psychiatric coverage in 1986. Only 6% of plans provided the same coverage for outpatient mental health as they did for other outpatient conditions in 1986 (Staton, 1989). However, the fastest growing health care cost is for mental health and substance abuse treatment. Payers typically spend 15 to 24 cents of every health care dollar for these services (Kenkel, 1990). Further restrictions seem likely, and any limitations and restrictions lead to increased referrals to public mental health facilities (Frank & Lave, 1985).

Managed Health Care

Managed health care, through prepaid health delivery systems and utilization of review organizations, is the fastest growing trend in modern health care (Sederer & St. Clair, 1989). These payers attempt to restrain health care expenditures by using price limits, offering third-party discounts, limiting provider selection, limiting the scope of benefits, and instituting utilization controls to limit hospital stays.

Initially, peer review organizations (PROs) were begun by Congress in an attempt to instill quality into the prospective Medicare payment system. The concept has become increasingly popular and most reimbursement sources now use some form of utilization review. The "management" of managed care reflects economic necessity as much as or more than it does clinical need, and it includes utilization of a variety of preferred provider organizations (PPOs), health maintenance organizations (HMOs), and case management/utilization review companies (Staton, 1989). Approximately 30% of the insured population has health coverage through HMOs and PPOs and this number is expected to at least double in the next 5 to 10 years (Kenkel, 1989). Unfortunately, most managed health care organizations resist providing mental health care, impose severe coverage limitations, and rely on risk-sharing physician–"gatekeepers" to reduce specialist referrals and inpatient treatment. Thus, managed care not only leads to limited psychiatric benefits for the population served, but also raises ethical dilemmas for physicians and administrators who participate in these rapidly growing organizations.

Proprietary Psychiatric Systems

For-profit health care systems grew by 8% to 10% per year during the 1980s (Staton, 1989). Causes were: the elimination of certificate-of-need laws for bed expansion per capita, psychiatry's freedom from diagnostic related group (DRG) reimbursement, less costly treatment operations, low capital investment, and the ability to transfer or reject patients who had no insurance or had exhausted their benefits. In addition, admissions and treatment in psychiatric units can be accomplished with minimal physician involvement. Investor-owned, multihospital corporations have financial, managerial, and marketing advantages and offer few unprofitable services. Proprietary hospitals tend to skim off the insured patients, leaving treatment of the uninsured or underinsured patients for public facilities, which are experiencing increasing financial disadvantages. There is increasing concern about the overhospitalization of insured adolescents in proprietary facilities (Butts & Schwartz, 1991). Several national organizations have prepared position statements regarding the appropriate use of hospitalization. Third-party case management/utilization review is also providing some constraint.

HOSPITAL REGULATION AND REVIEW

It is becoming increasingly important for clinical administrators to be very familiar with the standards for care developed by various accrediting bodies.

Joint Commission on the Accreditation of Healthcare Organizations (JCAHO)

The JCAHO accredits approximately 75% of the nation's hospitals, including almost all of those with more than 50 beds (Senior, 1989). General hospital psychiatric programs are asked to meet Hospital Accreditation Program (HAP) standards and residential programs are asked to meet standards from the *Consolidated Standards' Manual* in order to gain accreditation.

Since April 1987, free-standing psychiatric, chemical dependency, and mental health programs have been asked to meet the HAP standards in order to gain accreditation. Not all hospitals or residential programs gain accreditation. Those least likely to gain it are the underfunded public institutions that treat the underserved. Lack of accreditation often means less reimbursement from outside sources and greater reliance on state funding.

Credentialing and Privileges

Physicians practicing in an inpatient setting must go through a two-step procedure to gain authorization to practice. The first step is receiving from the state a license to practice; the second is the credentialing and privileging process of the health care facility. The hospital medical staff includes fully licensed physicians and may include other licensed individuals who are permitted, by law and by the hospital, to provide patient care services independently in the hospital (Joint Commission on the Accreditation of Healthcare Organizations, 1989). Hospital-specific criteria for clinical privileges help to ensure that physicians admitting and treating psychiatric patients meet appropriate training and performance requirements. Admission to psychiatric units and inpatient treatment of children and adolescents should be done only by those psychiatrists who have specific clinical privileges to admit and treat patients in this developmental age group. The JCAHO's standards for children's hospitals require that all individuals responsible for the assessment, treatment, or care of patients be competent in obtaining information regarding the patient's developmental needs, in a knowledge of growth and development, and in an understanding of the range of treatments that are age-appropriate (JCAHO, 1989). In addition, at the time of application or reapplication for clinical privileges, the physician must be considered on the bases of experience in providing inpatient treatment to children and adolescents, competence as judged by monitoring and evaluation activities and peer review, health status, and documented continuing education.

Quality Assurance

The term *quality assurance* (QA) is most commonly thought of as one of the requirements for JCAHO accreditation. However, organizations such as professional review organizations (PROs) and the Health Care Financing Administration (HCFA) also require some form of quality assurance. The required JCAHO standard is for an ongoing QA program "designed to objectively and systematically monitor and evaluate the quality and appropriateness of patient care, pursue opportunities to improve patient care, and resolve identified problems" (JCAHO, 1989). This includes operational linkages between clinical risk management functions and QA functions.

Patient care monitoring review (PCMR), an integral part of a mental health facility's ongoing QA process (Silverman, Comerford, & Stoker, 1988), involves review of and direct consultation on problematic cases by the professional staff, either upon request or when a certain indicator such as length of stay, lack of discharge plans, or excessive use of seclusion or restraint identifies a case for review. By following a number of problematic cases over time, PCMR personnel can observe patient care trends and, thus, improve patient care. The QA process may appear to function only to fulfill an accreditation requirement, but creative indicators can identify problem areas and trends and measure the success in ameliorating them.

NEED FOR PLANNING

Strategic planning and marketing are gaining increasing importance in the successful delivery of mental health services. Some administrators fear that these techniques have the potential for manipulation of the marketplace. However, if the goal of planning and marketing is to help patients make informed decisions in meeting their needs, the process should help both mental health consumers and providers to reach their goal (Gibson, 1984). Strategic planning "determines the overall mission and goals of the institution and the public image to be exhibited, identifies competitive and pinpoints potential markets, which when developed can contribute significantly to hospital growth and fulfillment of community needs" (Domanico, 1981). Marketing involves efforts to "retain and attract new patient populations by serving and satisfying their needs by providing appropriate services in a manner that is consistent with professional standards of practice and is financially viable" (Gibson, 1984).

The marketing planning process asks three basic questions:

1. Where are we now? (Analyze both the external and the internal environment of the organization.)
2. Where do we want to go? (Evaluate the opportunities, threats, and realistic, measurable goals.)
3. How do we get there? (Develop a strategy of operational planning, formulated objectives, and targeted marketing.)

The most important portion of this process is the continual reevaluation of these three basic questions and appropriate adjustment of the strategies.

ETHICAL CONSIDERATIONS

The demands of the competitive mental health environment create a number of ethical dilemmas for both the mental health administrator and the practitioner delivering the service (Webb, 1989). The health care professional is ethically bound to serve the best interest of his or her patients. However, unless the professional's practice or health care organization stays financially viable, the patient will not be able to receive the needed clinical care.

Ethical conflicts are raised when the health care professional is asked: "Whom do you work for—the patient or the organization?" In managed care organizations, professionals serve as gatekeepers, utilization reviewers, and, through risk sharing, financial partners (Sederer & St. Clair, 1989). Patient confidentiality is eroded by the reporting requirements of the judicial system, third-party payers, and the state and federal government. At times, patients may not be fully informed regarding for whom the practitioner is working.

The health care administrator faces ethical dilemmas when deciding the distribution of scarce resources. How should the uninsured and underinsured be served? What about the poor and minorities or the high-risk, chronically mentally ill patient? Under what conditions should those without financial resources be treated for their mental illness without reimbursement? What about abandonment, when the resources run out? We have not yet acknowledged that the rationing of mental health care and the lower mental health benefits in most reimbursement programs are creating a two-tiered system of health care in which those with comprehensive insurance, or any insurance at all, may receive more rapid, higher quality care than those who are uninsured or underinsured and must rely on an overburdened public system.

Marketing and advertising may help patients to access the service they need but may also create a need not previously recognized and may misrepresent the results of treatment. Financial incentives offered to practitioners, administrators, and advertisers also create ethical dilemmas when considering whether the patients' best interests are being served.

Another potential ethical dilemma involves the demands for teaching, research, and service (Reece, 1989). At times, patient care may appear to be sacrificed in the interest of providing a training opportunity. However, the necessity of training programs is obvious if continuing, up-to-date patient care is to be provided. Excessive preoccupation with research can also compromise patient care but a lack of research may also present a threat to quality patient care.

CLINICAL LEADERSHIP

In response to the multiple pressures to provide cost-effective, ethical medical care, it is increasingly important for clinicians to assume administrative roles and become "the champions of quality care for the mentally ill and restore clinical imperative to their treatment planning" (Rodenhauser

& Greenblatt, 1989). Clinical administration requires leadership and knowledge, to help synthesize the various tensions in a mental health organization and to form a common and coherent formulation and plan (Harper & Geraty, 1987).

Historically, mental health professionals have arrived at administrative leadership roles as a result of recognized skills as clinicians, researchers, or educators, not as administrators. This background does not usually provide the management information necessary in the current competitive marketplace in such areas as planning, finance, cost control, management, employee relations, medicolegal issues, the political process, and public relations (Silver & Marcos, 1989). In fact, the reflective, nondirective approach of a therapist may be detrimental where action and clear leadership are needed (Hirschovitz, 1971).

Silver and Marcos (1989) identified the following five distinct factors, the interplay of which leads to the development of a clinical administrator:

1. Individual personality traits such as creativity, high energy, intelligence, motivation, perseverance, and tolerance for ambiguity;
2. Clinical psychiatric training and clinical competence;
3. Administrative training;
4. On-the-job administrative experience;
5. A mentor relationship.

However, in one survey of psychiatric administrators, only 27% had formal administrative training, although 73% thought it was important. Only 59% actually had a mentor, although 91% thought it was important (Silver, Akerson, & Marcos, 1990). Clinician–executives should consider learning management theory and business techniques and incorporating them into their administrative practice (Silver & Marcos, 1989).

An appreciation of the organizational structure of a mental health system or institution is essential for an effective leader. A formal structure has written definitions of the roles of and relationships among the individuals within an organization. An informal structure has actual but unwritten lines of communication and of the relationships that exist functionally within the organization. Many clinical problems within a mental health organization can result from a lack or ambiguity of formal structure or from tension between the formal and informal structures (Harper & Geraty, 1987). The formal structure may appear confusing; many mental health institutions have a matrix model of organization, in which an individual has organizational accountability within a service (e.g., a hospital unit) and within a discipline (e.g., nursing, social work). It is uncommon in most mental health institutions, especially hospitals, for an individual to be accountable in one hierarchical line to a single service chief (Harper & Geraty, 1987).

Leadership style is an important aspect of effective clinical administration. In different situations, a variety of styles may be effective (Gardner, 1986). An authoritarian or charismatic leader may do well when the group needs clear leadership and is willing to follow. A process-oriented leader who works with the organization to set goals and achieve them may do well when the group is highly motivated and able to work independently. A laissez-faire leader gives others freedom to do what they want, to facilitate creativity, but the result may be chaos if clear direction is needed instead. Examination of one's own leadership style and needs is an important part of being an effective clinical administrator. What leadership style is needed and expected in the organization at its present developmental level? Personal needs, cultural expectations, and previous experience are a few of the factors that can influence the success of the match between the leader and the organization.

To develop the number of clinical administrators needed in the health care marketplace, training programs should give increased emphasis to this area. Several possibilities exist (Silver et al., 1990). An "administrative track" could be offered, or a separate fellowship, or an administrative rotation. The training program could provide management theory and supervised administrative experiences in which clinical administrators serve as mentors. Other possibilities are to assign a senior clinical administrator to serve as a mentor for each trainee, or to develop a relationship between the training program and an MBA or MPA program. Prospective clinician–administrators could develop their business and management knowledge and skills and earn an advanced degree upon completion.

PROBLEMS OFTEN ENCOUNTERED IN CLINICAL ADMINISTRATION

Administrative Constraints

Cost effectiveness is a financial reality in the running of any hospital. To be cost-effective in a child and adolescent psychiatric hospital poses some special problems. The critical issue is: At what point does the effort to reduce costs undermine therapeutic effectiveness? The constraints placed on clinical administrators by government agencies and private hospital corporations may also result in such poor clinical care that referrals of patients to those hospitals cease.

In their cost-saving effort, some child and adolescent psychiatric services tend to hire therapists who have not been trained to treat children. They hire professionals who cost them less, instead of hiring a well-trained child and adolescent psychiatrist, to indicate to the community an effort to provide the best treatment possible and a knowledgeable management of psychotropic medications. Maintenance on each unit of a core patient-care staff who can educate new staff and facilitate aspects of the milieu programs as patient census increases becomes essential to effective and cost-effective patient care. It is important, in the face of a low census, to have contingency plans in place to maintain core staff. They may have to work different shifts on other wards or fewer hours, or float between wards, but their availability is critical to good care.

Inservice education to staff and allotment of time for staff supervision to enhance staff treatment effectiveness are rare because they are thought to be too expensive. Evidence is contradictory: the more educated and self-aware the staff becomes in dealing with difficult patients, the more effective and *less* costly the milieu treatment program will be.

Another cost issue of some importance is the school program the hospital offers. Some hospitals maintain that since patients' stay is brief, a token school program is all that is required. It has been our experience in both private and publicly funded hospitals that an active and educationally effective program is essential to patient progress. Such a program focuses on tasks that need to be accomplished to make up for the usual academic failure. An effective educational program tends to help the young person and the family recognize that the hospital program seeks to help patients to overcome problems in every sphere of living and to enhance competence and a sense of self-worth. An objective, task oriented school program also enables the teachers, aides, and milieu staff assigned to the school to develop close, nonthreatening relationships as a prelude to close relationships and bonding with other staff.

Prejudice in the Clinical Administrator

Like most human beings, administrators have racial and status prejudice which, in many ways, may make their work more difficult. Unconscious prejudices may lead the administrator to view black, Hispanic, and native American people as fit only for maintenance or kitchen jobs. Thus, even when they have had good training, the administrator may not believe minorities to be competent in bookkeeping, accounting, patient services, and other administrative areas. This prejudice often results in underemployment of minority professionals in clinical positions for which they are qualified. Some administrators accommodate the Affirmative Action directives by hiring qualified minority workers, but they then keep them from advancement.

Unconscious prejudice against minority cultures is even more pervasive against women. Thus, top executive and clinical positions are often not offered to women despite their clear competence and suitability. Or, a token woman is given token assignments and authority so that the woman's position cannot elicit notice and favorable comment.

These prejudices usually lead to formation of an "old boy network" in which "belonging," not competence and innovative skills, results in being hired. The institution is then cheated of the creativity necessary in today's competitive hospital market to provide excellent patient care and financial solvency.

The Role of Power in Clinical Administration

Some administrators, when they use their administrative authority, find themselves dealing with their unconscious drives for power; they act authoritarian and omnipotent. For most of these persons, being all-powerful and all-knowing, rather than providing leadership in collaborative efforts to serve patients well, is necessary for their sense of well-being. They describe having their ideas questioned and challenged as a sign of disrespect and an undermining of authority and perceive any questioning of their authority as a threat.

One administrator, when questioned about an unannounced firing of a department head, became adamant about his prerogative to fire employees, despite the fact that it circumvented reasonable and historic protections in hiring. This unexpected, unilateral firing foreshadowed a number of incidents in which responsible persons were let go without much discussion and with no consideration of their functioning or of how they could have functioned more effectively. This pattern of hiring and firing without consultation unfortunately became imitated by others in the administrative hierarchy.

Unchecked decision-making power and omnipotent and authoritarian conduct clearly indicate a lack of self-confidence in one's capabilities, talents, and leadership and discourage collaboration and discussion in decision making. A competent clinical administrator is able to encourage collaboration and discussion of administrative decisions without giving up accountability and the final decision-making role.

CONCLUSION

The successful clinical administrator must learn the essential principles of hospital administration through training and experience. Familiarity with and understanding of current health care economics and policy, hospital regulations, strategic planning, effective leadership styles, and the ability to work effectively with others in the administration of the hospital are essential. Practices in today's health care marketplace raise difficult ethical dilemmas that need to be resolved in a clinically sound yet financially viable manner.

REFERENCES

Abramowitz, K. S. (1986). The future of health care delivery in America. *Bernstein Research,* 16–17.

Butts, J. A., & Schwartz, I. M. (1991, in press). Access to insurance and length of psychiatric stay among adolescents and young adults discharged from general hospitals. *Journal of Health and Social Policy.*

Domanico, L. (1981). Strategic planning vital for hospital long-range development. *Hospital and Health Services Administration, 25,* 25–50.

Frank, R. G., & Lave, J. R. (1985). The impact of Medicaid benefit design on length of hospital stay and patient transfers. *Hospital and Community Psychiatry, 36,* 749–753.

Gardner, J. W. (1986). *The nature of leadership: Introductory consideration.* Washington, DC: Independent Sector.

Gibson, R. W. (1984). Strategic planning and marketing of mental health services. *Psychiatric Annals, 14,* 846–850.

Harper, G., & Geraty, R. (1987). Hospital and residential treatment. In R. Michaels & J. O. Cavenar (Eds.), *Psychiatry* (Vol. 2, ch. 64). Philadelphia: Lippincott.

Hirschovitz, R. G. (1971). Dilemmas of leadership in community mental health. *Psychiatry Quarterly, 22,* 102–116.

Joint Commission on the Accreditation of Healthcare Organizations. (1989). *Accreditation Manual for Hospitals.* Chicago, IL: Author.

Kenkel, P. J. (1989, November 17). Meeting the challenge of managed care in hospitals. *Modern Healthcare,* pp. 52–53.

Kenkel, P. J. (1990, January 29). Utilization review takes toll on mental health units. *Modern Healthcare,* p. 42.

Kim, H. (1990, April 23). Sicker psych patients could help hospitals. *Modern Healthcare,* p. 28.

Office of Technology Assessment. (1989). Analysis of trends in coverage and preliminary estimates of the effects of an employer mandate and Medicaid expansion on the uninsured: Background paper. Washington, DC: U.S. Government Printing Office.

"Preliminary analysis of adolescent health insurance status." (1989). In *Analysis of trends in coverage and preliminary estimates of the effects of an employer mandate and Medicaid expansion on the uninsured.* Washington, DC: U.S. Congress, Office of Technology Assessment.

Reece, R. D. (1989). The new medical ethics and mental health administration. *Psychiatric Annals, 19,* 428–431.

Rodenhauser, P., & Greenblatt, M. (1989). Transformations in mental health system management: An overview. *Psychiatric Annals, 19,* 408–411.

Sederer, L. I., & St. Clair, R. L. (1989). Managed health care and the Massachusetts experience. *American Journal of Psychiatry, 146,* 1142–1148.

Senior, N. (1989). Regulation and review of psychiatric services in the United States. *Psychiatric Annals, 19,* 415–420.

Sharfstein, S. S., & Beigel, A. (1984). Less is more? Today's economics and its challenge to psychiatry. *American Journal of Psychiatry, 141,* 1403–1407.

Silver, M. A., Akerson, D. M., & Marcos, L. R. (1990). Critical factors in the professional development of the psychiatrist–administrator. *Hospital Community Psychiatry, 41,* 71–74.

Silver, M. A., & Marcos, L. R. (1989). The making of the psychiatrist–executive. *American Journal of Psychiatry, 146,* 29–34.

Silverman, W. H., Comerford, R., & Stoker, T. (1988, October). Patient care monitoring review at a psychiatric hospital for adolescents. *QRB,* pp. 307–310.

Staton, D. (1989). Mental health care economics and the future of psychiatric practice. *Psychiatric Annals, 19,* 421–427.

Webb, W. L. (1989). Ethical psychiatric practice in a new economic climate. *Psychiatric Annals, 19,* 443–447.

CHAPTER SEVENTEEN

Some Principles of Clinical Administration Derived from Therapeutic Insights

Irving N. Berlin

The administrator who is clinically trained tends to be sensitive to the feelings of others and aware of their general state of tension or relaxation. From experiences in working with patients and with clinical staff, the administrator becomes aware of the transference manifestations that his or her personality elicits and recognizes his or her countertransference reactions to certain staff and patient behaviors and personality characteristics. The administrator can use this awareness to facilitate administrative practices.

Settings where patients and families from various cultures are treated require special awareness. Sensitivity to important cultural values and to attitudes toward mental illness, hospitalization, the use of medication, and treatment in general allows these issues to be dealt with in a culturally relevant way. An administrator who has this awareness will be inclined to select competent staff members who are from various indigenous cultures or who have worked extensively and effectively with minorities. Clinical experience affords to those clinicians who later administer child and adolescent inpatient and outpatient facilities familiarity with the problem areas in both patient care and staff effectiveness. The administrators can then anticipate difficulties before they become serious.

In this chapter, I have tried to recapture the various clinical therapeutic experiences which, over 30 years, enriched my understanding of clinical administration and slowly emerged as principles of clinical administration.

EARLY LESSONS

One of my earliest experiences as an administrator occurred shortly after I became training director in the child psychiatry training program at Langley Porter Children's Service at the School of Medicine, University of California—San Francisco. We had been warned about a new Fellow, Dr. X, by the General Psychiatry program. He was described as very bright and talented but chronically tardy to seminars and in his paper work. He continued these behaviors on the Child Psychiatry service, even though the committee, during the interviews for the Fellowship, had warned him of the need to change. Since I was supervising Dr. X, I kept reminding him that he would have to mend his ways. No change occurred. About one month after Dr. X came on our service, the Director of Child Psychiatry, Dr. S. A. Szurek, called me in and asked why Dr. X was always late to his seminar. I replied that this was an old problem and that we were working on it. The director commented, "I don't want him to be late again to my seminar. See to it." My dilemma was how to alter this Fellow's character problems quickly. I did not want to face the director's annoyance, nor did I want to fail, in his eyes, as the recently appointed training director.

The next time I met with Dr. X, who came late to supervision, I told him he would have to come on time to all meetings or I was prepared to recommend to Dr. Szurek and to the department chairman that he be dropped from the Fellowship. Dr. X became livid with anger. He explained that he was working on the problems in his analysis, and accused me of being out to ruin his career. My response was, "Either meet your obligations as a child Fellow or you force me to act. I do not intend to have the director angry with me because of your behavior; is that clear?" Dr. X kept up his angry tirades in supervision for some weeks, but he did come on time to Dr. Szurek's seminar and in a few weeks he was on time for all of his conferences and began to catch up on his paper work. At a party several months later, his wife thanked me for being so firm. Dr. X, despite his angry tirades at me, had gradually become more responsible at home, with a great reduction of tension (Berlin, 1967; Szurek, 1967).

Out of these experiences, I evolved my first and second principles of administration. First, firmness and unambivalent fairness with one's colleagues who hold subordinate positions helps them to carry out their obligations and keeps superiors off one's back. Second, being in analysis does not excuse anyone from carrying out responsibilities or from performing assigned learning and clinical responsibilities as a trainee or faculty member.

I also learned at Langley Porter how to avoid being spit on. Sally, a 6-year-old girl, mounted watch at the front door of the children's ward and would, with unerring skill, spit into the face of all who entered. Somehow, Dr. Szurek had escaped being a target. Since I had gotten my share of spittle, I was determined to use my observational skills to study Dr. Szurek's technique. Rather than rushing through the door, in the vain hope of avoiding the spit, Dr. Szurek slowly opened the door and carefully looked at Sally with a serious expression on his face. He did not dare her to spit nor avoid her spitting. My emulation of this stance brought a great reduction of being spit upon and helped to formulate my third principle of administration. No matter how distasteful the problems that must be confronted, one needs to gather all the data one can and then face them directly, nonpunitively, and promptly (Szurek, 1950).

Another lesson that Dr. Szurek helped me to learn centered around the treatment of a young adolescent schizophrenic boy, Joe, who was over 6 feet tall and very destructive. It became clear to me that, because of his size, he received very few direct signs of physical affection. One day I mentioned to Dr. Szurek that I was going to feed Joe with a baby bottle, hoping he would feel more cared about. Dr. Szurek's response was that if I thought it was therapeutically relevant to the treatment, it was worth trying. I had observed Joe mouthing objects but not sucking on them. I also knew he had had little nurturance from his physically ill mother and guessed he had not had much sucking experience. Since Joe was irritable, large, and occasionally aggressive, I wondered if he would react favorably to an opportunity to suck from a baby bottle. The staff agreed it was a good idea to try and made the dayroom available to me. The next day, many of my colleagues, trainees, and ward staff peeked through the dayroom window and saw me on the couch with Joe's head in my lap, feeding him juice from a baby bottle. His large frame was draped over the entire couch, and his feet dangled over the end. I was aware of the tension I felt and the incongruous picture we made. However, Joe relaxed, sucked contentedly, emptied the bottle, and was less destructive that day. Other ward staff were encouraged and began to interrupt Joe's tantrums with an offer of milk or juice from a baby bottle. Tantrums and destruction were reduced, and nurturant contact between patient and staff was markedly increased. In time, Joe sat, with the staff person's arm on his shoulder, and drank milk or juice from a glass.

It was characteristic of Dr. Szurek to gently explore with faculty and trainees why they wanted to try a new approach. He was always supportive of others' intuitions if they were based on some clinical data. In Joe's case, I had reservations and very mixed feelings about looking silly and about the possibility that the effort would not work. Dr. Szurek's encouraging acceptance of my intuitions as being worth a try gave me the support I needed to proceed with staff discussions and the trial attempt.

The principle I derived from this experience was that one should trust intuitions and gut feelings at least enough to try them, if sufficient self-examination has been given to clarifying their motivation. The corollary was that one should respect the intuitions of others and, where possible, be supportive.

Concomitant lessons were learned in collaborating with Dr. Szurek on a number of publications. When I wrote a clinical vignette, he would sometimes say events could not have happened in that way. After my indignation abated, I came to recognize that he was concerned because the sequences did not fit together to make dynamic sense. In our discussions of the details of the therapy, I found myself recalling the missing interactions. At another level, there were occasions when Dr. Szurek and I disagreed on a theoretical issue. Dr. Szurek always invited me to write my own version and even to publish versions that openly stated the differences in points of view. These attitudes obviously promoted very close examination of clinical work. Finally, the encouragement to describe in detail my theoretical ideas, even if they were not in agreement with the director's, provided the opportunity, in Dr. Szurek's words, of "self-examination." He maintained that writing down one's ideas was second only to free association in self-learning (Szurek, 1950; Szurek & Berlin, 1964).

This attitude promotes more openness in examining one's own and others' theoretical positions. It also frees one to be receptive to varying theoretical points of view and enables one to learn from others and to use what seems useful.

The administrative principle I evolved from these experiences was: Encourage and be receptive to disagreement and various points of view.

Otherwise, they often become covertly expressed ideas and lead to acting-out. Openness to another point of view does not mean one has abrogated the responsibility for decision making (Hardy, 1970).

LESSONS FROM THE PRACTICE OF COMMUNITY PSYCHIATRY AND MENTAL HEALTH CONSULTATION

Skills from individual psychotherapy need to be combined with community consultation principles and with innovative thinking that can be applied appropriately to community processes. A particular instance stands out as validation of that statement.

While I was consulting with a superintendent and his administrative staff in a suburb of a large metropolis, the problems originating from a particular housing project were brought to my attention. The project was built for Appalachian families who were being resettled after their home sites were submerged under the waters created by a new dam. These families, who had had no preparation for living in apartments, were having trouble keeping the project clean. Their children were experiencing serious learning problems in school, but most disconcerting to school authorities were the high rate of truancy among the boys and the many hysterical episodes seen among the junior and senior high school girls—mostly hysterical paralyses of upper and lower limbs, which kept them out of school. Clearly, these displaced Appalachian people felt anger at their displacement and universal discrimination from the new community.

The superintendent and his staff, with my help, began examining the factors that might be contributing to the overt behavior of the adolescents. In the process, we became more conscious of how unfriendly and biased the older, established community was toward the newcomers. They had strange customs and accents, and they behaved oddly in social situations. Besides, they threw their garbage out of the window. Thus, these newcomers were ostracized by the upper-middle-class residents. Their children were academically far behind their peers and dressed shabbily. To resolve these various problems, the help of a large part of the community would be needed.

Community groups found it difficult to understand the very serious stresses being suffered by the newcomers as a result of being dislocated from a home community, separated from relatives in nearby towns, relocated on essentially foreign soil, and placed into a strange and frightening environment. They had been uprooted from their poor homes and subsistence living in their little towns and transferred without preparation to a high-rise federal housing project in a densely populated suburb of a large city where employment was difficult to find because of the Appalachian adults' poor writing and reading skills.

This phenomenon is a core issue. I had come to understand it during attempts to develop collaborative programs with Plains Indians. Tribes that had been moved from their hunting grounds to reservations could not accommodate to the displacement, especially when no hunting was possible and no way was available for the adults to become economically self-sufficient.

A number of discussions with the superintendent and staff produced agreement that the community had to be more welcoming to these newcomers. The junior and senior high school administrators agreed to keep the sewing rooms and the woodworking and auto shops open in the evenings, on a trial basis. They obtained volunteer instructors who invited mothers and daughters to learn how to make dresses and fathers and sons to work on cars or furniture making. Within a few months, the school was seen as a more familiar and more friendly place. Several of the school nurses paid visits to the homes of the most troubled girls, invited them to work together, along with their mothers, on sewing dresses in the evening, and introduced them to the volunteer teachers from the community. The school nurses became confidants to these girls, who needed help with a variety of health problems. Some students volunteered to help the girls with their schoolwork. Besides a decrease in hysteria among the girls and truancy among the boys, the school's outreach had other effects. The parents' involvement with the school in the evenings made it easier to approach them about the hygiene problems around the housing project. They were helped to plant gardens by elderly members of a local garden club, who appeared less threatening to the parents. Thus, what was first described as a clinical therapeutic problem of disturbed and disturbing adolescents turned out to be symptomatic of a community mental health problem and required involvement of the school and the entire community. In minority communities, some serious problems that lead to hospitalization of children and adolescents stem from community mental health problems—problems related to displacement, unemployment, loss of traditional values and the resulting widespread alcoholism, and chaotic family life and its inevitable child abuse and neglect.

The principle derived for administrative application was to dare to try new and different approaches to problems so long as they are based on sound clinical thinking and experience. In this instance, knowledge and clinical experience urged an enhancement of self-image and a sense of self-worth, which was critical to behavioral change (Argyris, 1962).

COKE MACHINE CONSULTATION

When one is fortunate enough to be involved in a movement at its beginning, as I was in the mental health center movement, one's name may be associated with certain events and experiences. My name became associated with "Coke machine consultation." I had been hired as a consultant to a juvenile probation department as part of a county consultation package to two school systems and the welfare and public health departments. It was immediately clear that the chief probation officer did not want a consultation. The office I used when I came to consult was in the basement and there was a sign-up sheet on the door for any probation officer brave enough to sign up. The sheet was always clean. Since no one came to consult with me, I left my office and spent the morning around the coke machine. Not many probation officers stayed very long to talk after they got their coke, but at least they got to know my face. However, many people did stop to chat—the janitors, the head motor pool mechanic, other mechanics, and various secretaries.

In a relatively short time, I understood the chief probation officer's reluctance to have a consultant. As my colleague, Sam Susselman (1969), so accurately wrote, people in agencies related to law enforcement have a tendency to distort the law by taking it into their own hands. Thus, I learned from the motor pool manager that county cars were being treated by the chief probation officer and others as their own personal vehicles. From the janitors I learned that, in certain offices, there were frequently whiskey bottles in the waste baskets. The secretaries told me that, in certain probation units, the tougher the juvenile was who was put on probation, and thus the more difficult and threatening to the probation officers who were required to regularly check up on the conditions of probation, the more rapidly a reason was found to return him to the correctional institution.

As I became acquainted with the probation officers, the members of one of the boys' probation units most frequently sought me out. It was clear that their unit chief sanctioned consultation with me and, in time, the chief himself sneaked into my office to consult. Many problems existed in supervising probationers in the department. This unit began to function more effectively as a result of surfacing and discussing its problems during consultation and being helped to problem-solve. In all units, there was a tendency to avoid confronting the very tough juveniles with their failures to obey the conditions of probation. Our discussions led to the awareness that everyone was uncomfortable with the threats of physical harm. Only when such a threat, no matter how offhand, was met with a promise of close vigilance and prompt reporting to the court did the probation officer become an effective deterrent to acting-out.

In one session, I described a personal experience of feeling afraid and being able to acknowledge it but also being firm about my duty. I had been transferred to be the new chief of a psychiatric ward in a general hospital in France during World War II. On my first rounds, a giant psychotic paratrooper confronted me. He said, "Doc, I've been running this ward, see, and if you know what's good for you, you won't interfere." As I looked around for support, I noticed my corpsmen had vanished. I was alone and scared to death. I said to this soldier, "I'm very frightened of you and what you could do to me, but this is my job. I'm going to run this ward with all the MPs on the base if necessary." For a long moment, the psychotic paratrooper glared at me. Then he turned around and said, "OK, Doc, have it your way." Being afraid and being able to verbalize it with those who are intimidating requires courage and also signals that one means business. Because the probation officers could openly admit to each other their fear of certain probationers, they could also discuss how to set limits and deal with threats. The effectiveness of this unit stood out, and the Juvenile Court judge investigated the problems that were seriously impairing the effectiveness of the other probation units. The investigation resulted in widespread changes of personnel and of ways of dealing with youth on probation.

I drew several administrative principles from my effective Coke machine consultation. First, don't just sit in an office. Circulate and become available to everyone. Second, as an administrator, be aware that every person in an organization may have important information that could be helpful in understanding some general organizational problems. Seize every opportunity to communicate to others that you are an interested and concerned human being. Third, share your own personal experiences in problem solving, to reveal your lack of omnipotence and your human frailties. Consultees and younger colleagues will be encouraged to face their own frailties, some of which may be obstructing the effectiveness of their work.

EXPERIENCES WITH THE INDIAN CHILDREN'S PROGRAMS

Some of my unique experiences in New Mexico came from working with the Indian Children's Programs and learning from and with my Indian Health Service (IHS) colleagues. One of the most valuable insights I gained was that different people, different cultures, and different groups within a culture deserve all possible attention, so that one can slowly learn about their uniqueness and their special problems.

In one incident, an IHS colleague and I were invited to the psychiatric ward at the Indian Hospital in Gallup. Two child psychiatry Fellows were with us as observers. We were invited to attend a family conference about a Navajo adolescent who was schizophrenic. The family consisted of the grandmother (the matriarch who made the decisions), the mother and her two sisters, and a Navajo translator. A Navajo sing had been held to relieve the patient of his illness; now we needed to convince the family that he should be placed on neuroleptics. The hope was that having a psychiatry professor there to endorse the medication would speed up the persuasion process. Every sentence spoken in English was translated into Navajo and vice versa. My careful observations of the grandmother, mother, and aunts gave me a strong feeling that they all understood English. However, at issue was our show of respect to the grandmother, the family, and the culture's very gradual way of arriving at a decision. For three hours, we talked quietly and patiently, after which the grandmother gave her consent to the psychotropic medication.

At the end of the family conference, our child Fellows were beside themselves. They asked us how we could sit so quietly and relaxed for so long. My reply was, "What alternative was there?" We had to reveal not only our concern for the patient but also our respect for the family and their culture. In other pueblos and reservations, our patience was repeatedly tested by particularly slow or complicated ways of obtaining permission to carry out educational or psychological tasks. Although these services had been requested previously by the tribe, the delays were a necessary precursor to collaboration and to being trusted to do one's work in a sensitive way. During the delays, we became aware of the particular traditions and values of these communities. It is important to remember that many tribes and pueblos have been exploited by observers for their own purposes and no community needs were served.

As therapists, we all know the importance of patience in all therapeutic work. As a clinical administrator, one needs to learn to be patient and to understand that certain processes take time. Too frequently, our impatience with others defeats our purpose (Parkinson, 1957).

THE CASE OF HAL

Hal, a depressed and obsessive 12-year-old, was under great pressure from bright, striving parents to be outstanding scholastically. Hal began to refuse to go to school. In our sessions, to bridge his apathetic and sometimes angry silences, I offered to play checkers with him. He was contemptuous of such a childish game and insisted we play chess. When he beat me easily, even predicting after the third move the outcome of the game, I found myself feeling angry at his derisive comments, although I could sense that his attitudes covered anxieties about his adequacy in other areas, especially his capacity for relationships with peers and adults.

I then insisted that we play checkers. This permitted a number of therapeutic interactions. First, checkers permitted handicapping the better player, who plays with fewer checkers. It also allowed me to express a variety of feelings with each move. Thus, I would loudly express my delight and even gloat when I made a good move. When Hal made a good move, I would moan and groan about losing. My rather dramatic expression of either glee at how great a player I was or distress at possibly losing a game was treated derisively by Hal, but, as time went on, his derision became gentler. Gradually, Hal expressed similar feelings of pleasure and anger with each move and each game. At first, his reactions were expressed quietly and anxiously. In time, he expressed them more openly. He was especially pleased when I appreciated and complimented him for his effective way of teaching me to play better checkers.

I dealt with my initial reaction of irritation at his contempt for the level of my ability to play chess and his derision at my efforts at checkers by recognizing the origin of my feelings as derivative of sibling experiences. I could then empathize with his anxieties about his need to be nurtured and cared about. As he began to talk while playing, he described his controlling parents and his anger at their expectations, which did not take his interests into account. It became clear that he was beginning to identify with me as a benign and concerned authoritative adult.

My initial reaction of annoyance or even anger at this bright adolescent's need to prove himself at my expense and his contemptuous attitudes toward me required careful attention. I came to understand that Hal's behaviors were defenses against his need to be cared about and his fear of being controlled.

As a psychiatric administrator, I have learned repeatedly that aggressiveness in very bright and sometimes derisive young colleagues often hides a need to be cared about and helped in finding their own areas of competence, without being controlled by the senior's advantage in position. As their growth is facilitated in nonthreatening ways, they become collaborators in mutually enjoyable and profitable enterprises, an outcome that gives continuous and unfailing pleasure.

CONCLUSION

There are a few principles of clinical administration that I have slowly worked through and can recommend.

Firmness and fairness in requiring others to carry out their obligations in training or on the job are helpful to their work and effectiveness. There are no good excuses for failure to carry out one's responsibilities, not even the fact that these problems are being worked on in one's analysis.

No matter how distasteful problems are, they need to be dealt with directly, promptly, and nonpunitively. One needs to follow clinical hunches and gut feelings; they are often correct. If one encourages open disagreement and can be tolerant of other points of view, opportunities are often created for new learning. However, the administrative responsibility for decision making cannot be abrogated.

In the community setting, work with professionals in fields other than mental health can yield clinical insights that can be translated into innovative community actions. Making oneself available to all others in an organization promotes exchange of information and often a new level of problem solving. Isolation solves nothing. These principles apply to clinical administration in many therapeutic settings.

In the politics of clinical administration, a slow and painful lesson is that no action taken will please everyone but the administrator must persist in actions supported by personal beliefs. Such commitment often serves integrative purposes.

Brashness, aggressiveness, and even derision from younger colleagues usually hide a need to be cared about and to be helped in finding areas of competence and effectiveness. Helping others to grow rather than controlling them leads to mutually satisfying and productive collaboration.

What one has learned as a psychotherapist, a mental health consultant, or a beginner in clinical administration can provide useful insights. Lessons may be out of awareness for a time and then become translated at moments of need into operative principles of clinical administration. Over time, one can put them into some framework and order.

To be an effective clinical administrator, one cannot be a therapist to those persons with whom one works. Therapy is an explicit arrangement between two persons, one of whom requests help and is the patient. However, an administrator can strive to be empathic and therapeutic. According to the dictionary, "therapeutic" means "to be helpful."

REFERENCES

Argyris, C. (1962). *Interpersonal competence and organizational effectiveness.* Homewood, IL: Dorsey Press.

Berlin, I. N. (1967). Some implications of ego psychology to the supervisory process. In S. A. Szurek & I. N. Berlin (Eds.), *Training in therapeutic work with children* (pp. 234–242). Palo Alto, CA: Science & Behavioral Press.

Hardy, O. B. (1970). Delegation: The administrator's challenge. *Hospital Administration, 15,* 8–20.

Parkinson, C. N. (1957). *Parkinson's law and other studies in administration.* Boston: Houghton Mifflin.

Susselman, S. (1969). Interrelationship of the correctional worker, the offender, and the legal structure. In S. A. Szurek & I. N. Berlin (Eds.), *The antisocial child, his family and his community* (pp. 134–148). Palo Alto, CA: Science & Behavioral Press.

Szurek, S. A. (1950). Emotional factors in the use of authority. In E. L. Ginsburg (Ed.), *Public health is people* (pp. 205–265). New York: Commonwealth Fund.

Szurek, S. A. (1967). Remarks on training. In S. A. Szurek & I. N. Berlin (Eds.), *Training in therapeutic work with children* (pp. 216–233). Palo Alto, CA: Science & Behavioral Press.

Szurek, S. A., & Berlin, I. N. (1964). Teaching administration in the training of child psychiatrists. *Journal of the American Academy of Child Psychiatry, 3,* 551–560.

CHAPTER EIGHTEEN

Evaluating Outcome in a Multicultural Inpatient Setting

Luis A. Vargas

Inpatient psychiatric treatment of children and adolescents from different ethnic groups raises serious epistemological, cultural, methodological, and ethical questions. Attempts to assess the outcome of such treatment face even more serious challenges simply because of the nature of inpatient treatment. This chapter addresses the problems in evaluating the efficacy of inpatient treatment in a multicultural population of children and adolescents and provides some solutions and strategies to overcome, at least in part, some of these problems. Before considering solutions and strategies that will make outcome studies more culturally sensitive, the general issues pertaining to psychiatric treatment of ethnically diverse populations in the United States are reviewed. The chapter then addresses methodological issues in the assessment of the efficacy of inpatient treatment of ethnically diverse children and adolescents. The suggested solutions and strategies acknowledge the difficulties in evaluating outcome in a multicultural setting.

PSYCHIATRIC HOSPITALIZATION AS A CULTURAL PRACTICE

Psychiatric hospitalization is a culturally derived solution for severe problems of living. Clinicians who use psychiatric hospitalization for some of their patients usually are guided by a medical model that postulates the existence of discrete disease entities that can be "accurately" diagnosed with "proper" training. Hospitalization is recommended when these mental disorders reach certain proportions, as assessed through the "clinical acumen" of an evaluating clinician who has been trained in this medical model. However, this clinical acumen may have been obtained with only limited experience with ethnic minority populations. The major premise of psychiatric hospitalization is that an intensification of psychiatric treatment, which the patient may have been receiving in a lesser amount on an outpatient basis, along with the additional inpatient benefits of environmental controls, will help the patient by alleviating the signs and symptoms of the mental disorder.

This entire premise makes sense only if we believe the epistemological assumptions of the medical model, which derive from our predominant and more pervasive Western epistemologies. For example, the medical model takes a dual view of the person wherein the mind is separated from the body. Thus, we have separate hospitals for physical illnesses and for mental illnesses. In a culture like that of the Navajo or the Pueblos, the dualism may seem ludicrous. American mainstream culture emphasizes the importance of the individual and separation of self from others and from the environment. One idea behind hospitalization is that the separation of the mentally ill individual from the family is essential to treating and alleviating severe emotional and/or behavioral problems. Yet, we often fail to notice that this is a very ethnocentric notion.

Only recently have investigators examined how psychiatric hospitalization in the United States is used for members of different ethnic minority groups. Snowden and Cheung (1990) reported national data on racial and ethnic differences in psychiatric hospitalization in state and county mental hospitals, nonfederal general hospitals (psychiatric units), VA medical centers, and private psychiatric hospitals. Their results showed that blacks and American Indians are much more likely than whites to be hospitalized. Asian Americans and Pacific Islanders are less likely than whites to be admitted but have considerably longer lengths of stay in state and county mental hospitals. Hispanics are only slightly more likely than whites to be hospitalized in state and county mental hospitals but are less likely to be hospitalized in other types of inpatient psychiatric settings. Snowden and Cheung also found ethnic and racial differences in diagnosis. Blacks, and Hispanics to a lesser extent, are more likely than whites to be diagnosed as schizophrenic, although this did not hold true at VA medical centers. Blacks and Hispanics were less likely than whites to be diagnosed as having an affective disorder. Large-scale studies have yet to address how different ethnic minority group members fare after inpatient psychiatric treatment.

CULTURAL CLASHES IN THE INPATIENT MELTING POT

Westermeyer (1985) noted that cross-cultural, or *etic,** diagnosis implies that a clinician from one culture can make a diagnosis for a patient from another culture. *Etic* approaches are cross-cultural and, consequently, use one general set of classification in diagnosis and, by implication, treatment. In an inpatient setting where patients are from different ethnic groups, an *etic* approach is illustrated in the implementation of the same treatment plan for the same type of disorder, regardless of the cultural background of the patients. Some investigators (Kleinman, 1977; Rogler, 1989; Westermeyer, 1985) have pointed out the necessity of taking an *emic* approach if treatment is to be culturally responsive. *Emic* approaches are intracultural and, consequently, will vary from culture to culture. The *etic–emic* distinction is easy to understand if we are dealing with ethnic groups within their countries of origin, for example, comparing depression among Germans in Germany and Peruvians in Peru. The distinction becomes blurred when we are dealing with ethnic groups, such as German Americans and Peruvian Americans, in a host culture. As a colleague (Canive, personal communication) put it: "It is very different being a Mexican in Mexico and being a

---

* *Emic* and *etic* are derived from the linguistic terms *phonemic* and *phonetic*. They have been used to describe two perspectives of cross-cultural research.

Mexican in the United States or a Mexican American." In other words, Mexicans in Mexico are not subject to acculturation stresses and related stresses that Mexicans and Mexican Americans face in the United States. These stresses—socioeconomic problems, prejudice, and language differences—combine to exacerbate pre-existing psychological vulnerabilities in ethnic group members in the United States.

The hospitalization of patients from different cultures in a setting that treats all patients (more specifically, all patients' disorders) the same demonstrates an *etic* approach to treatment. The problem encountered in an inpatient setting is how to provide an *emic* approach when dealing with the "melting pot dilemma," the presence of multiple ethnic patient groups simultaneously. In dealing with ethnically diverse patients in the United States, it becomes unclear how "true to the original culture" an ethnic minority patient is. A Mexican American patient who may be seen as very unacculturated may be dismissed as too Americanized by his Mexican counterparts. In a unit that has patients from several ethnic minority groups— for example, Mexican American, black, Chinese American, Navajo, and Pueblo—how is an *emic* treatment approach defined and accomplished? The melting pot dilemma presents a significant obstacle in attempting to assess the efficacy of treatment in a multicultural setting within the dominant culture.

An even greater complication related to the melting pot dilemma in an inpatient setting is that ethnic minority children and adolescents who present to the hospital often come from dysfunctional families that are not typical of their ethnic groups. These young patients and their families may not be representative of the culture exemplified by their psychologically healthier or more functional counterparts from the same community.

DIFFERENTIAL THRESHOLDS IN DEFINING PSYCHOPATHOLOGY

Noting the ethnocentricity of our theories of individualism in psychology, Sampson (1988) emphasized that psychology needs to consider alternatives to the mainstream American conceptualization of individualism and recognize other indigenous psychologies as equally viable. Although Sampson did not take a clinical view, it is easy to see the potential damage of imposing our views about the importance of culturally based values pertaining to developmental processes, such as separation–individuation, on children and adolescents from different cultures. Marsella (1980) suggested that individuals from cultures that have metaphorical languages and encourage imagistic mediation of reality may not psychologize their experiences. Consequently, the risk of certain phenomenological experiences associated with depression in Western cultures, such as isolation, detachment, separation, and alienation may be reduced. The WHO study of depression (Sartorius et al., 1983), which employed cross-culturally the WHO Schedule for Standardized Assessment of Depressive Disorders (SADD), had some findings that appear to corroborate Marsella's contention. For example, despite similar patterns of depressive disorder in the different cultural groups, 68% of the Swiss sample and only 32% of the Iranian sample reported guilt feelings.

A large body of literature addresses the issue of cultural definitions of abnormality. However, the hospitalization of ethnic minority patients within a dominant society presents a challenge to the determination and measurement of psychopathological and normative behaviors. What do we use as a criterion, whether in a clinical interview or in assigning a numerical value on a structured interview schedule or questionnaire, to define abnormal versus normal behavior, or behavior warranting hospitalization, or sufficient improvement to warrant discharge? The idea that we are defining behavioral or emotional problems of someone from a very different culture according to what constitutes our culturally based criteria for mental health is most disturbing. At worst, one is left to wonder whether, for someone from a very different culture, the basis for discharge from the hospital is not, as may have been empirically demonstrated, an alleviation of signs and symptoms but rather the patient's quick learning in a harsh lesson of acculturation.

Manson, Shore, and Bloom (1985) developed a modification of the Diagnostic Interview Schedule (DIS) (cf. Robins, Helzer, Croughan, & Ratcliff, 1981) called the American Indian Depression Schedule (AIDS), for use with the Hopi. The AIDS captures five discrete Hopi illness categories related to the Western notion of depression. Such efforts demonstrate a willingness to adjust Western diagnoses to cultural nuances in the manner in which a psychiatric disorder is manifested. Marsella, Sartorius, Jablensky, and Fenton (1985) noted that, even if certain types of psychiatric disorders are shown to have a biochemical basis, an individual experiencing one of these disorders must still interpret the abnormal experience, translate the experience into behavior, and respond to the social reaction to that behavior.

Draguns (1977) indicated the need to establish (a) clear, unambiguous standards of mental disorders that are cross-culturally acceptable, at least for the purposes of comparative research; (b) operational measures that embody these concepts in a manner applicable across cultures; and (c) demonstrations of equivalence of these measures in different cultural settings. Marsella (1979) advocated conducting empirical studies of the conceptualizations of mental health and disorders in different cultures. He suggested the development of research matrices for investigating problems, causes, and treatment interactions in different cultures. One of his primary concerns was that most researchers have been neither willing to acknowledge nor responsive to cultural differences in defining normality and abnormality; instead, they have chosen to impose Western standards. The suggestions of Marsella and Draguns are reasonable for purposes of cross-cultural research, but those engaged in inpatient treatment outcome studies of ethnically diverse populations within the dominant society face two significant obstacles:

1. Cross-cultural research of this type may not be reflective of the psychological and acculturation-related struggles that ethnic minority patients experience in a hospital within the dominant culture.
2. There is still insufficient data regarding the incidence of different disorders in ethnic minority groups within the United States. This has implications for both culturally sensitive measures of psychopathology and culturally sensitive and accurate diagnosis of disorders that constitute a sufficient basis for hospitalization.

Using data from the NIMH Epidemiologic Catchment Area (ECA) Project, Robins et al. (1984) reported differences between blacks and whites in lifetime prevalence of 15 specific disorders. Of the five ECA sites, only three (New Haven, CT, Baltimore, and St. Louis) were reporting data. Only four of 45 black/white comparisons were significant at levels the investigators considered trustworthy ($p<.001$). Blacks were significantly higher in simple phobia and agoraphobia than whites in Baltimore. Blacks were significantly higher in simple phobia and cognitive impairment than whites in St. Louis. Less reliable differences, due to marginal levels of significance ($p<.05$), were found in Baltimore, where blacks were more likely to suffer from schizophrenia and drug abuse/dependence than were whites.

Karno et al. (1987) compared ECA site data from Los Angeles on lifetime prevalence between Mexican Americans and non-Hispanic whites. Mexican Americans had rates of disorder similar to those of non-Hispanic whites as well as to samples from the three other reporting sites (New Haven, Baltimore, and St. Louis). Non-Hispanic whites reported far more drug abuse/dependence and major depressive episodes than Mexican Americans. Mexican American women had a very low lifetime prevalence for drug and alcohol abuse/dependence. Dysthymia, panic disorder, and phobia were somewhat more prevalent among Mexican American women over age 40 compared to non-Hispanic white women and Mexican American women under age 40.

So far, results from the ECA data are inconclusive in regard to the question of ethnic differences in psychopathology, and reports from the ECA institution-based survey are still forthcoming. However, other studies have epidemiological relevance to the question of ethnic differences in psychopathology. Sue and Morishima (1982) noted that Asian Americans are more likely than other ethnic groups to present with somatic complaints. This led Snowden and Cheung (1990) to suggest that such symptom presentation may lead Asian Americans to go to medical settings rather than psychiatric ones. From a review of the treated case method to estimate prevalence of psychopathology in Asian Americans, Sue and Sue (1987) concluded that Asian Americans seek treatment only when their psychiatric disorders are severe and that those with milder disorders do not turn to the mental health system. Sue and Sue underscored the results of various studies that highlight the amount of stigma and shame that is associated with emotional problems in the Asian American population. Like Snowden and Cheung, these authors believe that Asian Americans conceptualize mental health problems differently and may feel that the problems are caused by organic factors, leading Asian Americans to avoid psychotherapy and seek medical treatment instead.

Neighbors (1984) reviewed two types of epidemiological studies—treatment rate studies and community surveys—and compared the rate of psychiatric morbidity between blacks and whites. On the basis of his review of community surveys, which he considered methodologically superior to treatment rate studies, Neighbors drew two general conclusions: (a) blacks tend to have higher levels of stress than do whites on most measures, and (b) when socioeconomic status is controlled, blacks either exhibit lower levels of psychological distress than do whites or they show no difference. Neighbors' first conclusion led Snowden and Cheung (1990) to suggest that a greater expression of psychological distress by blacks might increase their chances of being hospitalized. Yet, does this mean they have higher rates or prevalence of psychopathology?

Of particular relevance to the issue of defining psychopathology in different cultures within a dominant culture is a study (Kessler, 1979) that Neighbors cited to elaborate his conclusions. Kessler had reanalyzed a certain data set by separating distress into two parts: (a) that due to differential exposure to stress and (b) that due to a differential response ("impact") to stress. Kessler did not find race differences in average distress, but his analyses of extreme distress showed some fascinating results. Blacks were twice as likely as were whites to report extreme distress because blacks were exposed to more stress than whites. Kessler also found that comparable levels of stress had more impact on whites than on blacks, yet this advantage was not sufficient to overcome the greater exposure of blacks to stress. Kessler and Neighbors (cited in Neighbors, 1984) suggested that, since, given exposure to comparable levels of stress, blacks were less affected than whites, blacks may have more effective coping strategies than whites. As a result of these findings, Neighbors (1984) argued for more epidemiological research on representative all-black samples, on discrete psychiatric disorders, and on the validity and reliability of the NIMH Diagnostic Interview Schedule (which was used in the ECA project) in order to better assess black mental health issues.

Neighbors' review serves to point out the difficulty of measuring psychopathology across racial/ethnic groups and how easily different investigators can derive very different conclusions. Using the *etic–emic* distinction, Westermeyer (1985) noted that the diagnostic problem cannot be understood in mutually exclusive terms. Rather, one needs to ask to what extent *emic* and *etic* perspectives apply. As Westermeyer phrased the question: "[T]o what extent do depressed patients from various cultures express symptoms differently, and to what extent do psychiatrists from different cultures recognize the same depressive syndrome?" (p. 800).

METHODOLOGICAL ISSUES

Having briefly reviewed various general issues pertaining to the hospitalization and treatment of ethnic minority patients within a dominant culture, let us consider the following methodological questions:

1. What variables do we use to measure improvement?
2. Do we impose one standard of improvement for all the cultural groups present in our inpatient population?
3. What are the construct validity issues in applying instruments developed in one culture on another in which the instruments were not developed?
4. What role does language translation play in developing and employing measures of change?
5. How does culturally biased methodology affect interpretation of outcome data?
6. How do we deal with the "package treatment" problem (cf. Institute of Medicine, 1989, citing Kazdin) wherein we are measuring the impact of the total hospitalization experience together with all of its many and varied components (e.g., individual, group, family, occupational, speech, and language therapies; medication; and special education)?

Determination of Relevant Variables

Rogler (1989) emphasized the importance of guarding against the "category fallacy," described previously by Kleinman (1977) and Good and Good (1985). The category fallacy develops when a construct, usually a diagnostic category, that is derived from one culture is applied *etically* without establishing the validity of the construct for the other cultural groups to which it is being applied.

Rogler pointed out that this fallacy is most evident in cross-cultural psychiatry in the use of the DSM-III and the MMPI on cultures for which these instruments were not developed nor intended. Rogler assumed that a construct developed from one culture cannot be applied to another without establishing the validity of that construct within the culture to which it is applied. However, this restriction may not be necessary as long as we do not assume that the phenomenon measured *means the same* as in the culture in which the construct was developed and validated. The fact that a discrete racial/ethnic group scores very high on measures of psychopathology, like the MMPI, does not necessarily mean that they have high degrees of psychopathology.

For example, Gynther, Fowler, and Erdberg (1971) gave the MMPI to 88 blacks in rural, isolated areas. They found that 41 of the respondents had T-scores greater than 80 on the F scale (unusual or atypical ways of answering the test items). The most frequent high-point scale for both males and females was Scale 8 (Schizophrenia). The next highest scale was Scale 9 (Hypomania) for males and Scale 6 (Paranoia) for females. The mean profile for this sample would have been classified as psychotic by most MMPI interpretive criteria. Yet, as the investigators pointed out, the MMPI was simply overpathologizing the group. Thus, the usual interpretive criteria could not be applied to this sample; high scores in the Schizophrenia scale did not *mean* what they typically do in American mainstream culture.

Rogler recommended that the pretesting phase in culturally sensitive research be expanded to include spending time within the culture to be studied, preferably using traditional ethnographic methods that involve participant observation and interviews with informants who are knowledgeable about the culture being studied. In assessing treatment outcome in a multicultural patient population, Rogler's recommendations, while undoubtedly illustrative of a culturally sensitive approach, are not feasible because of the length of time such research would take.

We need to develop an alternative, more feasible strategy that answers the need for short-term results under less than optimal research circumstances. In an outcome study of a multicultural inpatient population for which we do not know the relevant *emic* classifications (i.e., culturally relevant variables), selection of variables for study of outcome could still be guided by efforts to be culturally sensitive. A central problem of hospitalization of ethnic minority patients is that the structure and function of the hospital are usually predicated on *etic* formulations developed from the dominant, mainstream culture. In other words, to draw from Manson et al.'s study (1985), the Hopi girl who presents with *un nung mo kiw ta* (which literally means "heart is broken" and refers to the despair or acute sadness arising from unrealized expectations or disrupted interpersonal relationships) may be diagnosed as suffering from dysthymia or depression and treated according to Western medicine approaches.

This is not necessarily as negative as it sounds. Part of the melting pot dilemma involves the accommodation of ethnic minority groups to the dominant culture. In mental health settings, we often see ethnic minority patients who have not been able to accommodate without adverse psychological effects, which undoubtedly might be better understood from an *emic* perspective. Yet, within the hospital setting, treatment staff must make important decisions about the ability of an ethnic minority patient to function in the dominant society. Such decisions illustrate the potential blurring of boundaries between *etic* and *emic* formulations, which we discussed earlier. Regarding the nonexclusiveness of *etic* and *emic* perspectives, Westermeyer (1985) argued that, for example, in the study of depression, *emic* depression scales have not been demonstrated to be better than well-translated *etic* depression scales, either for clinical or research purposes. *Etic* scales like the Hamilton Rating Scale for Depression have been shown to have very high intercultural validity in other countries (Fava, Kellner, Munari, & Pavan, 1982). I would like to take this thinking a step further: This issue of *etic–emic* distinction becomes even more blurred—more precisely, it becomes interactive—when dealing with psychiatric disorders among diverse ethnic minority groups within one country.

In the case of the Hopi girl, the treatment team may ask: Are we really being culturally sensitive if we treat this girl's condition *emically,* which may mean recognizing that her condition might be seen as either less or more pathological in her culture than in our clinical assessment of her in the unit? The accuracy of the clinical assessment is dependent on the breadth of training and experience of the clinical staff, who may have variable or little experience with the Hopi. To complicate matters further, what does the treatment team do if this child is shown to have either a very serious or very mild mental disorder on a standardized semistructured interview or a very high or very low level of impairment on a behavior rating scale? More specifically, what should be done when the more standardized and "objective" measures yield scores that may be widely discrepant from the frequency and extent of the presenting problems as given by the patient, family, and/or referral source? Those of us in the dominant culture who are striving to be culturally sensitive can be immobilized by such efforts. We get stuck within the meanings we impose on the results of our assessments (clinical or "standardized") or measurements of certain presumed psychiatric disorders. Assessment of behavioral or psychological symptoms in our culture assumes a limited number of reasons as to why a child or adolescent cannot function adequately. In the case of an ethnic minority child, the reason for the low or high scores on measurements of psychopathology may be one *not* considered in the dominant culture. This might range from the Hopi girl's *un nung mo kiw ta* to acculturation-related stresses or to the presence of different coping strategies not present in members of the dominant culture, as suggested by Kessler and Neighbors (cited in Neighbors, 1984).

If we do not know the *emic* formulation of the behavioral or psychological signs and symptoms, we might take a utilitarian approach of helping the ethnic minority patient, among other goals, to function adequately in the dominant society and we might avoid making inferences about what the signs and symptoms mean. In other words, we may note that the Hopi girl has a particular score on a rating scale of depression but then not impose the meaning that she is depressed at the 98th percentile when compared to her dominant culture peers or that such a score is typical of a certain type of person from the dominant culture. The score serves either to compare the girl to her peers in the same ethnic group or to provide a baseline against which to compare her later measurements.

This approach of looking beyond our culturally defined meaning of psychiatric disorders might be referred to as a strategy of *cultural transcendence in measurement*. Note that this strategy is not an *etic* approach. It refers to the need to hold in abeyance interpretations that have meaning within a culture, because we do not know the meaning of the numbers we have obtained in measurement. *Etic* approaches impose what is assumed to be a universal meaning on particular phenomena. However, these numbers can be used to make comparisons among the same ethnic group in which the instrument was used, as long as we do not impose interpretations on the numbers outside the culture in which the instrument was developed and validated.

The problem of evaluating outcome with *emic* sensitivity under the conditions of *etic* diagnostic and treatment formulations may require us to engage in cultural transcendence in measurement as a strategy in assessing treatment outcome in multicultural populations. With regard to the cultural manifestation of *etically* derived signs and symptoms, patients from ethnic minority groups who are admitted to the hospital must reach a certain level of functioning as measured by these *etic*, dominant-culture constructs, in order to be discharged as improved and capable of functioning better in the dominant culture. Thus, aggressiveness and depression, as measured by the Child Behavior Checklist (CBC) (Achenbach, 1981), may be dominant-culture constructs with a long history of importance and salience in Western European and American cultures. Yet, for an ethnic minority patient living in the American mainstream society, these constructs begin to take on a different and particular significance.

Often, when ethnic minority children are hospitalized, their families or community members in their ethnic group believe that the children have emotional or behavioral problems too severe to be handled in the home or community. Let us consider an extreme, if also unlikely, case to illustrate the strategy of cultural transcendence in measurement. It does not matter that the amount of aggression expressed by a Navajo boy whose family has recently moved to the city is not considered as severe on the reservation as it is in an urban setting. The fact that the Navajo boy has been hospitalized for aggression implies a need to reduce that aggression to levels that are more manageable in the setting of urban, dominant-society schools, one of which he will be attending after discharge. This is said not to promote a political or moral stance or to detract from the need for the dominant society to be culturally responsive to its ethnic minority constituents. Rather, it is said to acknowledge the impact of the dominant society on defining psychopathology and on developing criteria for adaptive functioning. It is also said to acknowledge that, as stated earlier, many ethnic minority patients may be experiencing greater psychiatric symptomatology (violence, suicidality, or depression), because of acculturation and related stresses that exacerbate predisposing psychological vulnerabilities, than their ethnic counterparts in their countries of origin.

The importance of cultural transcendence in measurement in assuming this utilitarian approach to establishing relevant variables for measurement cannot be overemphasized. The fact that we choose to measure ethnic minority children and adolescents on hyperactivity and oppositionality on the ACTeRS (Ullmann, Sleator, & Sprague, 1985) or depression on the Children's Depression Inventory (CDI) (Kovacs, 1983) does *not* mean that we can interpret the scores as they are interpreted for the dominant society, for which the scales were developed. For example, if American Indian children score higher than other ethnic groups on hyperactivity, it does not necessarily mean that they are more active. Cultural transcendence in measurement requires that we use the instrument without the typical meaning given to the scale or subscales. Remember Westermeyer's (1985) point that different ethnic groups might express symptoms differently and observers from different ethnic groups may not assess a particular disorder or syndrome (in our example, hyperactivity, oppositionality, and depression) similarly. Thus, the numerical values from our measures are just that: numbers; but we must now make use of culturally sensitive *interpretation*, a topic that is discussed in a later section. However, the numerical values derived from these various measures become important in establishing culturally sensitive standards of improvement for each ethnic minority group in the patient population.

Establishing a Standard of Improvement

Once the relevant variables for study (hyperactivity, aggression, or depression, for example) are chosen, the primary problem in assessing treatment outcome in a multicultural patient population becomes the determination of a standard of improvement. Consider this question: Is passivity in an American Indian child as dysfunctional as passivity in a Mexican American child or in a child from the American mainstream? The standard of improvement issue in this case is that what the hospital treatment team may establish as the desirable goal for developing assertiveness in a American mainstream child may, in fact, be undesirable in an Indian child who is returning to a nonurban setting. It is crucial to address the context for a behavior (i.e., being passive on the reservation or in the *barrio* versus being passive in the dominant-society school) and the respective cultural norms for that behavior.

Context of Behavior and Inter-Rater Reliability. Development of an adequate strategy requires awareness that an ethnic minority child may need to learn where to be passive and where to be assertive, in order to function more adaptively in his or her bicultural world. This awareness obviously underscores the need to assess the child's ability or capacity to show what are considered adaptive behaviors in their appropriate contexts. With regard to measurement of these abilities as demonstrated in their appropriate cultural contexts, we need to be careful to whom we administer the instruments. For example, we might not want to administer a CBC to a Pueblo grandmother of a child whom the treatment team sees as depressed and lacking sufficient initiative to function adequately in school and whom the grandmother sees as defiant, if we want to get "a good measure" (speaking in full recognition of the cultural context in which initiative is desirable) of the alleviation of the depression. A treatment staff person or teacher may be a better respondent regarding school, and the grandmother may be a better respondent to assess the alleviation of the defiance and oppositionality in the home.

This strategy may be considered by some readers to run counter to "good methodology" or to deny the purpose of the inter-rater reliability values presented in the manuals or articles for the instruments we are using. The inter-rater reliability scores of a particular instrument may show the instrument to be very reliable across respondents. However, if we adhere to the belief that a child or adolescent may be capable of showing certain desirable behaviors in culturally appropriate contexts but will not show them in contexts in which the same behaviors are culturally inappropriate, then we should take a measurement of those behaviors in the cultural context in which they are both appropriate and, consequently, likely to be manifested.

Cultural Norms and Their Effect on Measuring Improvement. Development of an adequate outcome study begins with establishing culturally sensitive treatment goals that have some basis on a continuum of behavior relevant to the ethnic minority group that is of interest or, if possible, of normative behavior for children and adolescents in that ethnic group. The measurement of improvement might be obtained in two ways. In the absence of any normative data on a particular ethnic group, one strategy is to measure improvement on the basis of change in target behaviors, using the patient's symptomatology at admission as a baseline measurement, as in the single case study method. Another strategy is to compute separate statistical means for a general set of symptoms and behaviors for discrete ethnic groups in the patient population and measure change on the basis of deviation from the intraculturally variant means. For example, suppose one of the general set of symptoms and behaviors selected for measurement is depression. A mean for American Indian patients, another for Mexican American patients, and another for American mainstream patients would be computed, and improvement would be measured against those means. This approach develops a continuum of relevant behaviors (e.g., the range of items endorsed by American Indian patients on the CDI) from the composite population of patients in the hospital who are from the same ethnic minority. The continuum can be used to measure change from the group means in order to carry out nomothetic analyses.

The first approach, which is a single-subject design and, consequently, idiographic, is well-recognized; it is most commonly used to assess behavioral interventions and can be applied to any patient regardless of race or ethnicity. The second approach has obvious problems, primarily deriving from its limited range of measurement (only patients are used to compute the means from which deviations are measured) and from its limitations in making cross-ethnic group comparisons.

A better variation of the second strategy is to request, if available, the means for the American Indian, Mexican American, and American mainstream children of the normative sample from the publishers of the instrument used to measure, in this case, depression. These means could then be used to determine how "depressed" a particular American Indian child is at the time of admission and how close to the mean for his or her ethnic group the child is at the time of discharge. The reason for putting depressed in quotes is that, since the construct of depression has not been validated in most American Indian populations using these instruments, we do not know what a particular score really means in the instrument we are using to measure depression in American Indian children and adolescents. Does this mean there is no point to using the instrument on American Indian populations? No. It means, though, that we cannot use the scores for comparison with other racial or ethnic groups. The scores are still useful for intracultural comparisons, that is, for comparing the score of an Indian child to the scores of other Indian children. As with the isolated blacks of the Gynther et al. study (1971), we cannot say that, because these children may have a higher mean in a measure of depression, they are more depressed.

To make this interpretation requires that the construct of depression, as measured by this instrument, be validated on particular American

Indian tribal groups. If the instrument is translated, equivalence of the instruments must be demonstrated. This method has certain *emic* advantages despite the fact that the construct of depression as measured by this instrument is *etically* derived. Another caution is needed: Among certain ethnic groups that are generally presumed to be similar, there may be significant differences. For instance, among American Indians, substantial differences might exist not only between, say, Pueblo and Sioux tribes but also within particular tribes like the Pueblos which can be culturally and linguistically very different from each other. Thus, investigators must decide, on the basis of their knowledge of the particular tribes of interest, whether means for "American Indians," which may be available from the publishers of the instrument being used, actually provide a more culturally sensitive approach.

The Cultural Context of Instruments to Assess Change

If the patient population comes from one ethnic group (for example, Americans of British descent) or similar ethnic groups (for example, Americans of Western European descent) that implicitly hold beliefs consistent with the American medical model of treating mental disorders, the evaluation of outcome may be as simple as choosing various well-recognized instruments. For example, the Schedule for Affective Disorders and Schizophrenia for Children and Adolescents (Kiddie-SADS or K-SADS) (Chambers et al., 1985) or the Diagnostic Interview for Children and Adolescents (DICA) (Herjanic & Campbell, 1977; Herjanic & Reich, 1982) can be used to define the presenting problems (i.e., to make the diagnoses or to define symptom groups) and instruments that are well normed within the United States, such as the CBC (Achenbach, 1981) for the children and the FACES III (Olson, Portner, & Lavee, 1985), a measure of family functioning, for the families, can be used to measure the progress of patients and their families at various time intervals. Although this is an oversimplification of treatment outcome evaluation, it illustrates an important methodological problem in assessing multicultural populations in a psychiatric hospital. In a patient population of Hispanic Americans and American Indians who differ in degree of acculturation, we cannot assume that the normative sample upon which the instruments are based adequately represents the type and degree of psychopathology of these particular ethnic minority patients. This section briefly addresses how construct validity is influenced by cultural context, and the issue of translation of instruments.

Construct Validity and Cultural Context. The question of construct validity remains even in the case of instruments that have included a normative sample that contained ethnic minority subjects in proportion to their numbers in the general population. The problem with using a proportional representation of ethnic minorities in a sample that largely consists of the dominant culture is that the constructs are usually developed by grouping the entire sample together, that is, treating the sample as one general group. Ethnic minority group differences then "wash out" because of their small numbers in the "representative sample." A greater problem is caused by applying an instrument that has been normed on a sample that had proportional representation. Because constructs from instruments using "representative samples" are derived from the whole sample's being treated essentially as one homogeneous group (for example, principal components analysis is conducted on the entire sample), the procedure may only *seem* to avoid the category fallacy. Instead, it remains. Even to apply the instrument *etically*, that is, cross-culturally, in an adequate manner, it would be necessary to determine whether the same constructs can be derived from *each* ethnic group sampled. For example, if certain "factors" emerge from a principal components analysis in the Anglo group, do the same "factors" emerge in each of the Mexican American, Cuban, or Pueblo groups? They should, if the instrument is going to be applied in an *etically* appropriate manner. If they do not, then we might conclude that the "factor" (representing some construct) does not mean the same in a particular ethnic group. This is essentially the point behind Rogler's (1989) caution about the use of the MMPI and the DSM-III.

Translation of Instruments.   Assuming that we are not in a position to employ the ideal strategies suggested by Rogler (1989), we are likely to face a decision on which instruments or measures to use and translate, if the publishers' translations are not available. If translations are available, we cannot assume that, for example, a Spanish translation of the instrument will work equally well with Mexicans, Cubans, and Puerto Ricans. There is considerable variety in the Spanish spoken by Hispanic groups, even when comparing Mexicans with Mexican Americans in New Mexico.

When instruments have not been translated, investigators must decide which instruments to choose and what translation method to use. Before selecting instruments, it is important to scrutinize them to determine which are more appropriate for use in the ethnic group of interest. For example, a family functioning questionnaire that has ethnocentric items, such as queries about whether the family attends church services weekly, may not be well-suited for use with traditional American Indians. Some instruments that are methodologically very sound and very well accepted for use in the American mainstream culture may not be even roughly adaptable to different ethnic groups because of their obvious ethnocentricity. Translation of these instruments will not be worthwhile.

After an instrument is chosen for translation, the investigator must decide which type of translation to use. The most commonly used method is the back translation—one translator translates the instrument from the original language into the language of interest, and a separate translator then brings the resulting instrument back to the original language. The back translation is compared to the original version, and the discrepancies are examined by the translators, to create a translation that is more natural from the standpoint of the language of interest.

However, in cultures with unwritten languages and more than one orthographic system, back translations may not be adequate. In Manson et al.'s (1985) Hopi translation of the DIS, their strategy was to modify the DIS by developing a sociolinguistically appropriate translation that approximated local English use. Their primary objective was to retain the intended meaning of the original structured interview questions, regardless of any ultimate relevance to the Hopi world view. As might be obvious, this was a challenging endeavor. For example, they noted that one DIS item combined the concepts of guilt, shame, and sinfulness. Yet, their Hopi informants clearly differentiated these concepts. Their solution was to create three different questions, each addressing a separate concept, to avoid confounding the Hopi respondents' answers.

A Caution About Interpretation

In attempting to assess outcome, the tendency may be to apply well-accepted instruments (e.g., K-SADS, CBC, or CDI). However, given the problems we have discussed, we must be careful not to make *emic* interpretations from *etic* applications. When assessing hyperactivity, oppositionality, and depression, *emic* interpretations under *etic* conditions may be evident if we are using various "well-normed" instruments when we do not know:

1. Whether these constructs would have emerged in the ethnic minority culture of interest as they did in the general sample;
2. Whether the ethnic minority group of interest would have the same distribution and group means if the same constructs did emerge.

If the same constructs do emerge in the ethnic minority group of interest and have the same distribution and group means, then the scale might be used with similar interpretation of the scores on the constructs. However, this is unlikely to happen. If the same constructs emerge but the scores have a different distribution and group means, then caution needs to be exercised in interpreting scores of the ethnic minority respondents. One might argue that comparing scores under these circumstances is best kept within each ethnic minority group. If different constructs emerge, then comparison across cultural groups on the constructs derived from the dominant group is invalid.

The solution I propose is to develop a standard of improvement from within each ethnic group. This approach is not immune to the problem of *etic* applications and *emic* interpretations. As I noted earlier, hospitalization is a culturally derived solution; we cannot escape certain values of the dominant culture. For example, the fact that suicidality in a particular American Indian tribe is high is not likely to lead us to set a criterion of improvement to accept a greater degree of suicidal behavior. The criterion of improvement in this case may be defined by the dominant culture's determination of what is acceptable with regard to manifestation of suicidal behavior in its society. (This statement is *not* to imply that particular Indian tribes have a greater acceptance of suicidal behavior; the tribes see suicidal behavior as unacceptable and those with high rates of suicide want to decrease it.) At issue here is what we use as criterion levels or what we set as acceptable levels of behavior or symptomatology. We can look at the homicide rate in the United States in much the same manner. We might impose a standard of improvement, based on the white homicide rate, on blacks, who have a much higher rate. Yet, by European standards, the homicide rate for whites in the United States is very high. Nonetheless, for the purpose of establishing a criterion of improvement to assess the efficacy of a program aimed at reducing homicidal behavior in males, the use of the white homicide rate makes sense. The criterion may then be applied *etically* across all ethnic minority groups in the dominant society.

Another issue relative to interpretation has to do with differential responses to treatment by ethnic minority groups. Many outcome studies assess what Kazdin (cited in Institute of Medicine, 1989) called the "treatment package," which simply asks: Has the entire package of hospitalization produced change? In addressing multicultural populations, it may be more important to invoke different strategies, such as some of those described by Kazdin and by the Institute of Medicine—applying them, however, to ethnic minority populations. These include:

1. The parametric strategy;
2. The dismantling strategy;
3. The comparative outcome strategy;
4. The process-outcome strategy;
5. The patient–therapist variation strategy.

The parametric strategy addresses the question: What changes can be made in a specific treatment to increase its effectiveness for particular ethnic groups? The changes may involve making cultural accommodations, such as incorporating aspects of the "talking circle" into group therapy for American Indian children (Joe & Miller, 1988). Or they may apply to doses of psychotropic medication. For example, Lin et al. (1989) showed that Asian schizophrenic patients required significantly lower doses of haloperidol than Caucasian schizophrenic patients for the optimal treatment of their disorders.

The dismantling strategy asks: What components are necessary, sufficient, and facilitative of therapeutic change in each ethnic group served? Different cultural groups may vary in their responses to particular types of treatment. For example, for some American Indians, the separation of the child from the family, which occurs during hospitalization, might be more traumatic and perhaps even more detrimental than for, say, the American mainstream group. On the other hand, the impact of particular treatments, for example, family and group therapies and special education, might be significantly more positive for some American Indians than for the American mainstream group. Measuring the total outcome, which combines the effects, both positive and negative, of all treatments received during hospitalization may lead us to make erroneous interpretive statements such as: The American Indian children benefited only minimally from inpatient treatment. In fact, what might have happened is that the negative effect of separating the American Indian child from his or her family offset the positive effects of the family and group therapies and special education. Furthermore, the general statement of minimal improvement may be misleading because, assuming the scenario described above, the best treatment for the American Indian child may have been day treatment, to take advantage of the types of treatment from which the Indian child was likely to benefit.

The comparative outcome strategy asks: What treatment is more or most effective for a particular problem in a particular ethnic group? Continuing our example of the American Indian child, we might find that family therapy, which defines the child's problem in the context of the extended family, and culturally accommodated group therapy, which makes use of certain tribal traditions, are most helpful.

The process-outcome strategy asks: What processes occur in treatment that enhance, contribute to, or are responsible for treatment outcome in each ethnic group served? For Hispanic children, these processes might include the participation of the parents in support groups, the organization, by the parents, of pot luck dinners or of baby sitting for each other's children, and the preparation of a discussion curriculum for the staff facilitator.

The patient–therapist variation strategy asks: Which characteristics of the ethnic minority child and family, the therapist, or the setting are necessary to make treatment for a particular ethnic group effective? For example, for an American mainstream child, a similarly mainstream therapist who is perceived as very professional and somewhat distant emotionally, who has a light complexion, and who does not speak with a third world accent may be most effective. On the other hand, for the Pueblo child, any therapist, regardless of ethnicity, may lead to a positive outcome provided that the child and family perceive the therapist and the unit staff to be emotionally warm, accessible, respectful, and genuinely interested in the child's and family's welfare. For the American mainstream child, a better outcome might be associated with a state-of-the-art hospital setting; for the Pueblo child, an open, campus-like setting that is not anything like a hospital unit might yield better results.

CONCLUSION

The issue of culturally sensitive outcome studies needs much more investigation and theory development. The solutions proposed in this chapter are intended to be applied in developing outcome studies, *given our current state of affairs.* Many of the proposed solutions are based on the premise that this is the best we can do currently. Some might argue that they are far from ideal or are inadequate. The problem many of us face in clinical work is the development of even a rough estimate of how our young ethnic minority patients are doing. Much more research on the most commonly used instruments, like the K-SADS or CBC, needs to be conducted, to address the question of how particular ethnic minority groups respond. Such research is necessary to help those of us who are interested in evaluating the outcome of psychiatric hospitalization for ethnic minority populations to understand how best to interpret their responses and scores.

Acknowledgments

I wish to express my most sincere appreciation to Irving N. Berlin, M.D., Joan D. Koss-Chioino, Ph.D., Robert L. Hendren, D.O., and Natalie Porter, Ph.D., for their critiques of earlier versions of this chapter.

REFERENCES

Achenbach, T. M. (1981). *Child behavior checklist for ages 4–16.* (Available from T. M. Achenbach, University of Vermont, 1 South Prospect St., Burlington, VT 05401.)

Chambers, W. G., Puig-Antich, J., Hirsch, M., Paez, P., Ambrosini, P. J., Tabrizi, M. A., & Davies, M. (1985). The assessment of affective disorders in children and adolescents by semistructured interview. *Archives of General Psychiatry, 42,* 696–702.

Draguns, J. (1977). Problems of defining and comparing abnormal behavior across cultures. *Annals of the New York Academy of Sciences, 285,* 664–679.

Fava, G. A., Kellner, R., Munari, F., & Pavan, L. (1982). The Hamilton Depression Rating Scale in normals and depressives: A cross-cultural validation. *Acta Scandinavia, 66,* 26–32.

Good, B., & Good, M. D. (1985). The cultural context of diagnosis and therapy: A view from medical anthropology. In M. R. Miranda & H. H. L. Kitano (Eds.), *Mental health research in minority communities: Development of culturally sensitive training programs.* Rockville, MD: National Institute of Mental Health.

Gynther, M. D., Fowler, R. D., & Erdberg, P. (1971). False positives galore: The application of standard MMPI criteria to a rural, isolated, Negro sample. *Journal of Clinical Psychology, 27,* 234–237.

Herjanic, B., & Campbell, W. (1977). Differentiating psychiatrically disturbed children on the basis of a structured interview. *Journal of Abnormal Child Psychology, 5,* 127–134.

Herjanic, B., & Reich, W. (1982). Development of a structured psychiatric interview for children: Agreement between child and parent on individual symptoms. *Journal of Abnormal Child Psychology, 10,* 307–324.

Institute of Medicine. (1989). *Research on children and adolescents with mental, behavioral, and developmental disorders: Mobilizing a national initiative.* Report of a study by a committee of the Institute of Medicine (Division of Mental Health and Behavioral Medicine), National Academy of Sciences. Washington, DC: National Academy Press.

Joe, J., & Miller, D. (1988, May). *Native American healing techniques: Their usefulness and implications for therapy.* Workshop presented at a conference on Psychotherapeutic Interventions with Hispanic and Native American Children and Families at the University of New Mexico School of Medicine, Albuquerque.

Karno, M., Hough, R. L., Burman, A., Escobar, J. I., Timbers, D. M., Santana, F., & Boyd, J. H. (1987). Lifetime prevalence of specific psychiatric disorders among Mexican Americans and non-Hispanic whites in Los Angeles. *Archives of General Psychiatry, 44,* 695–701.

Kessler, R. (1979). Stress, social status, and psychological distress. *Journal of Health and Social Behavior, 20,* 259–272.

Kleinman, A. (1977). Depression, somatization and the "new cross-cultural psychiatry." *Social Science and Medicine, 11,* 3–10.

Kovacs, M. (1983). *The Children's Depression Inventory: A self-rated depression scale for school-aged children.* Unpublished manuscript, University of Pittsburgh School of Medicine.

Lin, K. M., Poland, R. E., Nuccio, I., Matsuda, K., Hathuc, N., Su, T. P., & Fu, P. (1989). A longitudinal assessment of haloperidol doses and serum concentrations in Asian and Caucasian schizophrenic patients. *American Journal of Psychiatry, 146,* 1307–1311.

Manson, S. M., Shore, J. H., & Bloom, J. D. (1985). The depressive experience in American Indian communities: A challenge for psychiatric theory and diagnosis. In A. Kleinman & B. Good (Eds.), *Culture and depression.* Berkeley: University of California Press.

Marsella, A. J. (1979). Cross-cultural studies of mental health. In A. J. Marsella, R. G. Tharp, & T. J. Ciborowski (Eds.), *Perspectives on cross-cultural psychology.* New York: Academic Press.

Marsella, A. J. (1980). Depressive experience and disorder across cultures. In H. C. Triandis & J. G. Draguns (Eds.), *Handbook of cross-cultural psychology, Vol. 6: Psychopathology.* Boston: Allyn & Bacon.

Marsella, A. J., Sartorius, N., Jablensky, A., & Fenton, F. R. (1985). Cross-cultural studies of depressive disorders: An overview. In A. Kleinman & B. Good (Eds.), *Culture and depression.* Berkeley: University of California Press.

Neighbors, H. W. (1984). The distribution of psychiatric morbidity in black Americans: A review and suggestions for research. *Community Mental Health Journal, 20,* 169–181.

Olson, D. H., Portner, J., & Lavee, Y. (1985). *FACES III.* (Available from D. H. Olson, Family Social Science, 290 McNeal Hall, University of Minnesota, St. Paul, MN 55108)

Robins, L. N., Helzer, J. E., Croughan, J., & Ratcliff, K. S. (1981). National Institute of Mental Health Diagnostic Interview Schedule. *Archives of General Psychiatry, 38,* 381–389.

Robins, L. N., Helzer, J. E., Weissman, M. M., Orvaschel, H., Gruenberg, E., Burke, J. D., Jr., & Regier, D. A. (1984). Lifetime prevalence of specific psychiatric disorders in three sites. *Archives of General Psychiatry, 41,* 949–958.

Rogler, L. H. (1989). The meaning of culturally sensitive research in mental health. *American Journal of Psychiatry, 146,* 296–303.

Sampson, E. E. (1988). The debate on individualism: Indigenous psychologies of the individual and their role in personal and societal functioning. *American Psychologist, 43,* 15–22.

Sartorius, N., Davidian, H., Ernberg, G., Fenton, F. R., Fujii, I., Gastpar, M., Gulbinat, W., Jablensky, A., Kielholz, P., Lehmann, H. E., Naraghi, M., Shimizu, M., Shinfuku, N., Takahashi, R. (1983). *Depressive disorders in different cultures.* Geneva, Switzerland: World Health Organization.

Snowden, L. R., & Cheung, F. K. (1990). Use of inpatient mental health services by members of ethnic minority groups. *American Psychologist, 45,* 347–355.

Sue, S., & Morishima, J. K. (1982). *The mental health of Asian Americans.* San Francisco: Jossey-Bass.

Sue, D., & Sue, S. (1987). Cultural factors in the clinical assessment of Asian Americans. *Journal of Consulting and Clinical Psychology, 55,* 479–487.

Ullmann, R. K., Sleator, E. K., & Sprague, R. L. (1985). Introduction to the use of ACTeRS. *Psychopharmacology Bulletin, 21,* 915–920. (Special feature: Rating scales and assessment instruments for use in pediatric psychopathology research.)

Westermeyer, J. (1985). Psychiatric diagnosis across cultural boundaries. *American Journal of Psychiatry, 142,* 798–805.

Part V

Conclusion

The final chapter deals with current issues and future directions in the psychiatric hospitalization of children and adolescents. It contains an overview of the impact on hospital care, and on less restrictive treatments for children, adolescents, and families, of (a) increasing population in minority groups, (b) increasing population at poverty level, and (c) increased mental health problems in infancy, childhood, and adolescence. Among these increasing serious mental health problems are substance abuse, physical abuse, neglect, and sexual abuse. The chapter also reviews the impact of insurance on shorter lengths of hospital stays and the related implications for effective treatment. The chapter ends with some recommendations for future directions in inpatient treatment of children and adolescents and their families.

CHAPTER NINETEEN

Current Issues and Future Directions for the Psychiatric Hospitalization of Children and Adolescents

Robert L. Hendren
Irving N. Berlin

The chapters in this volume have described the special sensitivity required to effectively treat children, adolescents, and families from minority cultures. With the populations of Hispanic, black, native American, and some Asian minorities rapidly increasing ("Beyond the melting pot," 1990), an ever larger number of children, adolescents, and their families from these cultures will need treatment. In all populations in this country, the continued increase of physical and sexual abuse, the steady escalation in the divorce rate, and the growing numbers of adolescent pregnancies forecast an ever larger population requiring mental health treatment, including inpatient and residential facilities (Berlin, 1990a, 1990b; Egeland, Sroufe, & Erickson, 1983; Weithorn, 1988).

The state and federal government support of training, research, and treatment of mental illness of children and adolescents continues to fall short of the need. In recent years, prevention of some mental disorders has become possible but there is no effort to finance the most effective methods of dealing with these disorders or to conduct extensive research in this area (Berlin, 1982, 1990a; OSAP, 1989; Ward, 1984).

We have not discussed alcoholism as such, but it should be clear from the various vignettes that alcoholism in adults, chaotic families, and depression are major etiologic factors in physical and sexual abuse in children and adolescents. The use of drugs, alcohol, and inhalants by depressed children and adolescents in our country is a major concern. Substance abuse leads not only to hospitalization for the underlying psychiatric problems in addition to the alcoholism, but is a major factor in the increasing incidence of violent deaths in the adolescent and young adult population (Lex, 1981; National Institute on Alcohol Abuse and Alcoholism, 1987; Van Winkle & May, 1986; Winfree & Griffiths, 1985). There is a large increase in fetal alcohol syndrome and fetal drug and inhalant syndrome in this country (Abel & Sokol, 1987; Hoffman, 1990; Little, Young, Streisguth, & Uhleland, 1984; May & Hymbaugh, 1988; Streisguth, 1990; Streisguth, Bookstein, Sampson, & Barr, 1989).

Thus, the future of the children and adolescents in our nation does not look bright. Despite the effective treatment now possible for some mental disorders, support for treatment is minimal. Inpatient treatment for severe psychiatric disorders of children and adolescents is ever more difficult to finance, yet we are faced with an increasing need for every modality of mental health treatment including inpatient care.

A number of forces have changed the way in which inpatient psychiatric treatment is practiced: improved evaluation and treatment methods, changes in treatment philosophy, increased use of less restrictive, community-based treatment settings, and pressures from payers to decrease or eliminate costly inpatient care. The results from these changes have been described as redefined goals for inpatient treatment, blurring of the boundary between the hospital and the social service system, a decreased focus on understanding the child, and a fragmentation of care (Jemerin & Philips, 1988). At least a few of the resulting changes may lead us to overlook some key elements of effective inpatient treatment. The pressure for shorter hospital stays often results in treatment units that only focus on diagnosis and very limited treatment goals for all of the young people admitted, regardless of their need. The needs of those children who require more extensive inpatient treatment often are overlooked until the insurance has run out and efforts are begun to find a longer-term treatment facility.

The pressures for shorter inpatient stays may result in less recognition of the importance of relationships in the evaluation and treatment process and among an effective treatment staff. This is especially a danger for the understanding and treatment of those children, adolescents, and families whose behavior, emotions, and expression of mental disorders have strong cultural influences. The role of the milieu has needed to evolve in order to continue to be an important part of the treatment process. The separation of the function of the milieu treatment from the individual, group, and family treatment, which occurred frequently in the past and continues in a few long-term programs (see Chapter 11), is not effective in most present-day inpatient treatment programs. Some programs continue to overlook milieu treatment as an essential ingredient in a successful program. Milieu treatment must creatively consider multiple ways of enhancing the formation and use of relationships, especially culturally sensitive ones, in effective short-, intermediate-, or long-term hospital treatment. A number of ways to do this have been suggested here.

The integrated, multidisciplinary treatment team is another important ingredient of a successful inpatient treatment program that present-day pressures may cause us to overlook. Efficient and effective treatment depends on a close working relationship among all members of the treatment team. The integration of all treatment staff helps them to sustain each other as they rapidly engage and disengage with young people who have increasingly complex disorders. To have a culturally diverse treatment team, it is often necessary to have a treatment team composed of individuals from a variety of disciplines who have varying levels of professional training and cultural backgrounds. The way in which the multidisciplinary, multicultural treatment team works together is often a good predictor of how effective and culturally sensitive the treatment will be for patients and their families. Continued training and supervision of milieu staff are critical variables in an effective milieu program.

RECOMMENDATIONS FOR FUTURE DIRECTIONS IN THE INPATIENT TREATMENT OF CHILDREN AND ADOLESCENTS

The forces that have shaped present-day inpatient treatment raise ethical dilemmas that should lead us to rethink our priorities and our efforts. How short can short-term treatment be and still be considered a useful intervention into the life of the child and the family? What is the most effective way to use our resources? What alternatives do we have? How should we direct treatment to meet the needs of the population in the next 10 to 20 years?

Sensitivity to Cultural Issues

Shorter and more focused hospital stays and an increasingly diverse cultural population make it increasingly important to assure that treatment is culturally sensitive and relevant.

Sensitivity to Parents and Family Members

We have learned that intensive inpatient treatment is most effective when family members are fully engaged in the treatment process. As the number of abused and neglected children increases, family issues become increasingly important. Resistances must be identified and worked with. In the past, longer-term stays allowed the hospital to reparent children and adolescents. Today's shorter stays require that resistances, including cultural resistances, be effectively addressed and family members drawn in as full participants in treatment. In addition, quick-cure expectations reinforced by certain hospital media promotions must be addressed early so that family members will have realistic expectations of the length of time and the degree of commitment necessary for effective treatment.

Prevention and Early Intervention

Increasing attention and support must be given to community-based, culturally relevant efforts at prevention and early intervention with young people who are at risk for emotional disorders. Because many of the previously strong supporting cultural institutions such as religious, community, and extended family support systems are currently less of an influence, we must consider directing our energies to bolstering the more viable support systems: our school systems, the primary health care system, and the nuclear family system. Our prevention and early intervention efforts should be directed to these areas. Alternatives to hospitalization that are available to young people before an emotional disorder becomes serious and are offered within their own geographic and cultural community must be funded and developed, if we are to make the most efficient and effective use of inpatient treatment.

Community and Government Education

Community and government leaders must be made more aware of important mental health issues that affect children and adolescents. Recruiting parents as advocates in this process is proving an effective way to gain support from these leaders. Issues such as equalization of access to mental health services, fair health insurance coverage of mental disorders, a community-based continuum of care, and support for prevention and early intervention should be given high priority by all community and legislative leaders through effective advocacy that involves not only parents, but also mental health providers, especially those who are concerned with the inequities experienced by the poor, the minority populations, and the increasing number of seriously disturbed youth. These mental health providers and parents must also demonstrate their commitment to a full continuum of concerned care rather than well-advertised brief treatment.

Research

The most effective way to gain support for any good program is through good research. Efforts should be directed toward the development of effective prevention, early identification, and early treatment of emotional disorders in children and adolescents. It is important that the research be culturally sensitive, as described in Dr. Vargas's chapter. Research should examine when and for whom short-, intermediate-, or long-term inpatient treatment is most effective and what alternatives to hospitalization are effective for certain patients at particular times.

CONCLUSION

This volume has aimed at demonstrating how sensitive multicultural inpatient care can be provided and how important the involvement of families and communities is in this process.

The seriousness of some of the illnesses requiring inpatient care should have become evident. Only when the mental health professions, parents, and interested citizen groups work together will we be able to influence legislators and governments to be seriously concerned with the increased need for trained mental health professionals, with increased access to a continuity of care, and with the desperate need to implement prevention and early intervention research and treatment efforts. The same forces must also make clear that research into the etiology and treatment of various mental disorders must be greatly accelerated if we are to make any impact on the mental health problems our nation faces.

In the course of writing and editing this volume, we became repeatedly aware of the effect that a large increase in mentally ill youth and families will have on our ability to provide sensitive and effective treatment. We appeal to our colleagues and to the parents of our patients and of all disturbed youth to become advocates of the mentally ill young people who might otherwise face their illness and the health care system at a great disadvantage. Our nation has an obligation to provide effective health care and continuity of care, responsive to the needs of an increasing number of severely psychiatrically disturbed children and adolescents and families from a variety of cultural backgrounds.

REFERENCES

Abel, E. L., & Sokol, R. J. (1987). Incidence of fetal alcohol syndrome and economic impact of F.A.S. related anomalies. *Drug and Alcohol Dependence, 19,* 51–70.

Berlin, I. N. (1982). Prevention of emotional problems among Native American children: Overview of developmental issues. *Journal of Preventive Psychiatry, 1,* 319–330.

Berlin, I. N. (1990a). The role of the community mental health center in prevention of infant, child and adolescent disorders: Retrospect and prospect. *Community Mental Health Journal, 26,* 89–106.

Berlin, I. N. (1990b). The history of the development of the subspecialty of child/adolescent psychiatry in the United States. In J. Weiner (Ed.), *Textbook of child and adolescent psychiatry.* Washington, DC: American Psychiatric Association Press.

Beyond the melting pot. (1990, April 9). *TIME,* pp. 28–31.

Egeland, B., Sroufe, L. A., & Erickson, M. (1983). The developmental consequences of different patterns of maltreatment. *Child Abuse and Neglect, 7,* 45–69.

Hoffman, M. G. (1990, April 27). Chemically dependent adolescents after treatment. Paper presented at 21st Annual Medical Scientific Conference, American Society of Addiction Medicine, Phoenix, AZ.

Jemerin, J. M., & Philips, I. (1988). Changes in inpatient child psychiatry: Consequences and recommendation. *Journal of the American Academy of Child and Adolescent Psychiatry, 27,* 397–403.

Lex, B. W. (1981). Alcohol problems in special populations. In J. H. Mendelson & N. K. Mello (Eds.), *The diagnosis and treatment of alcoholism* (2d ed., pp. 89–187). New York: McGraw-Hill.

Little, R. E., Young, A., Streisguth, A. P., & Uhleland, C. N. (1984). Preventing fetal alcohol effects: Effectiveness of a demonstration project in mechanisms of alcohol damage in utero. *CIBA Foundation Symposium 105* (pp. 113). London: Pittman.

May, P. A., & Hymbaugh, K. J. (1988). A macro level fetal alcohol syndrome prevention program for American Indians and Alaska natives: Description and evaluation. *Journal of Studies on Alcohol, 49,* 324–334.

National Institute on Alcohol Abuse and Alcoholism (NIAAA). (1987). *Alcohol and health.* Sixth Special Report to the U.S. Congress. Washington, DC: Government Printing Office.

OSAP. (1989). *Twenty prevention programs—project summary.* Washington, DC: Alcohol Abuse and Mental Health Administration.

Streisguth, A. P. (1990). Seriousness of fetal drug syndrome and fetal inhalant syndrome. (Prepublication personal communication to Irving N. Berlin.)

Streisguth, A. P., Bookstein, F. L., Sampson, P. D., & Barr, H. M. (1989). Neurobehavioral effects of prenatal alcohol: Part III. PLS analyses of neuropsychological tests. *Neurotoxicology and Teratology, 11,* 493–507.

Van Winkle, N. W., & May, P. A. (1986). Native American suicide in New Mexico 1967–1979: A comparative study. *Human Organization, 45,* 296–309.

Ward, J. A. (1984). Preventive implications of a Native Indian mental health focus on suicide and violent death. *Journal of Preventive Psychiatry, 2,* 371–386.

Weithorn, L. A. (1988). Mental hospitalization of troublesome youth: An analysis of skyrocketing admission rates. *Standard Law Review, 40,* 773–838.

Winfree, L. T., & Griffiths, C. T. (1985). Trends in drug orientations and behavior: Changes in a rural community 1975–1982. *International Journal of Addictions, 20,* 495–508.

Author Index

Aardema, V., 170
Abel, E. L., 314
Abramowitz, K. S., 265
Achenbach, T. M., 299, 303
Adams, P., 67
Aichhorn, A., 104
Akerson, D. M., 272
Alessi, N. E., 76
Ambrosini, P. J., 303
American Academy of Child and Adolescent Psychiatry, 41, 178
American Psychiatric Association, 41, 178
Anaya, R. A., 32
Anderson, C. M., 156
Anderson, L. T., 77, 144
Arciniega, M., 68
Argyris, C., 283
Arnoff, M. S., 222
Asarnow, R. F., 77
Attneave, C. L., 134
Axline, V., 113

Bachelard, G., 94, 110
Bachman, D. L., 76
Ballenger, J. C., 77

Bandler, R., 109
Barker, P., 5
Barr, H. M., 314
Barrengos, A., 223
Beavers, W. R., 151, 155
Bedi, I., 190
Beigel, A., 265
Beitch, L. M., 76
Benalcazar-Schmid, R., 223
Berlin, I. N., 5, 25, 95, 109, 134, 169, 211, 213, 216, 223, 280, 281, 314
Berman, J. R. S., 146
Bettelheim, B., 163, 212, 224
Bion, W., 104
Birch, H. G., 67
Blank, G., 115
Blank, R., 115
Bleiberg, E., 222
Bloom, J. D., 293, 305
Blotcky, M. J., 8, 58, 177
Boatman, M. J., 211
Bonier, R. J., 212
Bookstein, F. L., 314
Bornholt, I., 70
Duszormeny-Nagy, I., 156

Boutin, P., 67
Bowen, M., 156
Bowlby, G., 70
Boyd, J. H., 294
Boyd-Franklin, N., 155
Bradshaw, C., 147
Budman, C., 183
Bulbrook, M. J. T., 240
Burke, J. D., 294
Burman, A., 294
Butler, J. A., 136
Butts, J. A., 6, 268

Campbell, M., 77, 303
Cantwell, D. P., 68
Carlson, C., 110
Caron, C., 67
Casaus, L., 68
Castillo, M., 68
Cervantes, J. M., 17
Chambers, W. J., 76, 303
Chang, C., 236
Cherniss, C., 254
Cheslow, D., 67
Chess, S., 67, 214
Cheung, F. K., 291, 295
Clark, T., 154, 156

Clarkin, J. F., 222
Cohen, I. L., 77
Cohen, P., 77
Comerford, R., 270
Conte, J. R., 77
Coppolillo, H. P., 140
Corn, R., 222
Cote, R., 67
Crawford-Brobyn, J., 120
Critchley, D. L., 95, 109,
    213, 216, 217, 255
Cromwell, R. E., 148
Croughan, J., 293
Curley, A. D., 165
Curran, C. R., 240

Davidian, H., 293
Davies, M., 76, 303
Delga, I., 77
Dell, P. R., 77
Delworth, U., 255
DiClemente, R. J., 188
Doherty, M. D., 223
Dolan, Y. M., 109
Domanico, L., 270
Draguns, J., 293
Dunn, L., 177

Edelson, M., 135
Egeland, B., 6, 314
Eisenhower, J. W., 77
Ekstein, R., 212
Erdberg, P., 297
Erickson, M., 6, 314
Ernberg, G., 293
Escobar, J. I., 294
Esman, A., 212
Evans, C. S., 237, 239,
    245

Falicov, C. J., 146, 150
Fava, G. A., 298
Feldman, M., 223
Fenichel, C., 163
Fenton, F. R., 293
Finkelman, A. W., 244
Fowler, R. D., 297
Fraiberg, S., 135
Frank, M., 114, 115, 267
Freud, A., 209
Freud, S., 131, 144
Friedman, R. C., 69, 222

Fristad, M. A., 77
Fritsch, R. C., 77
Fu, P., 306
Fujii, I., 293
Fuller, J. S., 120

Gardner, J. W., 273
Gardos, G., 189
Gastpar, M., 293
Geraty, R., 5, 6, 7, 266,
    272, 273
Gibson, R W., 270
Ginzberg, E., 240
Glaser, G. H., 223
Goetz, R., 76
Good, B., 296
Good, M. D., 296
Goodrich, W., 77
Gossett, J. T., 8, 58, 155,
    177
Grayer, E. D., 247
Green, A., 96
Green, H. A., 129
Green, J., 182
Greenberg, L., 212
Greenblatt, M., 272
Greenson, R., 129
Griffiths, C. T., 314
Grinder, J., 109
Gruenberg, E., 294
Gualtieri, C. T., 68
Gulbinat, W., 293
Gutierrez, M. J., 18, 157,
    158
Gynther, M. D., 297, 302

Haiman, S., 212
Haley, J., 151, 156
Haller, L., 255
Halperin, D., 212
Hammerschlag, C. A., 20
Hanrahan, G., 133
Hardy, E., 255, 282
Haring, N. G., 163
Harper, G., 5, 6, 7, 73, 131,
    133, 181, 266, 272, 273
Harris, T., 236, 241
Hartley, D. E., 179, 188
Hathuc, N., 306
Heinssen, R. K., 77
Helzer, J. E., 293, 294
Herjanic, B., 303

Hernandez, P., 148
Hewett, F. M., 163, 166
Hicks, R. E., 68
Hines, P. M., 155
Hirsch, M., 303
Hirschovitz, R. G., 272
Hobbs, N., 163
Hoffman, M. G., 314
Hooper, S. R., 165
Hough, R. L., 294
Howard, K., 222
Hoza, J. A., 68
Hughes, J. M., 215
Hurt, S. W., 222
Hymbaugh, K. J., 314

Imber, R. R., 223
Institute of Medicine, 296,
    306

Jablensky, A., 293
Jemerin, J. M., 5, 17, 315
Jilek-Aall, L., 147
Joe, J., 306
Joint Commission in
    Accreditation of
    Healthcare
    Organizations, 269
Joint Commission on
    Accreditation of
    Hospitals, 178
Joyce, P. A., 133

Kalojera, I. J., 190
Kaplan, L., 222
Karno, M., 236, 294
Kauff, P., 115
Keith, C., 222, 223
Kellner, R., 298
Kendrick, E. A., 237
Kenkel, P. J., 267, 268
Kent, J. J., 177
Kerlinsky, D., 110
Kernberg, O., 209
Kernberg, P. F., 69, 76,
    209, 222
Kessler, R., 295, 299
Kielholz, P., 293
Kim, H., 266
King, J., 76
Klein, M., 209
Kleinman, A., 291, 296

Kohut, H., 222
Kovacs, M., 300

La Fromboise, T., 144, 146, 147, 148
La Liberte, M., 252
Lauro, G., 212
Lave, J. R., 267
Lavee, Y., 303
Law, W., 76, 77
Lee, E., 183
Lee, J. H., 189
Lefley, H. P., 7
Lehmann, H. E., 293
Leighton, A., 215
Lenane, M., 67
Leonard, H., 67
Lerner, H., 69
Levy, L. P., 133, 134
Lewis, D. O., 223
Lewis, J. M., 237, 239, 245
Lewis, M., 42, 155
Lewis, S. K., 245, 246
Lex, B. W., 314
Lifton, N., 114
Lin, K. M., 306
List, J. A., 133
Little, R. E., 314
Loganbill, C., 255
Lomax, J. W., 237
Lopez, S., 148
Ludolph, P., 69
Lupatkin, W., 76

Maduro, R., 9
Magen, J., 76
Mahler, M. S., 222
Mahron, R. C., 222
Mandelbaum, A., 212
Mandersheid, R., 177
Manson, S. M., 225, 293, 297, 305
Marchi, M., 77
Marcos, L. R., 272
Marsella, A. J., 292, 293
Martini, P. P., 68
Masterson, J. F., 147, 222
Matsuda, K., 306
May, P., 215, 314
Maziade, M., 67
McDaniel, K. D., 77
McGlashan, T. H., 76

McGoldrick, M., 144
McKenna, S., 188
Meyer, A. D., 190
Millazzo-Sayre, L., 177
Miller, D., 306
Mindell, A., 108
Minnick, A., 240
Moffic, H. S., 237
Montalvo, B., 18, 157, 158
Moreau, D. L., 77
Morishima, J. K., 295
Mull, D. S., 9
Mull, J. S., 9
Munari, F., 298
Muscone, F., 212

Naraghi, M., 293
Nardolillo, E. M., 165
National Association of Private Psychiatric Hospitals, 63
National Institute on Alcohol Abuse and Alcoholism (NIAAA), 314
Neighbors, H. W., 295, 299
Nielson, G., 222, 223
Nocolis, G., 108
Norbeck, J. S., 252
Noshpitz, J., 223
Nuccio, I., 306
Nurcombe, B., 70, 181, 212

Offer, D., 222
Olson, D. H., 303
Orvaschel, H., 294
OSAP, 314
Ostrov, E., 222

Paez, P., 303
Palfrey, J. S., 136
Palmer, A. J., 131, 133
Parkinson, C. N., 286
Parmalee, D. X., 178
Pattak, S., 114, 115
Pavan, L., 298
Paz, O., 15, 17, 23, 24
Pearson, G., 153
Pelham, W. E., 68, 76
Peplau, H., 251
Perel, J., 76

Perlmutter, R. A., 38
Perry, R., 177, 189
Petti, T. A., 69, 76, 77
Philips, I., 5, 315
Phillips, E. L., 163
Phillips, V. A., 155, 177
Pincus, J. H., 223
Pinderhughes, E., 122, 155, 156
Poland, R. E., 306
Ponton, L. E., 179, 182, 183, 188
Popper, C., 100
Portner, J., 303
Post, R. M., 77
Pothier, P. C., 236, 252
Prigogine, I., 108
Puig-Antich, J., 76, 303

Quattrone, D. F., 169
Quintana, F. L., 9

Rappoport, J. L., 67
Ratcliff, J. S., 293
Rebhan, J., 212
Red Horse, J., 69
Redl, F., 5, 96, 163, 212
Reece, R. D., 271
Regier, D. A., 294
Reich, W., 303
Reid, K., 237
Rieus, J. I., 77
Rinsley, D. B., 157
Rivinus, T. M., 131
Roberts, M. J., 240
Robins, L. N., 293, 294
Rodenhauser, P., 271
Rogh, L. H., 64
Rogler, L. H., 291, 297, 304
Rosenthal, D., 70
Rosenthal, P. A., 223
Rossi, E. L., 108
Rossman, P. G., 95, 213
Roth, E. A., 64
Ruffino, S., 69
Ruiz, R. A., 148
Rutter, M., 77

Sacco, F. C., 154
Sampson, E. E., 292, 314
Sander, D., 11, 69, 78
Santana, F., 294

Sartorius, N., 293
Sax, P. R., 247
Schacht, A. J., 110
Schachter, B., 212
Schamess, G., 114, 116
Scheidlinger, S., 114, 115
Scheper-Hughes, N., 9
Schnabolk, J., 212
Schuerman, J. R., 77
Schwartz, I. M., 6, 254, 268
Sederer, L. I., 267, 271
Senior, N., 268
Shanok, S. S., 223
Shapiro, T., 95, 100, 101
Shapiro, V., 135
Sharfstein, S. S., 177, 265
Sheimo, S. L., 211
Shimizu, M., 293
Shinfuku, N., 293
Shockley, E. L., 254
Shore, J. H., 293, 305
Silver, M. A., 272, 273
Silverman, W. H., 270
Simmons, J., 42
Simpson, G. M., 189
Singer, J. D., 136
Skinner, K., 252
Slavson, S. R., 113
Sleator, E. K., 300
Small, A. M., 177, 189
Smalley, S. L., 77
Smolen, E., 114
Snowden, L. R., 291, 295
Sokol, R. J., 314
Spencer-Brown, G., 109
Spense, M. A., 77
Spitz, R. A., 70
Sprague, R. L., 300
Spurlock, J., 42
Sroufe, L. A., 6, 314
St. Clair, R. L., 267, 271
Stanton, A. H., 254
Staton, D., 266, 267, 268

Stengers, I., 108
Stern, D. N., 222
Stewart, D., 9, 156
Stewart, P., 76
Stewart, R., 129
Stewart, S., 144
Stoker, T., 270
Stonequist, E. V., 17
Streisguth, A. P., 314
Stroul, B. A., 62
Sturges, J., 68
Su, T. P., 306
Sue, D., 295
Sue, S., 144, 147, 148, 151, 158
Sun Bear, 15
Susselman, S., 284
Sussewell, D. R., 145, 147, 158, 159
Swedo, S. E., 67
Szurek, S. A., 134, 211, 280, 281

Taba, H., 169
Tabrizi, A., 76, 303
Takahashi, R., 293
Taylor, F., 163, 166
Thivierge, J., 67
Thomas, A., 67, 70, 214
Thomas, J. N., 77
Timbers, D. M., 294
Trafimow, E., 114, 115
Tramontana, M. G., 165
Trimble, J. E., 147
Tudor, G., 254
Tyler, F. B., 145, 147, 158, 159

Uhleland, C. N., 314
Ullmann, R. K., 300
Ulrich, D., 156
United States Department of Commerce, 265
United States Department of Justice, 234

Van Winkel, W. W., 215, 314
Varanka, T. M., 77
Varela, F. J., 109
Vargas, L. A., 148
Vasquez, F. H., 23
Vela, R. M., 69, 76

Walker, D. K., 136
Walker, J. L., 68
Wallerstein, J., 212
Ward, J. A., 314
Warner, V., 77
Watson, W. N., 190
Webb, W. L., 271
Weissman, M., 77, 294
Weithorn, L. A., 314
Weller, A. A., 77
Weller, E., 77
Westen, D., 69, 77
Westermeyer, J., 291, 296, 298, 300
White, A., 120
Williams, B. E., 132
Williams-McCoy, J., 145, 147, 158, 159
Wineman, D., 163, 212
Winfree, L. T., 314
Winnicott, D., 115, 214, 222
Wishik, J., 76
Wiss, F. C., 69
Wolf, J. R., 242, 248
Woolston, J. L., 73, 133, 214
Wynne, L. C., 155

Yager, J., 236
Yalom, I. D., 114, 115
Yates, B. T., 77
Young, A., 314

Zalis, T., 154
Zane, N., 144, 148, 151
Zinn, M. B., 148
Zowbok, B., 189

Subject Index

Acting out, 59, 68, 76, 115, 198
Acting-up behavior, 76
Action-reflection spectrum, 199
Acute care inpatient units, 7
Adaptive ego defenses, 109
Administrative
  authority, 275
  constraints, 273
  issues, 265
Admission criteria, 63, 178
  screening, 41, 42
Adult
  authoritative, 287
  benign, 287
  concerned, 287
  effective, traditional, 225
Advocacy, 181
Affect modulation, 95, 96, 100
Aggressive behaviors, 190
Alcoholism, 68, 225, 314
Allied therapists, 73, 173
Alter egos, 77
Altruism, 60
American Indian, 10, 23, 134, 141, 144,
  146, 150
American Indian cultures, 146, 148
American Indian families, 68, 69, 129
Anger, 222

Anger and contempt in staff members,
  215
Anger management, 120
Anti-Hispanic comments, 229
Antisocial behavior, 68
Antisocial personality disorders, 77
Applied behavioral analysis, 163
Art therapy, 69
Attachment, 70
Attention deficit disorder, 67, 76
Autism, 76
Autonomy, 222

Bad touch, 123
Behavior changes, 74
Behavioral consequences, 96
Behavioral constraints, 225
Behavioral expectations, 74
Bewitched, 78
Biopsychosocial model, 70
Biscochitos, 26
Black families, 156
Blaming, 30, 215
Borderline personality, 69, 76, 77, 222
Boundary intrusions, 155
Brief hospitalization, 177
Broken taboos, 78
Burnout, 199, 238

Career ladders, 237
Case managers, 252
Chaotic family units, 230
Character problems, 279
Child and Adolescent Service System
    Program (CASSP), 6
Child-care worker, 240, 245
Childhood schizophrenia, 67, 76
Children's Depression Inventory, 300
Cholo, 17
Chronic physical illnesses, 163
Civil commitment, 19
Clan matriarch, 19
Clan patriarch, 30
Classroom structure, 167
Clinical supervision, 217, 251, 253
    as learning, 256
    versus consultation, 256
    versus therapy, 256
Cognitive and affective mastery, 123
Community
    consultation principles, 282
    processes, 282
Conduct disorders, 69, 76
Confidentiality, 94, 95
Conflict resolution, 120
Conning, 229
Consequences, 75
Construct validity and cultural context, 303
Context of behavior, 301
Continuing education, 245
Convergent ethnic validity, 145
Coordinators of services, 252
Core team, 16
Counterphobia, 50
Countertransference, 21, 73, 99, 131, 208,
    212, 216, 223, 239, 247, 258, 259
    to parents, 210
Couples therapy, 201
Credentialing, 269
Criollos, 23
Crisis
    hospitalization, 177
    supervision, 260
Cross-cultural diagnosis, 291, 294
Cross-ethnic group comparisons, 302
Cultural, 21, 286
    anarchy, 18
    biases, 21
    concepts of death, 27
    consultants, 183
    consultation, 97
    context of instruments, 303

definitions, 293
expectations and values, 70
healing, 11
responsiveness, 15, 16
taboos, 30
transcendence, 299, 300
Culturally
    based criteria, 293
    diverse staff, 24
    sensitive, 290, 291
Curanderismo, 9
Curanderos, 68, 78
Custody determination, 64
Cyclothymic disorders, 77

Death's aftermath, 27
Defense mechanisms, 59, 198
    denial, 59, 198
    displacement, 60
    humor, 60
    identification, 59
    isolation of affect, 60
    primitive, 198
    project the bad introject, 223
    projection, 59, 223
    rationalization, 60
    reaction formation, 59
    regression, 59, 113, 197
    repression, 60, 210
    splitting, 59, 198, 199
    sublimation, 60
    suppression, 60
Defensive attitudes, 67
Degree of acculturation, 68
Depression, 67, 69, 76
Developmental
    assessment, 70
    level, 58
    line, 70
    problems, 222
Diagnostic Interview of Children and
    Adolescents, 303
Diagnostic Interview Schedule, 296
Discharge
    phase, 187
    planning, 68, 83
Disempowerment, 30
Disruption of bonding, 70
Divergent ethnic validity, 145, 146
Dominant culture, 15
Double bind, 26
Drawing of pictures, 120
Drug abuse, 113

Eating disorders, 77
Economics, 265
Education, 317
Educational assessment, 165
Efficacy of inpatient treatment, 290
Ego building experience, 75
Ego functioning, 114
Emic, 291, 298, 306
Emic sensitivity, 299
Empathy, 125
Empowerment, 29, 30
Enhancement of self-image, 283
Enmeshment, 25
Environmental
    controls, 290
    design, 163
    stress, 68
    treatment components, 251
Epistemological, 290
Eriksonian moratorium, 195, 200
Ethical considerations, 270, 290
Ethnic
    child, 27
    family, 29
    identity, 121
Ethnocentricity, 27
Etic
    diagnostic and treatment, 299
Evaluation phase, 186
Evil spirits, 78
Expressive therapies, 69, 164, 169
Extended family, 19, 22, 29, 68

Family
    component, 154
    systems theory, 132
    therapists, 144
Fetal alcohol syndrome, 162
Fire setting, 76
Fixated, 222
Focal problem, 181
Follow-up care, 32
Foster families, 68

Gatekeepers, 114
Generational boundaries, 120
Genetic factors, 67, 70
Goal-oriented treatment planning, 70, 181
Goals of treatment, 75
Goodness of fit, 67, 70, 73, 97
Good touch, 123
Governmental policy, 266
Grandiose and omnipotent fantasies, 199

Group
    analysis, 201
    as transitional object, 115
    behavior management, 113
    contagion, 114
    supervision, 231
    therapy, 113, 114, 119, 188

Hamilton Rating Scale for Depression, 298
Hate, 222
Healing ceremonies, 16, 69, 78, 80
Helplessness, 222
Hiring criteria, 239
Hispanic, 9, 134, 141
    families, 68, 150
Holding environment, 195
Holistic world views, 100
Hostile
    aggressive child, 222
    and noncaring environment, 227
    introject, 223
Human sexuality unit, 171

Identification with the aggressor, 120
Impulse control, 95, 96, 100
Incestuous thoughts, 195
Indian Child Welfare Act, 83, 153
Indigena, 23
Individual supervision, 103
Individuation stages, 69, 195
Initial planning meeting, 136
Inservice training, 173, 247
Instructional module, 171
Insurance, 267
Intake, 80
Integration of interdisciplinary treatment, 94
Interdisciplinary team, 73, 94, 215
Intermediate term inpatient treatment, 7, 73
Interpersonal patterns, 114
Interpersonal process, 114, 251
Interpretations, 115, 116, 305
Inter-rater reliability, 301
Interstaff conflicts, 261
Interventions, 27, 29
Intuitions, 281

Japanese clients, 147
Joint Commission on the Accreditation of Health Care Organizations (JCAHO), 268
Juvenile diabetes, 163

K-SADS, 303

Latin American families, 146
Leadership, 271
Learning disability, 165
Legal processes, 123
Leisure time skills, 171
Length of stay, 177
Level system, 74
Limit setting, 114
Long term inpatient treatment, 77
Long term psychotherapy, 200
Losing face, 226
Losses of caretakers, 120
Low riders, 18

Machismo, 68, 224
Major depressive disorder, 76
Managed health care, 267
Management issues, 190
Manic depressive, 68
Marketing, 270
Matrilineal, 24, 69
Medicaid, 266
Medical model, 290
Medicine man, 80
Methodological issues, 296
Mexican hierarchy, 23
Milieu, 24
  and school programs, 76
  management, 243
  safety issues, 103
  staff, 73
  teamwork, 95
  therapy, 76
  treatment, 251, 315
Modeling of social skills, 119
Morale, 248
Mourning, 69
Multicultural atmosphere, 16
Multicultural program, 183
Multidisciplinary treatment team, 73,
  94, 315
Multiple personality disorder, 77

Narcissistic, 124
  children, 222
  hurt, 96
  personality disorders, 69, 77
National Alliance for the Mentally Ill
  (NAMI), 6
Native healers, 30, 68
Native mental health workers, 79

Natural therapists, 25
Navajo, 69
  sing, 285
  social worker, 79
  taboo, 27
  translator, 285
Neurointegrative disturbances, 70, 75
Neurological anomalies, 162
Nurses, 245
Nursing role, 251

Object constancy, 223
Obsessive-compulsive disorders, 67, 68
Occupational therapist, 173
Operant conditioning, 163
Operational measures, 293
Oppositional disorder, 76
Organizational structure, 272
Orientation curriculum, 245
Outcome
  research, 84
  studies, 290
Outreach services, 130
Outreach team, 32, 84, 117

Pachuco, 17
Paradoxical intervention, 108
Parametric strategy, 306
Patient care, 279
Patient-therapist relationship, 306
Perpetrators, 122
Personality
  development, 70
  disorders, 69, 76
Pharmacologic interventions, 67, 94, 95, 189
  antidepressants, 76, 81
  lithium, 77
  neuroleptics, 76
  stimulants, 67
Physical abuse, 5, 70, 77, 228
Physical restraint, 226
Play therapy, 69
Possession by evil spirits, 78, 97
Posthospital treatment, 69
Post Traumatic Stress Disorder, 77, 123
Poverty, 30
Power struggles, 30, 197
Prejudices, 22, 225
Prevention, 316
Priests, 68
Primitive defenses, 198
Problem-solving, 284
  approaches, 16

computer games, 172
skills, 115, 120
Process-outcome strategy, 306
Professional ethics, 258
Professional identity, 258
Professional staff development, 255
Projective identification, 198
Protective limits, 114, 115
Psychiatric nurse-administrator, 254
Psychoanalytically oriented therapy, 196
Psychoeducation, 95
Psychopharmacologic agents, 5, 68
Public Law 99-660, 6
Pueblos, 69
Puppetry, 120

Quality assurance, 269

Rapprochement
crises, 222
phase, 222
Reality testing, 196
Recent onset adolescent schizophrenia, 76
Recreation therapists, 171
Recruitment issues, 236
Regressive acting-out, 197
Regressive play, 113
Repressed, 210
Research, 317
Resistance, 26, 64, 80, 154
Restraint teams, 226
Restructuring the physical environment, 251
Retention, 248
Risk management, 97
Role playing, 115

Safety, 103, 119, 123
Satanic involvement, 113
Scapegoating, 114
Schizophrenia, 67, 76
SCOAP, 169
Secondary process, 196
Secure treatment, 222
Seductive
adulation, 223
behaviors, 224
Seizure disorders, 75, 163
Sensorimotor functions, 19, 173
Separation-individuation, 222
Sex education, 123
Sexual
abuse, 5, 68, 77, 195
aggressive responses, 195

issues group, 122
knowledge, 123
Shalakos, 164
Short-term
hospitalization, 73
inpatient treatment, 178
milieu treatment, 212
treatment, 177, 181
Shutdown, 103
Single-subject design, 302
Social supports, 32
Socioeconomic status, 295
Specialty wards, 183
Stabilization phase, 185
Staff
education, 183
effectiveness, 279
development, 244, 251
interventions, 74
meetings, 217
members, 208
orientation, 244
prejudices, 79
split, 222
supervision, 246
supportive structures, 216
Storytelling, 69
Strategic planning, 270
Strategies in work with multicultural
parents, 137
Substance abuse, 314
Suicide attempts, 76
Superego projections, 199
Superior mestizos, 23
Supervision, 103, 173, 255, 257
definitions, 255
individual, clinical, 103, 173
participant, 257
Supportive psychotherapy, 94
Symbiotic relationship, 222, 223

Task group, 74, 118
Task-oriented, 79
instructional program, 164, 174
Tasks of daily living, 67
Temperamental influences, 67, 70
Therapeutic culture, 95
Timberlawn Study, 155
Time-out room, 167, 168
Token reinforcement principles, 166
Traditional cultural values, 109
Transference, 131, 208, 218, 247, 259, 279
Transference projections, 223

Translation of instruments, 304
Treatment
  alliance, 65, 69
  failure, 212
  models, 7, 114
  philosophy, 180
  planning, 67, 70, 181
  priorities, 94
  program, 68
  staff prejudice, 215
Tribal advocate, 225
Tribal social service, 69

Unconscious cultural biases, 99
Unconscious reactions, 210
Unit safety, 103

Video tapes, 257
Violent assaultive behavior, 224, 230
Vulgar mestizos, 23

Welcoming environment, 16
Western epistemologies, 290
Western healing, 11
Witched, 78, 135